THE DISASTER SURVIVA

D0618731

ABOUT THE AUTHOR

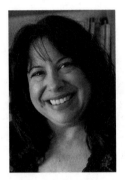

Marie D. Jones is the best-selling author of over fifteen nonfiction books, including *Demons, the Devil and Fallen Angels; The Power of Archetypes; Viral Mythology;* and *Mind Wars.* She is also a screenwriter and novelist and owns her own production company where she is developing projects for film and television. She has written for dozens of magazines and publications and is a regular guest on radio shows all over the world, including *Coast to Coast A.M.* Marie has appeared on the History Channel's *Ancient Aliens* series. She is a fully trained member of CERT, Community Emergency Response Teams, in San Diego County, and is a licensed amateur radio operator (KI6YES).

THE DISASTER SURVIVAL GUIDE

How to Prepare for and Survive Floods, Fires, Earthquakes, and More

Marie D. Jones

VISIBLE
INK
PRESS

Detroit

THE DISASTER SURVIVAL GUIDE

Visible Ink Press®
43311 Joy Rd., #414
Canton, MI 48187-2075

Visible Ink Press is a registered trademark of Visible Ink Press LLC.

Most Visible Ink Press books are available at special quantity discounts when purchased in bulk by corporations, organizations, or groups. Customized printings, special imprints, messages, and excerpts can be produced to meet your needs. For more information, contact Special Markets Director, Visible Ink Press, www.visibleink.com, or 734-667-3211.

Managing Editor: Kevin S. Hile
Art Director: Mary Claire Krzewinski
Typesetting: Marco Divita
Proofreaders: Larry Baker and Carleton L. Copeland
Indexer: Shoshana Hurwitz

Cover images: Shutterstock.

Library of Congress Cataloging-in-Publication Data

Names: Jones, Marie D., 1961– author.
Title: The disaster survival guide: how to prepare for and survive floods, fires, earthquakes, and more / by Marie D. Jones.
Description: Canton, MI : Visible Ink Press, [2018] | Includes index. |
    Identifiers: LCCN 2018015075 (print) | LCCN 2018015776 (ebook) | ISBN
    9781578596850 (ebook) | ISBN 9781578596737 (pbk. : alk. paper)
Subjects: LCSH: Survival. | Disasters. | Emergencies. | Emergency management.
Classification: LCC GF86 (ebook) | LCC GF86 .J664 2018 (print) | DDC
    631.6/9—dc23

LC record available at†https://lccn.loc.gov/2018015075

Printed in the United States of America.

10 9 8 7 6 5 4 3 2 1

DISCLAIMER

Some of the information in this book includes advice relating to medical procedures such as what to do when choking or how to deal with accidental poisoning, among other issues. However, this is not meant as a substitute for medical advice from a qualified physician. It is meant for educational and informational purposes only. If you have any questions about a medical problem, please seek help from a healthcare professional.

ALSO FROM VISIBLE INK PRESS

The Handy Math Answer Book, 2nd edition
by Patricia Barnes-Svarney and Thomas E. Svarney
ISBN: 978-1-57859-373-6

The Handy Military History Answer Book
by Samuel Willard Crompton
ISBN: 978-1-57859-509-9

The Handy Mythology Answer Book
by David A. Leeming, Ph.D.
ISBN: 978-1-57859-475-7

The Handy New York City Answer Book
by Chris Barsanti
ISBN: 978-1-57859-586-0

The Handy Nutrition Answer Book
by Patricia Barnes-Svarney and Thomas E. Svarney
ISBN: 978-1-57859-484-9

The Handy Ocean Answer Book
by Patricia Barnes-Svarney and Thomas E. Svarney
ISBN: 978-1-57859-063-6

The Handy Pennsylvania Answer Book
by Lawrence W. Baker
ISBN: 978-1-57859-610-2

The Handy Personal Finance Answer Book
by Paul A. Tucci
ISBN: 978-1-57859-322-4

The Handy Philosophy Answer Book
by Naomi Zack, Ph.D.
ISBN: 978-1-57859-226-5

The Handy Physics Answer Book, 2nd edition
By Paul W. Zitzewitz, Ph.D.
ISBN: 978-1-57859-305-7

The Handy Presidents Answer Book, 2nd edition
by David L. Hudson
ISB N: 978-1-57859-317-0

The Handy Psychology Answer Book, 2nd edition
by Lisa J. Cohen, Ph.D.
ISBN: 978-1-57859-508-2

The Handy Religion Answer Book, 2nd edition
by John Renard, Ph.D.
ISBN: 978-1-57859-379-8

The Handy Science Answer Book, 4th edition
by The Carnegie Library of Pittsburgh
ISBN: 978-1-57859-321-7

The Handy State-by-State Answer Book: Faces, Places, and Famous Dates for All Fifty States
by Samuel Willard Crompton
ISBN: 978-1-57859-565-5

The Handy Supreme Court Answer Book
by David L Hudson, Jr.
ISBN: 978-1-57859-196-1

The Handy Technology Answer Book
by Naomi E. Balaban and James Bobick
ISBN: 978-1-57859-563-1

The Handy Texas Answer Book
by James L. Haley
ISBN: 978-1-57859-634-8

The Handy Weather Answer Book, 2nd edition
by Kevin S. Hile
ISBN: 978-1-57859-221-0

PLEASE VISIT THE VISIBLE INK PRESS WEBSITE AT WWW.VISIBLEINKPRESS.COM

ACKNOWLEDGMENTS

I would like to thank my superwoman agent and dear, dear friend, Lisa Hagan, for making this happen and for always believing in me as a person and a writer. I would also like to thank the amazing staff at Visible Ink Press, starting, of course, with publisher Roger Jänecke first and foremost. Thank you for allowing me to write this very important and much-needed book and for making it look fantastic long after I turned the manuscript in! Your staff is wonderful to work with, and I am so proud to have my name on your books. Kevin Hile, thank you for being an awesome editor to work with!

Thank you to my mom, Milly, my dad, John, who is watching from the heavens, and my sister, Angella, and brother, John, for being my amazing and supportive family. And thank you to my good friends, my extended kin, and to everyone who has ever purchased one of my books, listened to me on the radio, or watched me on TV and engaged with me to tell me that you enjoy what I do and learn from it. Without you, I am just a writer with no voice.

Thank you to San Marcos CERT, the San Marcos Fire Department, the San Marcos Amateur Radio Club, the Red Cross, Burbank Police and Fire Departments, and everyone who helped train me in disaster preparedness and response over the years.

Most of all, thank you to my sun and moon and stars, my son, Max, who makes all the hard, hard work worthwhile every time he calls me "Mom."

CONTENTS

Photo Sources

Abasaa (Wikicommons): p. 73.
Air Accident Investigation Branch, United Kingdom: p. 66.
Alex Alishevskikh: p. 38.
Max Andrews: p. 191.
Boston Post: p. 68.
Celestis (Wikicommons): p. 92.
Dan Craggs: p. 88.
Federal Communication Commission: p. 91.
Flydime (Wikicommons): p. 52.
Jet Propulsion Laboratory, NASA: p. 321.
Mliu92 (Wikicommons): p. 77.
NASA: p. 41.
Oxfam East Africa: p. 19.
Polytechnic University of Milan: p. 49.
David Rydevik: p. 31.
Shutterstock: pp. 5, 7, 14, 17, 27, 30, 44, 47, 55, 58, 63, 71, 79, 81, 83, 96, 100, 105, 107, 110, 113, 116, 118, 124, 125, 128, 131, 134, 137, 140, 142, 146, 153, 157, 158, 161, 168, 170, 172, 174, 175, 178, 181, 183, 186, 194, 196, 199, 201, 203, 206, 210, 213, 216, 219, 220, 223, 225, 231, 233, 239, 240, 243, 245, 249, 252, 254, 256, 259, 262, 263, 266, 275, 278, 280, 283, 284, 288, 290, 293, 295, 298, 301, 305, 307, 310, 314, 316, 325, 326, 332, 334, 339, 340, 345, 349, 357, 359, 362, 364, 369, 373, 375.
Rick Singh: p. 273.
U.S. Air Force: p. 329.
U.S. Army: p. 34.
U.S. Geological Survey: p. 23.
U.S. National Park Service: p. 343.
U.S. Navy: p. 10.
Public domain: p. 121.

INTRODUCTION

Every year, disaster strikes. Somewhere in the world, people struggle to survive earthquakes, volcanic eruptions, superstorms, blizzards, and flooding, as well as man-made disasters such as terrorist bombings, nuclear plant meltdowns, and plane crashes. For those of us lucky enough to never have dealt with a major disaster, we still deal with the threat of smaller disasters lurking all around us. From active shooter situations to camping emergencies to bridge collapses, disasters are all around us.

There is an old adage that says, "It pays to be prepared." When catastrophe strikes, no matter how big or small, being ready and knowing how to respond can be the difference between the loss of life and survival. Even if our lives aren't threatened, our property may be, and there are many ways to be prepared for protecting what we have worked hard to obtain.

It's only human to not want to think about disasters, catastrophes, and major emergencies, but they do happen. Chances are high we will all be affected at least once in our lifetimes—if not by a nearby volcano bursting a pyroclastic flow or a tsunami hitting our beach community, then at least by other forces of Mother Nature. Such forces, because of climate change, are becoming harder and harder to predict or pin down.

Just as important as learning how to survive the worst is learning how to survive everyday emergencies such as bee stings, snakebites, house fires, gas explosions, poisons and toxins, and perhaps even the errant bear confrontation while camping in the woods. It's all important, and it's all in this comprehensive guide.

Surviving an emergency involves three parts. First, it helps to understand what potential emergency situations we might be exposed to based upon where we live and work and what the past has to teach us about natural and manmade disasters.

Second, we need to be ready, to be prepared, and with so many products and tips and tools at our fingertips, thanks to the Internet and prepper shows on television, we have no excuse for being caught unawares.

Finally, we need to learn how to react and respond when disaster does strike because knowledge is power. We might still panic, but once we catch our breath, the information we've absorbed about what to do first, where to go, how to get the proper news about evacuations and shelters, and what we need to bring with us should we leave the comfort and safety of our homes and offices could keep ourselves and our loved ones alive. Disaster preparedness is critical, but perhaps even more so is how we respond when it happens and how we plan to stay alive and thriving in the days, weeks, and months to come.

As a trained CERT (Community Emergency Response Team) member, I have the benefit of years of training through the Department of Homeland Security and FEMA (the Federal Emergency Management Agency). I am trained in all areas of preparedness and response and how to work in my home, neighborhood, and community to assist first responders in a disaster. More importantly, if no first responders are available, I know what to do to help my family, my neighbors, and myself. We were once told to have only seventy-two hours' worth of food and water stored for an emergency. Remember those days? Now we are told to have a minimum of *two weeks* worth of food, water, and medications because our infrastructure in a major disaster might be crippled enough that goods cannot get to our ports, across our highways, and into our stores for weeks.

I learned these things via CERT and also Red Cross training, but not everyone has that luxury, although I highly recommend getting this free training if it's offered in your community. That is why a book like this can be a huge help in giving the reader plenty of solid information to put to use if and when it's needed.

If writing this book can help just one person survive a disaster, I as an author and CERT member will be thrilled. My hope is that it helps a lot of people think hard about getting over those "Oh, I'll do it next week" excuses and preparing NOW for what might be right around the corner. The last thing we want to do is be caught off guard, having promised ourselves and our families we would come up with an emergency plan when we had time.

The time is now.

This book is divided into four sections that cover past disasters and what we learned from them, as well as current threats we face, preparing for any disaster, responding when it happens, and valuable resources to get prepped and ready. Don't have a bug-out bag or emergency kit? Check! Not sure how to get news during a major disaster? Check! Wondering what to do if you're on the road when something happens? Check! From tick bites to nuclear fallout, tornado outbreaks to terrorist bombings, chemical spills to flash floods, and everything in between, this book will give readers plenty of tools to increase your odds of staying safe. Whether you travel or camp or hike or stay home, there is ample information on how to take care of yourself and your loved ones if anything out of the ordinary should happen. Because if watching the news or going on social networking for an hour has proven anything, it is that something *will* happen.

There are a lot of lists in this book. Lists upon lists. Lists are a wonderful way to convey information in a structured manner for the brain to absorb. Lists are repetitive, and repetition is the mother of, well, of something. So be ready for lists, including some very helpful lists in the appendix section you can fill in yourself.

There is also a lot of sheer common sense in these pages. You may read it and say, "Did I really need to buy a book to hear this?" But apparently many people still do not use common sense when it comes to the potential for an emergency that could disrupt their normal, day-to-day routines. They want and need to be told exactly what to do over and over again until it sinks in and becomes a habit. The subconscious needs to be programmed before the conscious mind recognizes the importance of having a plan.

Life will never be emergency- or disaster-free. There will always be challenges to overcome, no matter where we call home or what we do for a living. Disasters don't pick and choose, they just happen. The onus of responsibility falls upon us to sit down and make the plans we keep putting off with our families and loved ones in order to survive.

Here is a challenge: Take one week out of your life and watch the nightly news for an hour. Every night. Then think about what you would do in each and every one of the disasters—natural or manmade—reported. Would you survive? Would you fall apart? Would you panic and become immobilized or jump up, take the lead, and save the world? The problem is that we don't really know *what* we will do until we are called upon to do it. But having plans helps. Having knowledge helps. Having options helps.

Think back on your life to when you had to go through something totally unknown and foreign to you. Were you terrified or elated? Maybe a bit of both? We wake up each morning under the false assumption that the day ahead of us will be pretty much the same as the day behind us, and most of the time we might be right. But on those days when all hell breaks loose, nothing goes as planned, and everything that *can* happen *does* happen, how do we respond? What is our default operating mode when something knocks us off our schedule and out of our routine?

It might behoove each of us to ask those questions and then ask, "Can I do better?"

There are no guarantees in life, but we can certainly guarantee that the more we know, the better our chances will be. It doesn't require thousands of dollars, or thousands of hours of time; it does require a commitment to making emergency survival a high priority because there are many things that can be put off in life for another day.

This is not one of them.

PART 1
THE THREATS: NATURAL AND MAN-MADE DISASTERS

The Worst Natural Disasters We've Faced

If we had a way to look far back in time to the birth of our planet, we might be horrified at the sheer level of destruction all around us. Our planet was formed because of one natural disaster after another, many of which still occur to this day. Imagine a world with no mountains or rivers or separate continents, oceans, and seas. No islands or caverns or vast forests. Millions of years ago, massive earthquakes, volcanic eruptions, and even asteroid and comet impacts molded, shaped, and formed the very ground we now walk on. Without such natural catastrophes, the planet might not have formed at all.

Luckily, humankind did not exist back then to deal with such extreme scenarios, although the other species that once walked the earth didn't fare as well. Just think of the dinosaurs, which died out approximately 64 million years ago during what is now called one of the five extinction-level events the planet has suffered through.

There are two kinds of disasters or emergency events we face. One is natural, caused by forces such as weather, wind, water, ground movements, eruptions, impacts by space objects, pandemics, and anything else Mother Nature might dish out. The other kind is man-made, such as infrastructure failures, war, nuclear accidents, hazardous waste mishaps, terrorism, mass murder, chemical leaks, and the like. We will start with Mother Nature, because the largest and worst disasters are those she delivers, and often one on top of another.

MASS EXTINCTION EVENTS

Over the course of Earth's history, there have been five "mass," or "great," extinction events, where millions of living creatures perished, whether on land or sea. These events are different from normal extinctions because they involve large numbers of species falling by the wayside and not just the demise of one or two.

Also known as "biotic crises," these mega jumbo disasters can literally change the face of species diversity and evolution itself by creating population bottlenecks that lead to genetic differentiation and limited breeding options. Extinction rates often don't take a direct and even course, but great extinction events do seem to happen on a somewhat regular basis, although this includes smaller events that may not have wiped out as much life, but changed some part of genetic history. Scientists actually measure the rate of mass extinctions by looking at marine fossils, which prove to be far superior as a fossil record than land animals because they are often better preserved on the ocean floor.

The causes of such great events can be long-term stressors to life, punctuated by a short-term situation such as an asteroid impact or a global ice age. All extinctions reshape the diversity of life on the planet, dictating the end of some species and the rise of others. Some could then say that extinction-level events have both positives and negatives when it comes to our planet's evolution.

Though the dinosaur extinction, the Cretaceous-Tertiary, or K-T, is the one most people know about, the complete list of such events is:

1. The Ordovician-Silurian is among the three largest extinction events in the planet's history, occurring approximately 440–450 million years ago. It was actually two events that were separated by hundreds of thousands of years but, combined, killed approximately 60%–70% of all species, including 27% of major "family" groups of living things. Possible causes are gamma ray bursts, global massive cooling, and a drop in sea levels.

2. The Late Devonian, during which three quarters of all species on Earth died out. There is some question as to whether this occurred over several million years, starting 375 million or so years ago, and may be what is called a series of extinction pulses that happen within a distinct time frame of an overall mass extinction.

3. The Permian-Triassic, or Great Dying, which happened approximately 252 million years ago, and is considered the greatest mass extinction event of all time. Over 96% of all species perished, including 96% of all marine life and 70% of all land species. This was the end of the trilobite and the end as well of reptile dominance on land. Vertebrates took 30 million years to recover from this event. Life on Earth today descends from the 4% or so of species that survived the Great Dying.

4. The Triassic-Jurassic, a three-phase extinction around 201 million years ago, wiped out about 75% of all species at the time, including most large amphibians. Climate change, flood basalt eruptions, and

even an asteroid impact are all possible causes for this event.

5. The Cretaceous-Tertiary, or K-T event, which drove all non-avian dinosaurs to extinction 65–66 million years ago along with 75% of all species on Earth. This was when mammals and birds emerged as the dominant animals on land and was the last extinction event before the one we are currently in. A possible and widely discussed cause is asteroid impact, but supervolcanic eruptions are also a possibility.

6. Yes, there is a sixth, the Holocene Event, also known as the Anthropocene because for the first time an extinction event is being caused by human activity. Though the Holocene is said to have begun in approximately 10,000 to 11,000 B.C.E., land and sea extinctions in this event are occurring at over a thousand times the background extinction rate since 1900 and showing no signs of stopping. Climate change is cause number one, along with overfishing, overhunting, deforestation, pollution and toxins, environmental degradation, and habitat destruction.

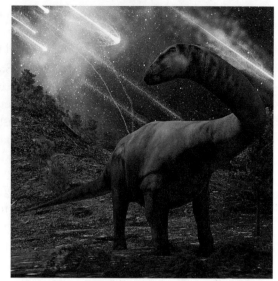

The mass extinction event with which most people are familiar is the one that occurred about 65 million years ago, when dinosaurs and many other animals and plants were wiped out by a meteor impact.

Though extinction events of this magnitude don't occur every day, the fact that we are facing our own possible extinction should be enough to drive every human on Earth to take positive action. In the meantime, though, we do face daily and yearly disasters and emergencies, whether at home or abroad, that we have more immediate control over.

THE MORE RECENT PAST

As humans fast approach a global population of over seven billion and urban and coastal growth skyrockets in many countries, including the United States, it's only natural that more people are being exposed to a variety of both natural and man-made disasters. According to the U.S. Disaster Statistics on the NOAA (National Oceanic and Atmospheric Administration) website, growing populations and infrastructures increase the exposure to hazardous situations. The strongest growth is found in coastal areas, where threats of flooding, cyclones, hurricane storm surge, rising sea levels, and tidal waves prevail. Yet in urban areas, there is also more to worry about in terms of flooding, landslides, and collapses of bridges, highways, and sinkholes. And the more people living in those areas, the more potential for damage to both lives and property.

The U.S. Natural Hazard Statistics, also a part of NOAA, stated that the top three disaster-related events involving the weather were flooding, hurricanes, and heat waves. Storms of every size are the biggest threat, responsible for an average of 12.69% of all disasters annually. Second in place are floods at 4.25% and wildfires at 1.76%. Between the years 1985 and 2008, the top ten natural disasters by type, year, and number of lives affected were:

Flood	2008	11,000,000
Storm	2004	5,000,000
Storm	1999	3,000,000
Storm	2008	2,100,000
Storm	1985	1,000,000
Wildfire	2007	640,000
Storm	2005	500,000
Epidemic	1993	403,000
Storm	2005	300,000

Of the lives lost, 90% were lost to storms, 4% to floods, 3% to wildfires, and 2% to epidemics. The economic damage totaled in the hundreds of millions of dollars. And these statistics are only for the United States. Add to that the losses of life and money from global disasters, and it becomes staggering.

In the year 2011 alone, there were 25 natural disasters in the United States. Only China had more that same year, with 29. In 2014, according to the Annual Disaster Statistical Review for the Centre for Research on the Epidemiology of Disasters, there were 324 natural disasters, the third lowest number reported in the last decade. Still, 7,823 people lost their lives.

The countries hit with the most natural disasters over the last decade are China, the United States, the Philippines, Indonesia, and India. These disasters included floods, earthquakes, landslides, megastorms, and droughts. The biggest disasters occurred in countries far from the United States, which may have a lot to do with much more modern U.S. infrastructure, building codes, and preparedness and response measures.

Other fascinating facts about disasters include:

- Between 2000 and 2012, natural disasters caused over $1.7 trillion in damage and affected the lives of over 2.9 billion people.
- In 2011, the world hit a record high of $371 billion in disaster damage and during that year recorded 154 floods, 16 droughts, and 15 extreme heat or cold events.
- The most widespread natural disaster is flooding, followed by wildfires. These disasters occur all over the world and are not limited to one region.

- In 2012, nearly half the reported fatalities from natural disasters involved flooding or hydrological events.

- Earthquakes are among the most severe natural disasters and can also trigger man-made disasters such as infrastructure collapses and gas explosions. Many people die in earthquakes because of gas fires and not the quake itself.

- Tornadoes can have a damage path of over one mile wide and 50 miles (80 kilometers) long.

- In 1975 there were 100 disasters. In 2005 there were 400.

- In the last decade, the number of people affected by disasters increased from 1.6 billion in the previous decade to over 2.6 billion.

- Tornado outbreaks in 2012 numbered over 930 in the United States, and that was a lower-than-normal year.

- Economic costs are fifteen times higher now than they were in the 1950s.

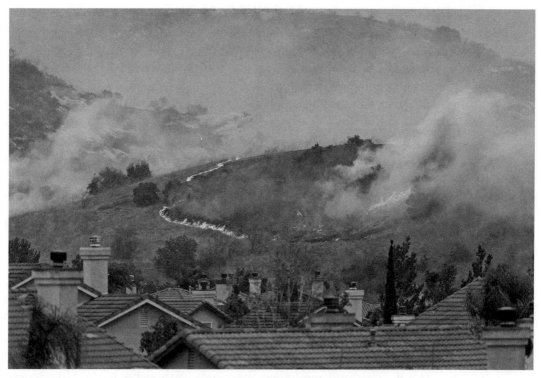

Climate change has resulted in more weather-related disasters recently. They are not only more common but also more damaging. For example, in Santa Barbara, California, fires were followed by rains that caused a rockslide, destroying homes and killing seventeen people in January 2018.

- The countries most exposed to multiple hazards are Taiwan, Costa Rica, Vanuatu, the Philippines, Guatemala, Ecuador, Chile, Japan, Vietnam, and the Solomon Islands, in that order, according to 2005 data from the World Bank.

Most major disasters reach catastrophic levels in terms of lives lost and property damaged based on their location. Obviously, those affecting urban and heavily populated areas are deemed far worse than those that occur in the middle of nowhere. But some areas are just plain prone to natural disasters. Floodplains, Tornado Alley, cyclone zones, any country that borders the notorious, seismically active Ring of Fire, close proximity to active volcanoes or rivers and dams with a history of overflow issues—it does often come down to location, location, location.

No one is immune, though, and with climate change now affecting weather patterns and creating its own disaster-prone scenarios, such as devastating droughts and massive flooding (sometimes in the same regions of the world), we have even more to become aware of.

ONE YEAR ALONE

In 2016 alone, the world suffered numerous major natural disasters. In the American Northeast, the Storm of the Century, also known as Jonas, left forty-eight people dead and large areas buried in record snowfall. Meanwhile, California was burning with a record number of wildfires, so many that over 10,000 firefighters were on the front lines of fourteen active fires, many started by arson, according to Cal Fire.

Louisiana was suffering at the same time from historic flooding that took the lives of thirteen people and caused billions of dollars in damage, with storms dropping over thirty inches (762 millimeters) of rain in some areas during a twelve- to fifteen-hour period. Hurricane Matthew dealt even more destruction with flooding in the southeastern region of the country, most notably in North Carolina.

Major earthquakes struck in central Italy, with a 6.2-magnitude temblor that took over 240 lives; Myanmar was hit with an even larger quake; there was a 7.8 monster in New Zealand's South Island that caused a tsunami; and a 7.7-magnitude quake hit the Solomon Islands.

So much can happen in a year, and 2016 set a North American record with 160 natural disasters, more than in any other year since 1980. And this doesn't include smaller disasters or those that happen in unpopulated areas. As the year 2017 got underway, there were large earthquakes in the Philippines; landslides in Indonesia killing 4; landslides in Nepal killing 2; Columbian mudslides leaving 254 dead; Cyclone Debbie, killing 2 in Australia; and a Japanese avalanche that took the lives of 8 people and injured dozens of others.

TOP DISASTERS GLOBALLY

The Internet and media are rife with lists of the top ten or twenty or fifty natural disasters to strike around the world, and it always seems that once a list is published, another, even bigger, disaster occurs worthy of being included. That is the nature of disasters. They often get worse over time and not better, mainly because, as we humans increasingly populate the planet, disasters take a higher toll of life. Huge disasters of yesteryear may have killed dozens, whereas today they kill thousands, even hundreds of thousands.

The following are some of the widely accepted mega-disasters of recent times as well as the loss of life incurred. This list does not include the hundreds of disasters that took fewer lives, ranging from a dozen dead in a wildfire to 90,000 dead in an earthquake.

Event	Location	Lives Lost
Yellow River flood	China, 1931	1,000,000 to 4,000,000 million dead
Yellow River flood	China, 1887	900,000 to 2,000,000 dead
Bhola cyclone	Bangladesh, 1970	500,000 to 1,000,000 dead
India cyclone	India, 1839	300,000 dead
Tangshan quake	China, 1976	650,000 to 800,000 dead
Haiyuan quake	China, 1920	240,000 dead
Indian Ocean quake and tsunami	2004	230,000 dead
Typhoon Nina	China, 1975	229,000 dead
Haiti quake	Haiti, 2010	160,000 dead
Yangtze River flood	China, 1935	145,000 dead
Great Kanto quake	Japan, 1923	143,000 dead
Bangladesh cyclone	Bangladesh, 1991	138,800 dead
Cyclone Nargis	Myanmar, 2008	138,000 dead
Messina quake	Italy, 1908	123,000 dead
Krakatoa eruption	Indonesia, 1883	120,000 dead
Ashgabat quake	Turkmenistan, 1948	110,000 dead
Kashmir quake	Pakistan, 2005	100,000 dead
Hanoi/Red River Delta flood	North Vietnam, 1971	100,000 dead

It's interesting to note that the largest losses of life due to natural disasters in recent times have involved water and earth movement, either in the form of superstorms, such as cyclones and floods, or earthquakes and even subsequent tsunamis. None of these events occurred in the United States or Europe, but mainly on the larger Asian continent. China and India are such heavily populated countries; disasters often result in massive numbers of lives lost.

Natural disasters are much worse when they strike vulnerable populated regions. Think about it: if an earthquake occurs in the middle of nowhere and no life is lost or buildings damaged, we probably would not categorize it as a disaster at all, just as an earthquake. When a naturally occurring event meets a

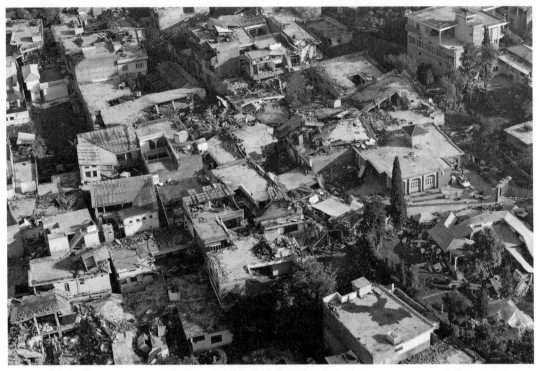

As a result of the 2005 earthquake in Kashmir, northern India, upwards of 100,000 people died because the area was heavily populated. When disaster hits unpopulated areas, we generally don't think of them as disasters.

hazardous location, and the lives of humans and even animals are at risk, along with the dangers to structures and roads, airports and bridges, factories and warehouses, offices and farms—then it becomes a disaster.

Yet to look at the loss of lives above is not to understand the bigger picture. As the following chapters will show, each different type of disaster takes lives and destroys environments and affects the local, regional, and even national economies where it occurs. And some of the biggest disasters of all are those so mind-bogglingly devastating that they result in the loss, not of millions of lives, but *hundreds* of millions. Those include famines, droughts, and plagues/pandemics. Such mega-disasters combine both natural and man-made causes and are the most devastating to life, whether human, animal, or plant. We will see just how shockingly catastrophic these events can truly be in a coming chapter.

ECONOMIC IMPACT

The financial impact from natural disasters is often crippling, depending upon where it occurs, what the infrastructure is like, and whether or not an initial disaster triggers something additional, as when a major quake triggers a tsunami. Usually the costs run into the billions of dollars, sometimes hundreds of billions, as money is needed to repair roads, dams, levees, bridges, homes, and buildings and assist survivors in getting the aid they need to rebuild or relocate. Further problems ensue when not all the damaged is covered by insurance.

In 2016 alone, disasters caused over $175 billion in damage, which was a four-year-high global cost according to Charles Riley's article "Natural Disasters Caused $175 Billion in Damage in 2016" for the January 4, 2017, edition of CNN.com. Ten billion dollars alone was allocated for the damage done by Hurricane Matthew.

According to "Top 5 Most Expensive Natural Disasters in History" by Bo Zhang on AccuWeather.com, the costliest disaster ever was the 9.0 earthquake and tsunami that struck the coast of Japan on March 11, 2011, and triggered a man-made disaster at the Fukushima Nuclear Power Plant. The World Bank estimates the damage at $235 billion, but the Japanese government claims the number is much higher, at $309 billion.

The other four on Zhang's list are (all estimates by the National Oceanic and Atmospheric Administration and the World Bank):

1. Great Hanshin or Kobe earthquake, 1995, Japan: $100 billion as per the World Bank

2. Hurricane Katrina, 2005, United States: $61 billion according to NOAA

3. Northridge earthquake, 1994, Southern California: $42 billion as per NOAA

4. Sichuan earthquake, 2008, China: $29 billion as per the World Bank (other lists estimate this at $100–140 billion)

Other lists include the 2011 Thailand floods, at $46 billion; the Christchurch, New Zealand, earthquake of 2011, at $40 billion; Hurricane Ike in 2008 in the United States, at $30 billion; the Yangtze River floods of 1998 in China, at $26 billion, and 1992's Hurricane Andrew in the United States, at $25 billion. Even wildfires can run into the billions of dollars of damage, as did the 2003 Cedar Fire in the United States, at $2 billion, and the 2011 Silver Lake wildfire in Canada at $1.8 billion.

Whether loss of life or property, environmental damage, or economic costs for recovery, natural disasters can have an impact that lasts decades after the actual event occurred.

The whole purpose of looking back at past disasters is to try to understand how we could have done a better job of being ready and responding in the manner most appropriate for survival. Emergency management professionals all over the world, as well as civilian groups involved in disaster preparedness and response, can examine the disasters that have happened in the recent past for clues to how communications, warnings, medical response, chain of command, emergency operations, and so many other things can be improved upon, not just for the populace at large, but for individuals and families.

For you, the reader, it helps to pinpoint what hazards exist in your area and gives insight as to the specific threats you and your family may face in the days ahead. Many people only know about major disasters from television shows and movies that sensationalize what really happens. Real information can be hard to come by, and many of us just don't have the time to do all the research required to separate fact from fiction.

With the advent of the Internet, disaster and emergency information is now at our fingertips, but again, it takes a great deal of time to search for every possible scenario. In the information age, it often helps most to have that information in one place—thus this book and others like it. It's a lot easier to grab a book when something happens than your computer, laptop, or tablet, and in some cases, there won't be the power to use those things, should the electrical grid go down.

The next chapters will look at specific disasters and also explore manmade disasters and emergencies, which can be just as dangerous to life and costly to property. The more you know about what you are facing, the more of an edge you have going into preparedness and response.

Avalanches to Wildfires: The Darker Side of Nature

When it comes to natural disasters, we face many threats no matter where we live or travel in the world. Some of those threats may even come from space. Though many of us will live a lifetime without ever experiencing some of these situations, they are a clear and present danger nonetheless. Though a natural disaster can be a simple storm that ravages a small area of land, the following are the larger threats, including those that made news headlines.

AVALANCHES

When we look at snow-covered mountains, our first thoughts may be of skiing and ski lodges or water sources for communities in the foothills. Rarely do we expect a mountain to turn on us, but avalanches are a danger to skiers and anyone living in the immediate vicinity. When a mass of snow, ice, and even rocks begins to slide down a mountainside, it takes everything in its path with it.

According to *National Geographic Online*, 90% of avalanches are triggered by human activity, such as skiing, snowmobiling, snowboarding, or mountain climbing. More than 150 people die every year all over the world. An avalanche might appear to happen suddenly, but there may be "sluffs," or small slides of dry, powdery snow, beforehand. An avalanche is far more likely to occur right after a storm when a foot or more of fresh snow is dropped. The reason for this is that the weight of the freshly fallen snow can fracture a weakened layer of snowpack below, but temperature, wind, steepness, and even the underlying terrain itself are all factors.

The National Snow and Ice Data Center states that the biggest months for avalanches are December to April, but there are some on record for every month of the year. The Data Center reports that a large avalanche could unleash approximately 200,000 cubic meters (7,062,933 cubic feet) of snow, which is enough to cover twenty football fields ten feet (three meters) deep! These larger avalanches are more often than not the result of natural rather than human factors.

There are three main zones: The starting zone is where the unstable fracture occurs and begins to slide. The track is the path the snow takes down the mountainside, and the runout zone is where the snow and the debris it picks up along the way finally come to a stop.

So what do you do if you are in the presence of an avalanche in the making? First and foremost, get off the slab as quickly as you can. If you are a skier or snowboarder, you have the gift of downhill speed to assist you and can veer out of the path by going in the opposite direction. If that is not possible, look for a tree to hold on to as the snow passes over. No trees, and it becomes a bit more difficult, as the human body will sink into the snow, so keeping a clear area under the snow by moving allows you to breathe until you can either punch your way out or help arrives. *National Geographic Online* states that about 93% of victims can survive if they are rescued within fifteen minutes. As time goes on, the survival rate plummets.

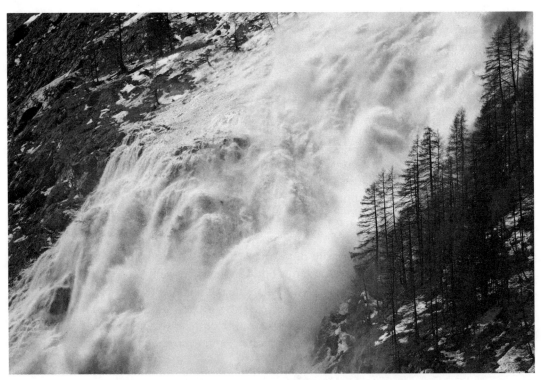

An avalanche similar to this one in the Italian Alps killed 10,000 people in 1916. Sometimes avalanches occur naturally, sometimes human beings set them off.

It's hard to believe, but all that snow speeding downhill can reach up to 80 miles per hour (129 kilometers per hour), making it difficult for anyone in its path to get out of the way in time.

Some of the deadliest avalanches in history include:

- 1970 Peru—Huascarán avalanche, which was triggered by the Ancash earthquake, killing approximately 20,000 people. The avalanche moved downhill at a speed of about 100 miles per hour (161 kilometers per hour) and consisted of over 80 million cubic feet (2,265,000 cubic meters) of snow, ice, mud, and rock. The 11-mile (18-kilometer) avalanche buried the nearby towns of Yungay and Ranrahirca.

- 1916 Italy—Tyrolean Alps avalanche. Over 10,000 were killed, including Austrian and Italian soldiers in World War I. The avalanche was caused by the detonation of explosives along with a heavy snowfall.

- 1962 Peru—The Ranrahirca avalanche. A storm the day before triggered an avalanche of 39 million feet (11.8 million meters) of snow and associated debris, killing over 3,500 people.

- 2015 Afghanistan avalanches—killed 310 people.

- 1950–1951 Austria and Italy avalanches—killed over 265 people.

- 2012 Afghanistan avalanches—killed over 200 people.

To give an idea of how often avalanches can occur, the World Avalanche Timeline on Google Maps shows six from January through March 2017. This includes two in Italy, one in Canada, one in Japan, one in Pakistan, and one in Afghanistan. Though deaths were considered low compared to other types of natural disasters, a total of over 100 people died in the Pakistan and Afghanistan avalanches. We most often think of Austria, Sweden, Canada, and other "snowy" countries as avalanche hot spots, but Middle Eastern countries like Pakistan and Afghanistan have their own mountains filled with dangerous snow.

BLIZZARDS

A blizzard is a type of snowstorm with sustained winds of 35 miles per hour (56 kilometers per hour) or stronger. The typical blizzard lasts over three hours, and some endure for days. The wind and snow in many cases cause zero visibility and cripple roadways and plane travel under a whiteout that can bring schools, businesses, and travel to a screeching halt. Though the only way to avoid a blizzard is to not be in a part of the country or world that has them, or to get out of town before one is predicted, the best way to survive one is to stay inside, shelter in place, and have already stocked up on food and water. Because electricity may not be available due to high winds, plenty of other means of staying warm, such as blankets and even fires in fireplaces, can help you ride out the worst of it.

Many people, sadly, freeze to death from being trapped in cars during a blizzard, often because they get stuck on a roadway and have nowhere to go. Hypothermia sets in, and unless cars are dug out from the several feet of snow they are buried under, time can be the killer. More on hypothermia later in the "Wilderness Survival" chapter.

There are actually two types of blizzards: regular blizzards, with winds accompanying falling snow, and ground blizzards, where snow already on the ground is blown about by winds, creating a blizzard condition that doesn't require currently falling snow. Winds in some blizzards can top 50 miles per hour (80 kph), and temperatures can plummet well below zero, with wind chill numbers that are low enough to cause frostbite for anyone caught outside. A regular blizzard requires cold air below freezing, moisture in the air, such as water vapor from air blowing across a lake or river, and warm, rising air. These are the prime conditions for a blizzard.

A type of blizzard or severe snowstorm well known in the United States is the nor'easter, which is named after the direction of its oncoming winds and mainly strikes the East Coast into Canada. These superstorms can include a major storm surge and high waves along the coastline. One of the worst blizzards in history was the 1888 Great Blizzard, which was considered a nor'easter and, before it was over, dropped over 50 inches (1.27 meters) of snow on the ground and created snowdrifts even higher. Four hundred people lost their lives, mainly in densely populated New York. This storm occurred in March and lasted four days, with winds well over 70 miles per hour (113 kph). Passengers on locomotives were stranded on the tracks, taxis and horse-drawn carriages were trapped in snow, and New York City came to a standstill. New York and the surrounding regions have suffered many blizzards since.

An even larger and deadlier blizzard occurred in Iran in 1972, causing over 4,000 deaths and covering villages with over 26 feet (8 meters) of snow. This remains the deadliest blizzard on record. Other noted blizzards include:

- The 2008 Afghanistan blizzard, the second deadliest on record, with a death toll exceeding 1,337 people. Temperatures plummeted below −30° Celsius (−22° Fahrenheit) as people froze to death in mountainous areas. Over 100 people had to have limbs amputated because of frostbite. In addition to human lives, over 415,000 sheep, goats, and head of cattle lost their lives.

- The 1993 "Storm of the Century" hit twenty-six states and most of eastern Canada, causing over $10 billion in damage and killing over 270 people in the United States alone. It struck in early March, with homes along the eastern shore of Long Island swept out to sea by mammoth waves. Many weather records were broken, and meteorologists claimed the storm had the same force as a Category Three hurricane.

One blessing: because of advances in storm prediction, many people were warned in advance and given time to prepare or find shelter.

- The 2008 Tibet blizzard, which struck Lhünzê County, with 59 inches (1.5 meters) of snow falling on some villages for over 36 hours. Seven died, and many buildings collapsed from the weight of the snow. Locals had to sell off or kill their domestic livestock and yak herds.

- The 1971 Eastern Canada blizzard was a March nor'easter that covered eastern Canada and ended up with over 20 deaths. A historical effect of this storm was the cancellation of the Montreal Canadiens hockey game, a first in Canada's history.

- The 1996 Monster Blizzard hit the East Coast with three days of harsh, wet snow and sleet. It hit New York City particularly hard, with over $1 billion in damage and dozens of people dead. Because New York City is so heavily populated, blizzards often cause more damage and death there than they would in a rural area.

An interesting factoid: blizzards are not as common as tornadoes or hurricanes but often result in as many deaths.

DROUGHTS

When a particular region of the world goes too long without precipitation, there is drought. Drought is more than just a dry spell. It is a period of time, perhaps even years, when usable water is scarce. Often accompanied by extensive heat waves and dry or extremely low humidity, droughts kill far more people than earthquakes, volcanoes, and most other natural disasters.

Major droughts have led to humanitarian crises of epic proportions as well as the decimation of animal and plant species that rely on rain and water coming off of snowy mountains to survive. The consequences of drought are harsh, with millions of living things dying as a result, because water is so necessary for survival. The causes of droughts are both natural and man-made, with three particular categories:

Meteorological drought—results from weather conditions such as prolonged spells without precipitation

Agricultural drought—causes crop failure and can be the result of weather or poorly planned agricultural practices

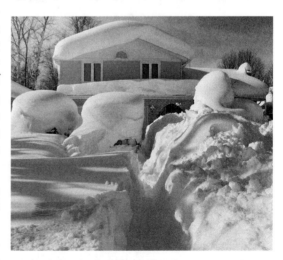

Blizzards can trap people in their homes or on the road, sometimes without electricity, heat, or water. If caught unprepared, a blizzard can prove to be lethal.

Winter Weather Advisories

When the cold winds blow, you may experience freezing rain—rain that freezes as it hits the ground and creates a slick coating of ice on roadways—or sleet—rain that freezes into ice pellets before it hits the ground but can also cause slippery roadways. Or you may be caught in a full-on snowstorm with freezing temperatures and high winds.

Wind chill is the temperature it actually "feels like" when you are outdoors, and severe wind chill can cause frostbite and hypothermia even if the actual temperature doesn't seem to be low enough.

Winter weather advisories are critical during snowstorms and blizzards because they provide critical information as to whether or not going outdoors is life threatening. Hazardous driving conditions should prompt people to stay off the roadways, or at least try to get where they are going quickly.

Winter storm watches are alerts that a winter storm is possible, with heavy snow, ice, hail, and other severe weather conditions. Monitor your local news and alert systems, and prepare to be indoors for a while.

Winter storm warnings mean that a storm in your area is imminent. Get indoors and stay indoors! Get off the roadways as soon as possible. Wrap up and get warm because the storm is about to hit. This does *not* mean run to the nearest store to buy the water and bread you should have already stocked up on during the advisories and watches.

Frost/freeze warnings mean that temperatures will plunge below freezing. Be ready to stay warm, but also be sure to bring in pets and sensitive plants.

Blizzard warnings mean that not only will there be severe weather but also high wind gusts and sustained winds of at least 35 miles per hour (56 kph). Visibility will be severely reduced, and major snowfall is expected.

Hydrological drought—when water reserves in lakes, reservoirs, and aquifers fall below a statistical average and stored water is used much faster than it can be replenished

Whatever their cause or type, droughts have major economic, social, and environmental impacts, yet are a part of the cycle of global weather conditions the planet undergoes over time. Droughts also trigger dust bowls, famine, malnutrition, mass migrations, even civil unrest and war as nations fight over scarce water and the rights to usable water sources.

Massive historical droughts have killed millions, especially when combined with famine, and the two often go hand in hand. One might say that famine is the man-made result of the natural disaster that drought is. A famine is described as a phenomenon involving a widespread lack of food and water that results in mass starvation. Often a number of factors occur before the stage is set for catastrophic famine, which usually occurs in highly populated third-world nations with weak and ineffective infrastructure. Not all of those factors are natural. One of the largest causes of famine is war and civil unrest that displace large groups of people.

Alleviating famine requires humanitarian aid such as food drops and refugee camps and often the supervision of the United Nations and governing bodies of many nations. Even with all the advances in food manufacturing, production, and distribution, the world recently faced the worst humanitarian crisis in decades when widespread famine occurred in Yemen, Somalia, Nigeria, and the Sudan, mainly due to wars and conflicts in these regions, leading to acute malnutrition of over 30 percent of children under the age of five, climbing mortality rates, increased rates of disease outbreaks, and even the potential for terrorism.

The only way to prevent famine is to take long-term measures to increase food production, protect crops and water sources, avoid war, and find new ways to store foodstuffs, including seeds. Agriculture must work with technology to find solutions to prevent famines, but once one occurs, it really becomes a response situation in which citizens and governments must take care of the situation.

The most devastating droughts and famines the planet has faced include:

- The Great Chinese Famine: from 1958 to 1961, this famine resulted in the deaths of approximately 43 million people.

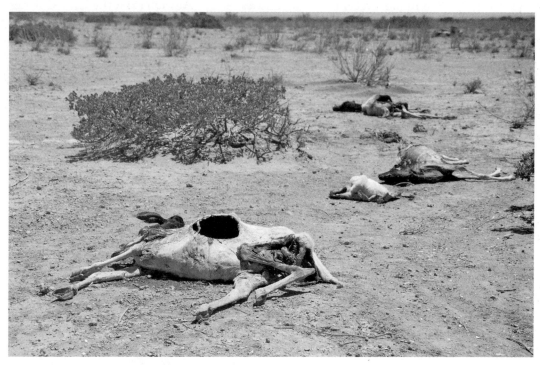

Dead livestock litter the desiccated ground in Somaliland during the 2011 Horn of Africa Drought. Millions of people died throughout the region, including in Kenya, Ethiopia, Somalia, and Djibouti.

- The Chinese famine of 1907 killed over 25 million people.
- The Northern Chinese famine of 1876–1879 killed over 13 million.
- The Doji Bara famine in India from 1789 to 1792 killed over 11 million.
- The Bengal, India, famine of 1769–1771 killed over 10 million—one-third of the entire population.
- The Soviet famine of 1932–1933 killed over 10 million.
- The Chinese drought of 1876–1879 killed millions of people and live-stock, making it one of the ten biggest natural disasters of all time.
- The African drought of 1981–1984: Twenty nations suffered severe drought, resulting in over a million dead.
- The Horn of Africa drought of 2011 killed millions throughout Kenya, Somalia, Ethiopia, and Djibouti.
- The Arduous March famine in North Korea from 1994 to 1998: Over 3,500,000 million were killed by a combination of famine and floods.
- The 2006 Chinese drought of Sichuan Province led to severe water shortages affecting over 8 million people and 7 million head of cattle.

In more recent years, countries such as Australia and the United States have suffered severe and ongoing droughts that have also led to massive wild-fires from the proliferation of dry brush, adding insult to injury.

EARTHQUAKES

"I feel the earth move under my feet," says a classic pop song, and if you've ever been in an earthquake, the feeling of having the ground beneath your feet, the very foundation you stand upon, rumble and tremble and shake is discon-certing, if not downright terrifying. We like to think that the earth beneath our feet is something we can depend on to be stable and solid and fixed, but it's not. Seismic activity that occurs along tectonic plates can be among the most dis-ruptive disasters we experience, especially when it occurs in major urban areas.

Also called tremors or temblors, earthquakes happen all over the world, although they are more prominent over known fault lines and areas that are highly active tectonically, like the Ring of Fire, which snakes up the western coast of South, Central, and North America and down the easternmost part of Asia and associated island nations. Basically, a quake occurs when the buildup of stress between two tectonic plates creates seismic waves that can be strong enough to level a city or weak enough to be barely perceptible. Quakes can also be triggered by volcanic activity, landslides, nuclear tests, and major mine blasts and can be as high as 9 and 10 on the Richter scale, which measures the mag-nitude of quakes, although it is entirely possible there might be a monstrous quake much higher in magnitude. Quakes can occur deep along fault lines, sometimes miles deep, or be much shallower, and it's the shallower quakes that cause the most damage to above-ground structures.

As more areas become prone to quake activity thanks to the appearance of new fault lines, and activities such as fracking that trigger quakes, it becomes harder to avoid them. There was a time when it was just a matter of staying away from key states such as California, known for its ongoing quake activity, but now many states and countries around the world are feeling the earth move under their feet. It used to be easy to never have to feel a quake in an average lifetime, but now everyone must be ready to respond and react accordingly. Gone are the days of getting under desks and beds, as many people have been crushed by falling debris during the initial shake and major aftershocks, some of which can go on for days, weeks, and months after the main shock.

We now know that it makes much more sense to get outside and away from buildings, power lines, and even trees, but if you're stuck indoors, getting in a doorway or crouching beside a bed or piece of formidable furniture can protect the body from falling debris. Those who live in high-rise buildings will certainly feel the swaying and shaking in a more pronounced manner, but often the most loss of life occurs in smaller and older buildings made of brick and not retrofitted for larger shaking. The key remains, though, to get out in the open, off of bridges and overpasses, away from glass and falling debris, and if near the ocean, to get inland and to high ground quickly to avoid a possible tsunami.

One of the biggest problems with earthquakes is the lack of warning they give scientists and laypeople alike. Earthquake prediction is not yet a science. Far from it. But there is progress being made. Sometimes there may be a small pre-shock, or perhaps pets and animals will react to the seismic waves we are unable to perceive yet. Or perhaps they are hearing sounds we cannot ear as the tectonic plates move together and create a stress fracture. But as of the present, earthquake prediction is not going to give us an hour or two to evacuate our belongings and get to firm ground, and though earth scientists can offer potential odds as to when a fault line might display noticeable activity, based on past eruptions or the visible buildup of stress, they still cannot pinpoint it to a day or time. So the best bet is to always be ready with a plan of response, escape, and survival. More on that later.

The three types of earthquakes are:

Normal—Displacement along the fault line is vertical, with one part of the fault dipping and one rising, causing quakes usually below magnitude 7.

Strike-slip—Displacement is horizontal along the two sides of the fault line, which push alongside each other after fracturing, causing quakes up to magnitude 8.

Thrust/reverse—Convergent boundaries actually shorten the crust and cause some of the most catastrophic quakes, up to magnitude 8 and over.

Just to give you an idea of how powerful a thrust-fault quake can be, imagine the energy released by 10,000 atomic bombs. That is the equivalent of an 8.6 magnitude quake. Other factors combine to increase or decrease the power of a quake, including how far down it occurs from the surface of the earth, and the maximum length of the fault line, as well as the dip angle of one side of a fracture on the fault. To measure a quake, you look for the seismic waves produced during the shaking, including longitudinal P-waves (P for Pressure), transverse S-waves, and surface waves.

Add any nearby volcanoes, and you have double trouble, as a quake can also trigger activity in a volcanic region—and vice versa. Swarms of quakes may also strike certain regions without any main shock. These quakes tend to be smaller in magnitude than a single large shock followed by sizable aftershocks.

The problem with earthquakes is that prediction has been a difficult goal to achieve, despite ongoing massive efforts by scientists and the United States Geographical Survey as well as global agencies that desire at least a short heads-up before the ground begins to move. Because prediction is still in its infancy, it's imperative to focus on being prepared and ready.

Larger quakes, especially in major urban areas, also produce a lot of equally disastrous effects, such as landslides, avalanches, gas explosions and fires, infrastructure damage to freeways and bridges, soil liquefaction, flooding due to the destruction of dams and levees, tsunamis, and building collapses.

Some of the largest earthquakes in recent history include:

1. The Valdivia quake in Chile in 1960 with a 9.5 magnitude
2. The Great Alaska quake of 1964 with a 9.2 magnitude
3. The Sumatra quake of 2004, with a 9.1 magnitude, which triggered devastating tsunamis
4. The Tohoku quake of 2011 near the east coast of Japan, with a magnitude of 9.1, which also triggered the largest nuclear disaster since Chernobyl when a partial meltdown occurred at the Fukushima Daiichi Nuclear Power Plant
5. The Kamchatka, Russia, quake of 1952 with a magnitude of 9.0
6. The Maule quake of 2010 in Chile with a magnitude of 8.8
7. The Ecuador/Colombia quake of 1906 with a magnitude of 8.8
8. The Rat Islands quake of 1965 in the Aleutian Islands with a magnitude of 8.7
9. The Assam quake of 1950 in Tibet with a magnitude of 8.6
10. The Northern Sumatra quake of 2012 with a magnitude of 8.6

Many of the larger quakes occurred along the Ring of Fire, with Sumatra, Indonesia, Japan, Alaska, Russia, Chile, Peru, Argentina, and the West Coast of the United States coming in with major activity.

China boasts some of the deadliest quakes, such as the Great Tangshan quake of 1976, which caused over 240,000 deaths. The 7.0 quake in Haiti in 2010 also caused over 200,000 deaths and left two million people homeless. The 2005 Pakistan quake, a 7.6, took the lives of over 75,000 people. The 2004 Sumatra quake, which spawned a tsunami in the Indian Ocean, measured 9.3 and, because it was an underwater fault quake, ended up in the deaths of over 225,000 as the tsunami hit eleven different countries. One million were left homeless.

In the United States, the areas other than Alaska that see the most quake activity are California and the Pacific Northwest, although fault lines exist in most of the fifty states. The United States has seen some "Great Quakes," with California leading the list in terms of deaths and destruction.

The 1994 Northridge, California, quake, with a magnitude 6.7, caused approximately 60 deaths and over $15 billion in damage to property. The 1989 Loma Prieta earthquake (south of San Francisco), a magnitude 6.9, killed 62 and caused over $6 billion in damage. The most famous California quake is no doubt the Great 1906 San Francisco quake, which measured a whopping 8.2 in magnitude and killed between 700 and 2,500 people. Between the quake and subsequent firestorm, much of the great city and surrounding areas were destroyed. Later quakes were at least confronted by more infrastructure and better response resources.

Other large U.S. quakes include:

- The 1811 Missouri quake along the New Madrid fault line, registering 8.1 on the Richter scale

- The 1868 7.9-magnitude Hawaii quake and tsunami, which killed over 77 people

- The 1933 Long Beach, California, quake, which measured 6.4 and killed 120 people

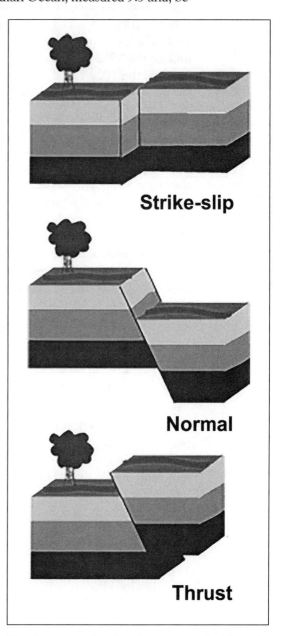

Strike-slip

Normal

Thrust

The three types of earthquakes are categorized depending on how rock and earth move along a fault line.

- The 1959 Montana/Idaho/Wyoming quake, with a magnitude of 7.5, which killed over 28 people
- The 1971 San Fernando quake in California, which measured 6.7 and killed 65 people

There have been a number of major swarms, including one as this book is being written, with over 300 small quakes reported at Yellowstone National Park, where one of the largest supervolcano calderas on the planet lies. Others include the 1962–1971 swarm in Denver, Colorado; the Reno, Nevada, swarm of 2008; the 2009 Oklahoma swarm that continues to this day; the 2004 Yellowstone swarm; and the 2012 Imperial Valley, California, swarm.

Though the largest and deadliest quakes occurred centuries ago, often killing well over 200,000 people—such as the 1138 Aleppo quake in Syria, which killed 230,000, or the Shaanxi, China, quake in 1556, which took over 800,000 lives as 60-foot-deep (18.29-meter-deep) canyons swallowed villages whole and the city of Huaxian lost every single building, mainly due to the types of homes people lived in at the time—more modern quakes rarely see that kind of loss of life in countries where there is ample retrofitting and infrastructure improvement. However, major quakes even today, if they happen in impoverished nations or urbanized regions, will take a big toll on life, and this will no doubt continue to be a risk as we urbanize and greater segments of the population move to the coastal regions and cities that are prime targets for major loss of life and property damage.

HEAT WAVES

Temperatures continue to rise around the globe thanks to climate change. Areas of the world that once rarely experienced warm spells now do so regularly, and it appears that global temps will continue to rise. This means more extended heat waves.

But even a normal summer can have disastrous results if people are not prepared and don't use common sense. Often major heat waves lead to drought and rampaging wildfires as the slightest spark tears through miles of dry brush and combustible fuels. High heat can also be accompanied by high humidity, which can make it feel even more uncomfortable, or extremely low humidity, which presents its own set of problems, especially dry throat and eyes and an increased chance of wildfires.

What truly defines a heat wave is often duration. If it's hot for a day or two, it doesn't qualify. But a week or more and you have a wave that can trigger a domino effect of related issues and often create a health crisis for the most sensitive among us: the elderly, the young, and the weak. When a prolonged heat wave also includes high humidity, it wreaks even greater havoc on the human body as well as on animals such as pets and livestock, whether indoors or not. Another associated problem is the excess use of air conditioners, fans, and energy in general, leading to power outages—not a good thing to have when it's sweltering to begin with.

In the United States, the National Weather Service defines a heat wave as more than three days in duration and gives the label "heat storm" to areas of low humidity (deserts) that experience skyrocketing temperatures. Heat advisories and heat warnings, which are more serious, occur when a heat wave is predicted and it's a danger even to be outside, let alone working and driving in such extreme temps.

According to Dr. Amanda Staudt, a climate scientist for the National Wildlife Federation, rising temps also lead to more pollution trapped over urban areas, which leads to increased levels of asthma, strokes, and heart attacks. The high heat does a number on the body and serves as a major stressor, and those who work outdoors are most at risk. In "Global Warming and Heat Waves" for

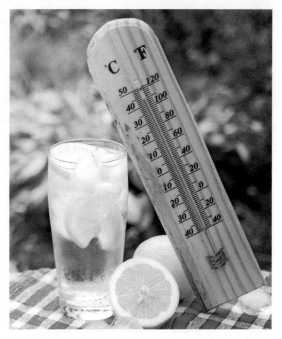

Heat waves—even normal ones not exacerbated by global warming—can lead to fires and health crises, especially among the elderly, the young, and the sick.

NWF.com, she states, "Global warming is bringing more frequent and severe heat waves, and the result will be serious for vulnerable populations." Not to mention the impact on agriculture and our global food supplies and the destruction of natural habitats vulnerable to the slightest changes in their ecosystems.

In the same article, Dr. Peter Wilk, M.D., who is the executive director of the Physicians for Social Responsibility, says, "Global warming is one of the gravest health emergencies facing humanity. It's life-threatening and it's affecting us now." Even normal summers can cause trouble if we don't prepare and respond accordingly—something that will be discussed later in this book. The issues we face today may be amplified to the point where we find every day is a challenge, not just certain seasons of the year.

As temps increase and the duration of heat waves lengthens, we are all vulnerable to the effects, and the after-effects, of a heat wave or heat storm. And when the temps don't drop much during the nights, things can really become deadly. Climate Communication states that, globally, extremely warm nights that once occurred maybe once or twice in twenty years *now* occur every ten years, bringing no cooling relief. In fact, Climate Communication also reported that heat waves claim more lives each year than hurricanes, tornadoes, lightning, floods, and earthquakes combined! An example of a deadly heat wave occurred in 2003 throughout Europe, when scorching temperatures created a drought, crop shortages, and major forest fires that later led to extreme flooding. Over 14,800 people died in France alone, with thousands more across the region, many of whom were in nursing homes and regular homes lacking air conditioning.

Each year we see new record-breaking temperatures all over the world as the summers get hotter and the winters grow milder, leading to water shortages such as the one that plagued the American Southwest for several years, before rains in 2016 and early 2017 alleviated some of the extreme drought warnings. But those droughts will no doubt come back as the hotter months once again scorch the earth, with little to no relief for weeks, even months, on end. "Extreme weather pummeled the United States this summer," Climate Communication writes, "but the next few years might see the most dramatic extremes occurring elsewhere around the world."

We are all at risk.

FLOODS/TSUNAMIS

Water is life, but when there is too much water, it can lead to catastrophic and deadly results. According to ScienceDaily's June 2017 article "Flooding Risk: America's Most Vulnerable Communities," of all the natural disasters, flooding kills the most people. Floods are also the most common natural disasters. Yet people still choose to live in both coastal and inland areas that are designated as flood zones. "Flooding is the most common and widespread disaster we face nationally, and the one that is easiest to alleviate by effective planning," states Richard Yuretich, director of the National Science Foundation's Dynamics of Coupled Natural and Human Systems Program. Increased research and education do help people become more aware of flood dangers, but it is still up to people to put that education into action.

Flooding is a major problem all over the world, whether in countries that traditionally get major rainfall or more arid climates that are seeing increased precipitation. A flood occurs when the dry land is saturated and can no longer absorb more water. Rivers, creeks, streams, and lakes may overflow into communities, threatening homes. Too much snow/ice melt from nearby mountains can result in flooding of foothill areas. Large storm swells and tsunamis can flood coastlines and send people inland to higher ground.

Even desert communities can experience flash flooding—quickly forming and fast-moving localized floods—during a major rainstorm. Flash floods are really a problem because they happen so fast, often leaving people stranded in cars or unable to pass on foot as water seeps over into the surrounding areas, called floodplains.

In the United States, the area most prone to deadly flooding is along the Gulf of Mexico, where hurricanes often strike. It is flooding that is responsible

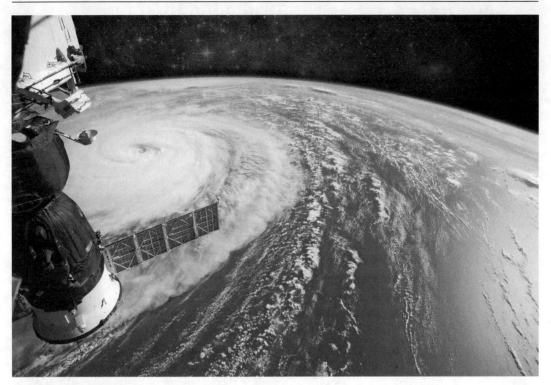

The size of Hurricane Harvey can be appreciated in this 2017 photo taken from the International Space Station.

for most deaths during hurricanes and superstorms, with storm surges taking the lives of those who are not aware of how powerful they can be.

Floods are usually classified in terms of how often they occur in any given time period. A "hundred-year flood" is a large event that occurs once every century, but thanks to global warming, even these rarer events are happening with greater frequency, and in many cases, parts of the world that never worried about major flooding from superstorms and storm surges now must deal with it on an annual basis.

The types of floods are:

- Flash floods—Can occur quickly, usually within a two- to six-hour period, and are usually the result of heavy rainfall, snowmelt, or the breaching of a river or rise of a lake that sends water downhill. They are so destructive and deadly because of the lack of warning, giving people little time to get to high ground or away from flood-prone areas.

- Rapid onset floods—Like flash floods, but take a bit longer to develop and only last for a day or two. There is a little time for people to get out of the area, at least as compared with flash floods.

A Case in Flooding History

As this book was being written, Hurricane Harvey made landfall along the Texas gulf coast on Friday, August 25, going from a Cat 4 to a Cat 3 as it hit the area around Corpus Christie, and began a super-slow crawl inland that would dump over three feet (one meter) of rain in some areas and up to 50 inches (1.52 meters) in others. Once it became a tropical storm, Harvey did even more damage to the area by drowning the area in record rainfall, including the city of Houston, which received over 50 inches (1.52 meters) of rain. This would make it the highest amount of rainfall ever to hit the state of Texas.

As streets and neighborhoods flooded, people who did not evacuate when told found themselves trapped in their homes or out in the streets. Images of cars up to their roofs in water, of adults rowing children in rowboats and kayaks through waist-deep and higher water, and of people slogging through standing water up to their chests and carrying their supply packs above their heads filled the news and social networks. In "Rescuers Pluck Hundreds from Rising Floodwaters in Houston," an August 27, 2017, article by Michael Graczyk for the Associated Press, the National Weather Service's alerts were ominous from the start, as it knew this type of weather pattern would cause a one-two punch with the catastrophic hurricane and massive flooding. "The breadth and intensity of this rainfall is beyond anything experienced before," the NWS said in a statement.

Houston mayor Sylvester Turner said more than two thousand calls came in to emergency services from people needing to be rescued from floodwaters. "I don't need to tell anyone this is a very, very serious and unprecedented storm.... We have several hundred structural flooding reports. We expect that number to rise pretty dramatically."

The rain fell at a rate of four inches per hour or more, creating higher water levels than any other tropical storm in the history of the area. There were videos of numerous rescues, many of which could have been avoided had people evacuated in the first place. Some places had water above chest-level—and more rain in the forecast.

Writing about flooding while watching the devastation live as it happened is humbling to say the least. Water is powerful, and too much of it coming too fast can kill.

- Slow onset floods—These occur as bodies of water flow over their banks and can last for days, even weeks, spreading out over floodplains for miles, especially in low-lying areas.

The United States does put a lot of effort into both predicting where a flood might occur and mitigation efforts, but even so, floods cause over $6 billion worth of damage and kill approximately 140 people each year, with much of that occurring along coastal areas. Globally, coastal flooding causes upwards of $3 *trillion* in damage and thousands of deaths each year, especially in countries like China, where flooding along the Yellow River Valley has caused millions of deaths in the last hundred years alone.

But it isn't just the water that causes all of the problems. Floods carry debris, silt, mud, and even trees and brush in their paths, and the water itself can contain contaminants such as hazardous waste, toxic chemicals, and untreated sewage. Floodwaters that sit for days, weeks, and months become havens for all kinds of disease-carrying mosquitoes and result in an increase of typhoid, West Nile virus, cholera, and other waterborne diseases.

Flooding can also undermine bases of steep slopes of hills and mountains and cause mudslides, which can travel at speeds up to 35 miles per hour (56 kph). Mudslides can carry debris along with them and become deadly to anyone in their path. Even objects as heavy as boulders, trees, and cars can be lifted up and carried on a mudslide path. Entire villages can be wiped away by a massive mudslide as it powers down a hillside or down populated streets located below the base of a large mountain.

Flooding is a natural occurrence, especially along river floodplains, but sadly, humans choosing to live close to rivers and coastlines that have a history of flooding must take part of the blame for deaths and damaged property. Increased developments near wetlands, which usually help to abate floods, also contribute to an increase in flooding that affects homes and lives. Flood insurance may help, but in high-occurrence zones the premiums can be outrageous. Yet floods can also have a beneficial side, as they help to carry nutrients to floodplains and farm fields.

The best way to deal with flooding is to pay attention when storms are predicted and be ready to evacuate if you must. A *flood watch* will be broadcast over television and radio when there is a chance of flooding. A *flood warning* means flooding is imminent and it's time to take action. These warnings will give instructions on what to do and where to go. Always have the basics ready to go if you live in a region prone to major storms and flooding. In the "Preparedness" section of this book, you can learn what you need to have ready for any situation.

In the case of a flash flood, there may not be time, so try to get to nearby higher ground if possible. If there is more warning, be ready to evacuate with the items you will need, and find out where the nearest shelter is. Also, when you leave, be sure to turn off all electrical appliances, gas, and lights. If you cannot leave, get up to a top floor, even the roof if you have to, if water is entering the main floor.

If there is time, drive to higher ground inland, but do not drive through rushing water. "Turn around, don't drown!" Many deaths occur because people think they can drive across a flooded street, only to be swept away by the powerful current. In fact, just two feet of water is all it takes to send your car rushing off with you in it. Try not to come into physical contact with floodwater to avoid contamination and disease. If you are stuck in your car and the water is *not moving,* leave the car immediately to get to higher ground on foot.

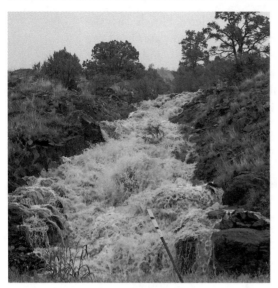

As the name indicates, flash floods come quickly, move fast, and arrive without warning. Therefore, whenever there is a flood warning of any kind, get to higher ground and plan for the worst.

If you are camping or outdoors when flash flooding begins, leave everything behind and get to higher ground. You can replace expensive camping equipment. You can't replace human lives. Try to avoid camping near streams, rivers, and lakes known to flood during heavy rains.

If you own your own home, plant trees and vegetation that can serve as a buffer and control erosion, especially if you live in a low-lying area or foothills. Retaining walls are a great way to divert floodwater, and make sure drains are all unclogged.

Once the problem has abated, wait for instructions from emergency personnel before returning home, and do not turn on electrical equipment until the gas and electric companies have cleared the home. You may think it's all dried out, only to find yourself facing more serious issues. If you set about cleaning the water out of your home yourself, be protected with the appropriate masks and gloves to avoid contamination.

The biggest natural disaster on record is considered to be the 1931 Yangtze River floods in China, which resulted from torrential rains that lasted from April to July. Five hundred square miles (1,295 square kilometers) were under water, and half a million people had to flee their homes. The destruction of rice paddies caused famine for months, and the flood also caused a rise in dysentery and waterborne diseases that killed thousands of people, adding to the approximately 3.7 million who died from the floods themselves. This doesn't take into account the loss of animal life and property.

In 1887, another river in China, the Yellow River, flooded and caused between one and two million deaths and left two million homeless as floodwater inundated over 50,000 square miles (129,500 square kilometers) of low-lying plains.

TSUNAMIS

Those people living along the coasts need to worry about another kind of flooding: tsunamis. Although they don't occur as often as flooding, tsunamis can have a devastating impact. We saw this happen in 2004 in Indonesia after a massive earthquake rocked the Indian Ocean, and again a few years later in 2011 when Japan was hit with a tsunami that submerged homes and cars, and destroyed a nuclear power plant, sending radiation into the waters of the eastern Pacific ocean.

A tsunami is basically an ocean wave that pulls away from shore and then moves back towards land again, moving further and further inland with amazing speed and power. Tsunamis are the result, generally, of major earthquake activity along the ocean floor, but can also be triggered by an asteroid impact or a massive landslide into the ocean. They can travel upstream in estuaries and rivers, bringing with them damaging waves that extend farther inland. Tsunamis can occur at any time of the year, day or night. In the past 224 years, 24 damaging tsunamis have hit the United States and its territories.

According to "Surviving a Tsunami in the United States," for *Emergency Management* magazine, there are two types of tsunamis:

Distant—A distant event originates at least 62 miles (100 kilometers), or more than three tsunami travel hours, away.

Local—A local event affects land within 62 miles (100 kilometers) of the "trigger point" and can take less than an hour to hit shore.

Distant tsunamis are "water events" that begin as a result of catastrophic undersea quakes. "If we have the 9.0 for up to five to 10 minutes, we're talking

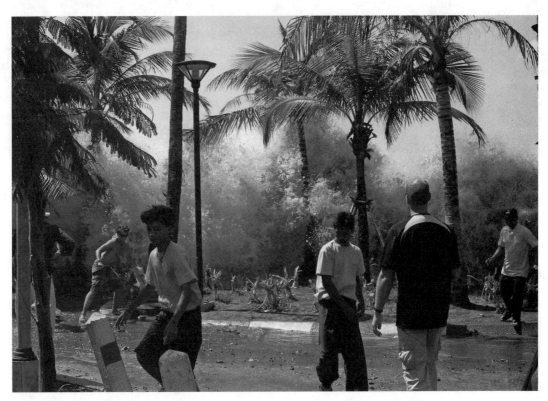

One man appears to stare at the wall of water heading towards him while everyone else runs from the tsunami striking Thailand in 2004. The devastating Indian Ocean tsunami resulted from a huge earthquake off the coast of Sumatra and killed nearly a quarter million people.

Tsunami Facts

Tsunamis are described as long-wave-length ocean waves that are produced by a sudden movement of large volumes of water, such as in an oceanic earthquake, asteroid impact, or landslide into the sea. The distance between wave crests in an open sea can surpass 62 miles (100 kilometers), with wave periods of between five minutes to one hour. Tsunamis can reach travel speeds of close to 500 miles per hour (805 kph)! Large tsunamis can wipe out entire coastal cities in minutes and often reach miles into landmasses. The most destructive tsunamis appear to follow earthquakes of magnitude 7.5 or greater.

Causes of tsunamis include earthquakes, landslides, volcanic activity, meteor impacts, and underwater explosions. The word is Japanese in origin and means "harbor wave."

Many people call tsunamis "tidal waves," but they are not the same thing. Tsunamis are not related at all to the ocean's tides. Nor are they "seismic waves," because an earthquake is not always required to trigger a tsunami.

Two of the largest and most devastating tsunamis in the last twenty years were the December 26, 2004, Indian Ocean tsunami, which followed a 9.1–9.3 magnitude earthquake off the coast of Sumatra and killed over 230,000 people; and the 2011 Tohoku tsunami, which occurred on March 11. The quake was between magnitude 9.0 and 9.1 and occurred deep under water. It was the largest quake ever to strike Japan and triggered a massive tsunami that, along with the quake, resulted in over 16,000 dead and over 273,000 buildings collapsed or destroyed. The worst thing about this event was the near destruction of the Fukushima Daiichi Nuclear Power Plant, which suffered a partial meltdown, sending radiation into the waters off the island and into the Atlantic Ocean. This is now considered the second largest nuclear disaster in history after Chernobyl, Ukraine, in 1986.

about infrastructure not standing in almost any scenario," states Matt Marheine, the deputy director of Oregon's Office of Emergency Management. This means mass evacuations away from the coast inland and to higher ground. Damage done by the initial quake will intensify once the tsunami hits, because the currents are so much stronger than a typical ocean wave.

In a tsunami, multiple long waves hit the shoreline. They can be shallow or form a wall 50 feet (15 meters) high or higher. Sometimes, it isn't the first wave strike that does the most damage. Each tsunami is unique, which requires a great deal of planning to account for all scenarios.

A major earthquake in Africa can cause a tsunami along the U.S. eastern seaboard, just as a major quake in Japan could cause a tsunami to hit Hawaii or even the coast of California. The West Coast and the Pacific Ocean experience much more tsunami activity than the East and the Atlantic. Though tsunamis are quite rare in the Atlantic, they do happen, and they also can happen along the East Coast, so no area can be considered immune.

You can survive a tsunami with adequate warning and by staying calm. The key is to watch or listen to the news to get alerts and instructions, especially after a large quake is reported nearby or across the ocean in coastal waters. Some communities have tsunami sirens and early warning systems in place, others rely on the Emergency Broadcasting System, but all recommend getting away from the shoreline and inland, to higher ground, as quickly as possible. The Pacific Tsunami Warning System in Honolulu, Hawaii, monitors all Pacific Ocean seismic activity, and public education in areas prone to tsunamis is a must to keep the public aware of the danger and instruct them how to act when one is on the way.

One of the biggest problems emergency personnel have is with a public that lacks the understanding that tsunamis can come in "waves" themselves and that it is critical to stay on higher ground until there is no longer any threat. Often, people go back down to their homes after the first wave has hit, unaware that another, possibly even bigger, wave can be coming.

The United States has not experienced a tsunami of catastrophic proportions, but it could happen, and emergency management services are looking to other nations that do experience them for guides to preparation and response.

PANDEMICS

Swine flu. Avian flu. Ebola. In recent years, global pandemics have made headline news even when they occur thousands of miles away. Contagious and infectious diseases are a disaster we will all face in some form in our lifetimes, and many of us already have. The outbreak of a viral or even bacterial agent that can kill can be one of the most terrifying disasters there is, because the enemy is invisible and often spreads through the air, water, and simple human contact.

The word "pandemic" comes from the Greek words *pan*, which means "all," and the word *demos*, meaning "people." When a virus emerges in the human population, it may start out as a smaller, community outbreak that can be contained easily if addressed quickly. But if the outbreak does spread, it can become an epidemic, which affects a larger area, albeit still one city, region, or country. If there is still no containment, and the disease is airborne or highly infectious, it can become pandemic, covering a large number of people on a national and possibly global scale.

The World Health Organization, or WHO, rates influenza pandemics (the most common) on a six-phase scale:

Phase 1—The virus is present in animals but not in humans.

Phase 2—An animal flu virus has infected humans.

Phase 3—Clusters are reported as well as human-to-human transmission, and a community-level outbreak is official.

Phase 4—Pandemic risk is present, but not yet certain.

Phase 5—The disease spreads among human populations in other countries and regions.

Phase 6—Other community-level outbreaks are reported in a WHO region different from that in Phase 5, and a global pandemic is now under way.

If not contained in time, millions of people can die from pandemics, especially if the virus is particularly virulent and the population is vulnerable, such as poorer nations with little or no medical infrastructure and limited access to clean water.

Past pandemics and smaller epidemics that have occurred include cholera, smallpox, typhus, malaria, Ebola, measles, yellow fever, tuberculosis, and Lassa. More recently, the concern has been with fast-mutating avian influenzas such as H1N1 and H5N1 as well as new and powerful antibiotic-resistant strains such as SARS, Zika, and MRSA. Even HIV and AIDS are pandemics. There is also the fear of biological warfare using weaponized viruses such as Ebola and Marburg, both of which are extremely virulent hemorrhagic fever viruses that cause brutal and painful deaths.

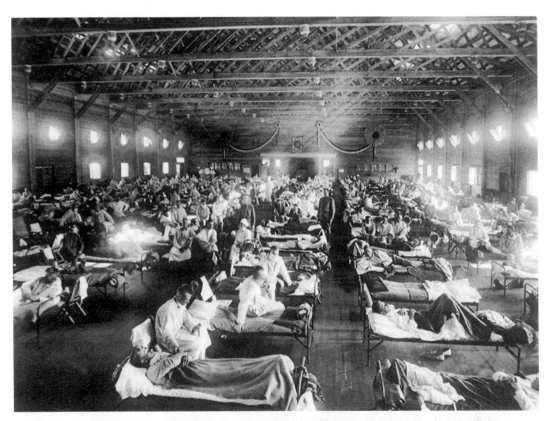

Soldiers sick with Spanish flu are quartered in the Camp Funston ward in Fort Riley, Kansas, in this 1918 photo. Tens of millions died worldwide from the pandemic.

The biggest pandemics in global history occurred in the distant past. In 1350, between 75 and 100 million people fell to the Black Death, a bubonic plague that lasted until 1453 and decimated Europe. It was, in fact, a series of plagues that struck Europe in the same time frame and recurred for centuries. China and India lost over 10 million to a plague pandemic in 1855.

In 1918 and 1919, the Spanish Influenza caused anywhere from 40 to 100 million deaths worldwide. It broke out in waves and spread through Asia, Europe, and into North America. More recently, we have seen HIV originate in Africa and spread into the United States between the years 1966 and 1972, killing millions, including a death toll of 90–100 million predicted for Africa alone by 2025.

Most pandemics are caused by what are called "novel" infectious diseases—new or mutated versions of diseases. Subtypes are viruses that humans either have no immunity against or very little and can be the most problematic to fight. Even with all the vaccines, antiviral drugs, and antibiotics to fight outbreaks, epidemics, and pandemics today, we would be in trouble because of the sheer number of people on the planet; the mobility that can spread an agent on planes, ships, trains, and other modes of transportation; and the lack of money, supplies, and infrastructure in smaller, less developed nations that would be needed to stop a viral attack from spreading.

The longer a pandemic or even an epidemic lasts, the more chance there is of humans developing an immunity to it. Some viral agents are specific to one part of the world but can be introduced into new populations via travel before quarantine can be enforced. Other diseases such as malaria are seeing a huge resurgence in existing areas as well as new areas of the world, because of global warming and changes in the environment that introduce the agent where it may never have thrived before.

The leading governing bodies that oversee and monitor the causes, spread, and prevention of infectious diseases are the World Health Organization (WHO), Centers for Disease Control and Prevention (CDC), and the Health Protection Agency of the United Kingdom.

The key to keeping yourself safe from a pandemic often comes down to common sense. Stay out of "hot zones" and, if told to, shelter in place (more on how to do that later!). Wash your hands often and avoid touching your mouth, nose, and eyes with your hands until you've washed them. Avoid standing water sources like the plague—pun intended. Pay attention to animals possibly carrying rabies and other diseases, and avoid them at all costs while hiking or outdoors. Avoid crowded places during an epidemic. Wear a face mask if necessary, and stay at least six feet (two meters) away from others. If you have to sneeze, cover your nose and mouth to prevent airborne spreading of the virus.

Most viral diseases have a contagion period of seven days, so once you are exposed, you are contagious for a week and continue to be until approximately twenty-four hours after symptoms disappear, whichever is longer.

If you are exposed, it is critical to get help immediately. Antibiotics, antiviral agents (which are about 70- to 90-percent effective in preventing illness or preventing it from getting worse), or a vaccine can be administered at a hospital or urgent care center. Right now, there are a handful of antiviral agents for fighting influenza within forty-eight hours of exposure in the United States, but when it comes to antibiotics, be aware that viruses mutate quicker than drug companies can pump out medications and vaccines. The overuse of antibiotics has created powerful strains of viruses that are resistant and are especially deadly for children, seniors, and those with compromised immune systems. So do what you can to prevent being exposed in the first place.

If you are sick, stay home from school or work. It's one thing to be sick yourself, but it's another to infect others, and then they in turn go home and infect their families. There is a lot to be said for the old-school advice of resting, staying hydrated, eating right, and taking it easy when sick.

Though we have come a long way in terms of preparedness and response to pandemics, we would be wise to pay attention to the words of Peter Palese, the chair of the department of microbiology at the Icahn School of Medicine at Mount Sinai. Palese stated in "Nightmare Scenario? A Flu Pandemic Is Coming, But When and How Bad Will It Be?" for the summer 2017 *Emergency Management* magazine. "In many ways, we are much better prepared than we were 100 years ago. Having said that, no one can really predict what a new pandemic would look like, when it would occur and whether it would be remotely as devastating as 1918 was."

While so many viruses and bacterial agents are out there waiting to attack, and more are being discovered all the time, we must focus on the most likely culprits, such as avian flu, and push our government representatives to keep the money flowing for research and response. With billions more humans, and chickens, alive on the planet now than in 1918, one can only imagine how bad it could get if we don't stay alert, get prepared, and continue to find ways to fight and stop pandemics before they stop us.

SPACE WEATHER

When it comes to threats from space, we often mean mass extinction events, such as a major asteroid impact or gamma ray bursts, that would pretty much end civilization as we know it. But smaller threats do occur, and we can be ready for them in the same manner as we would for a major storm or earthquake.

The earth is always having near misses with asteroids of varying sizes. On July 23, 2017, Asteroid 2017 001 was detected by the ATLAS-MLO telescope in Hawaii, and it came within 76,448 miles (123,000 kilometers) of Earth, which is about a third of the distance between Earth and our moon. It would not have been big enough to wipe out the planet, but it would have caused untold deaths, depending on where it struck. The largest actual impact in recorded history was in 1908, known as the Tunguska event. A meteoroid exploded over Siberia and caused an amazing amount of destruction, still evident in tree-growth patterns today. That impact had the same level of destruction as a small nuclear detonation, flattening approximately 80,000 trees. Luckily, there were no human deaths because of the remoteness of the area.

In 2012, an asteroid known as 2012 TC4 came within 4,200 miles (6,760 kilometers) of Earth, which is very close, since the moon is approximately 239,000 miles (384,633 kilometers) away. That asteroid measured between 30 and 100 feet (9–30 meters) long and about 7,000 tons (6,350 metric tons), which is about the same size as the one that struck in Chelyabinsk, Russia, in 2013. Damaging, but not the end of the world.

Most asteroids burn up in our atmosphere and never impact, or they break apart and land in tiny pieces. NASA is looking at a defense program to ward off the larger asteroids that could pose a greater problem in the future.

"Impact events" encompass anything that could collide with our planet, including asteroids, meteors, comets, and even space debris. Without impact events, our solar system may not have evolved as it has, so these are important events that create and shape landforms on Earth as well as other planets. Impact events were also instrumental in how life itself formed and how water originated on Earth. Our concern is, will Earth be threatened with a major impact in our lifetimes? And if so, can we push the object out of our orbit? And if we cannot, how do we survive, if survival is even possible?

In 2013, the Chelyabinsk meteor event occurred, considered the largest impact event since Tunguska, resulting in a large number of injuries. This was a superbolide that entered Earth's atmosphere over Russia on February 15, 2013, at approximately 40,000–43,000 miles per hour (64,375–69,200 kph). The light was brighter than the sun and could be seen miles away. No one was directly killed, but the event caused damage to over 7,200 buildings and injured approximately 1,500 people. Because the object first appeared so close to the sun, it went undetected until it was almost upon Earth!

This is one of the most frightening aspects of space impact events. They often happen suddenly because they may not be detected with enough time to send out emergency alerts. Because most impact events are small, they do limited damage, if any, to structures and even people. But now and then, on a scale of millions of years, we do experience one that literally changes the face of the planet and is considered an extinction-level event. Just ask the dinosaurs.

In the case of a large asteroid or other object hitting us, we look to NASA to monitor the event and alert the public. As NASA and other agencies look for ways to defend our planet against such impact events, the best we can do is be ready in case we learn that an object is on a collision course with Earth and stay on top of news reports that may require us to evacuate, get underground if possible, or shelter in place (we will go through the steps for doing just that later).

Space weather is a term used to describe situations that occur on the sun and in space that can influence the earth. Solar and geomagnetic storms are capable of shutting down our electrical grids and hammering technology into submission. In fact, during a strong enough solar storm, we could experience a catastrophe that would plunge humanity back into the Stone Age if it went on long enough.

Think about days, weeks, even months, with no power, no computers, no electricity, telecommunications, GPS, air traffic control, and all those things interrelated. Though most solar storms are not that disruptive, they can still cripple nations with widespread blackouts.

When it comes to space weather, the sun is our biggest enemy. A CME is a coronal mass ejection of plasma and electromagnetic energy that can cause problems here on earth. The same goes for solar flares, which are sudden bursts of radiation. In fact, the sun emits everything from ultraviolet rays to X-rays to energetic particle storms that can damage aircraft and satellites orbiting the planet. Though most of this activity would take days to reach us, giving us some time to prepare, and would have to be specifically directed towards Earth, we do face the threat of another "Carrington Event."

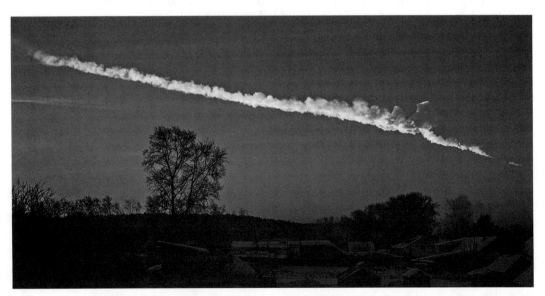

A trail of smoke remains in the sky, marking the path of the 2013 Chelyabinsk meteor that injured 1,500 people in Russia.

In 1859, amateur British astronomer Richard Carrington discovered that the sun's surface was dotted with gigantic dark spots and clusters. Within minutes the fireballs would vanish, and hours later the earth felt their impact in the form of electrified gas particles and subatomic particles that hit the earth, shutting down telegraph systems all over the world. The night sky was filled with auroras so bright that many people thought it was daytime. Known from then on as the "Carrington Event," if it were to happen today, the planet would go dark, and computers, mobile phones, satellites, even cars with computers, would all be rendered powerless. Electrical grids could be knocked out for days.

Imagine no Internet—for days! There would also be radio blackouts and shutdowns of financial systems and banking as well as cargo deliveries and air traffic. Any car with a computer, and that means most cars on the road nowadays, would be useless, sending us back to horse-and-buggy days or forcing us to walk to get the food, water, and other items we need—if we can find them. There won't be cargo coming in and out of our ports to fill store shelves.

In the event of an EMP—an electromagnetic pulse—which not only comes in the form of a solar surge, but can also be triggered by humans as a nuclear detonation in the atmosphere, the power could be off for months, even a year, as global infrastructures crumble and chaos and anarchy rule the streets.

Another large space weather event happened in March of 1989, when Canada was hit with a major blackout caused by a strong geomagnetic storm. Over six million people were without power for hours, and transformers melted as far away as New Jersey. Luckily, that event was over in just nine hours.

If an EMP were to occur, we would have some warning that solar activity was intensifying for a big storm from scientists watching all over the world (not the case for a terrorist act involving a nuclear detonation). NASA is working on ways to detect coming solar storms (they occur in eleven-year cycles, but it's hard to predict with accuracy how strong they will be on any given day) and build up infrastructure to be able to deal with a major event. The National Oceanic and Atmospheric Administration is also working on space weather issues at their Space Weather Prediction Center.

Because we have become so dependent on technology, space weather is a threat that we worry about more now than in the past. With so much of our lives intertwined with our computers and gadgets, and with the comforts of electrical power flowing into our homes and workplaces, it would take a solar or geomagnetic storm to remind us how our more primitive ancestors must have lived. Sometimes less is really more.

Geomagnetic storms are also associated with a number of other phenomena, such as SEPs, or Solar Energetic Particles; GICs, or Geomagnetically Induced Currents; ionosphere disturbances; and aurora displays, which can now be seen much further south than in the past, thanks to changes in the overall climate.

Space Weather Scales

Just as with most potential natural disasters, space weather is measured on a scale of intensity. Geomagnetic storms, which are disturbances in the geomagnetic field caused by solar winds blowing past the earth, are measured from minor to extreme, with G1 being the most minor and G5 as the most extreme.

Solar radiation storms are rated the same, S1 being the most minor and S5 the most severe.

Radio blackouts, which are disturbances in the earth's ionosphere caused by solar X-ray emissions, are rated from R1, minor, to R5, extreme.

Solar flares are rated by class, with A class being the weakest, followed by B, C, M, and the strongest, X class. C class and smaller do not affect the earth's atmosphere at all.

When it comes to space weather, preparation and response focus on a cascading number of events that would occur due to the loss of power:

- Loss of drinkable water
- Loss of wastewater removal systems
- Loss of food
- Loss of medications
- Loss of communications systems
- Loss of transportation
- Loss of fuel delivery and distribution
- Loss of electrical systems with no backup power

As a homeowner, one of the most important things you can do is have a generator for backup power along with stored food and water and medications for those who need them. In the preparedness and response sections, there are detailed lists of what to have and where to keep it during a power outage, which can require special planning if the event is of a long duration. Some of the things that can help you survive an extreme space weather event include having a landline phone that will work if the power goes out, but it must be non-broadband or VOIP; keeping extra batteries not just for flashlights, but for cell phones as well, should they get up and running; knowing how to use a ham radio for when cell towers are down; having alternative methods of transportation, such as a bicycle, in the event of an EMP, when computerized cars are immobilized; and making sure all electronics are shut off to avoid surge issues when the power does come back on.

Most important is to keep an eye on the news once an alert has gone out, which might be days before the largest event would occur. Luckily, our planet's atmosphere and magnetosphere would protect us from the harmful radiation from these events, although aircraft flying at high altitudes and of course astronauts are at high risk of such hazards.

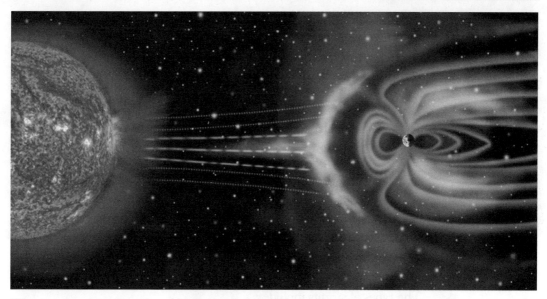

When a strong surge from the sun's solar wind strikes the earth's magnetosphere, the result can be a geomagnetic storm. Such storms can take out electrical and communications systems across large regions of the planet.

So, while getting hit by an asteroid or having a flyby with a comet is ever-so-slightly possible, the bigger threats are those that happen more frequently. And among the biggest threats we face during any of these events are our fellow human beings, which is why emergency management personnel across the United States have come up with incident action plans to deal with things like total solar eclipses, which can cause fear and panic for some, not to mention too much partying and celebrating for others. Known as the Great American Eclipse, the total eclipse of August 21, 2017, was the first total solar eclipse to cross the United States from coast to coast since 1918. Two hundred million Americans lived within its path. Millions of those people were expected to be celebrating.

Luckily, the event was met with much joy, celebration, and curiosity as people filled streets, parks, and even football stadiums to view the eclipse. No deaths were reported, and there were no apocalyptic riots in the streets. People cheered and even cried in awe, and everyone went back to school and work and their normal lives the next day. But had there been any trouble, authorities would have been ready!

Eclipses don't pose a threat to our survival, but there were still many concerns about how people would respond, based on how people react after a major sporting event, when celebration can get out of hand, especially if alcohol is involved. Fortunately, the event proved to be positive all the way around. Had the event been an asteroid impact or gamma ray burst instead, we might not have fared so well.

STORMS AND SUPERSTORMS

When warm, light air rises quickly into colder, higher air, you get storms, unstable updrafts that can reach over 100 miles per hour (161 kph). A storm is the result of lower pressure developing with a system of higher pressure surrounding it, creating high winds and cumulonimbus clouds or other types of stormclouds filled with rain, hail, lightning, and winds—even tornadoes if the conditions are right—that can cause localized and even regional devastation. The bigger the storm, the more potential for damage, including floods and mudslides.

The planet is riddled with thousands of storms making their way over the surface at any given time, many of them relatively mild, but some extremely powerful. Many occur over the oceans and create storm surges along the coastlines and choppy, often violent, waves for those on ships and boats. Some make landfall as powerful hurricanes, then dissipate into tropical storms that flood the area with sustained rainfall.

The types of storms include:

Blizzards—Gale-force winds and heavy snow along with cold temperatures below –10° Celsius (–14° Fahrenheit).

Cyclone—A tropical storm system with a warm core of air and a closed circulation around a center of low pressure. Similar to hurricanes and typhoons.

Dust devil—A localized updraft of rising air over an area with dirt, sand, and other easily lifted materials.

Gale—An extratropical storm with sustained winds of 39–55 miles per hour (63–89 kph).

Hailstorm—Usually occurs during severe thunderstorms, creating chunks of ice that can range from tiny to over two inches in diameter, even the size of a softball, causing great damage to property.

Hurricane—A massive storm system that forms over water and moves onto land, called a "typhoon" in the north Pacific Ocean and "cyclones" elsewhere in the world. Hurricanes can bring storm surge, high winds, heavy rainfall, flooding, and even spawn tornadoes.

Ice storm—Combines freezing and below-freezing temps with a thick layer of above-freezing air aloft, turning rain into ice upon impact with the ground. Ice storms create dangerous driving conditions, especially on unheated roadways, where they make the surface slick.

Lightning storm—Storm clouds with lightning that produce no rain. Also referred to as "electrical storms." When the lightning is cloud to cloud, it is beautiful to watch, but when the lightning is cloud to ground, it can spark fires and structural damage.

Squall—A sudden onset of increased winds that is sustained for longer than a minute.

Thunderstorm—A storm that generates thunder and lightning, often including heavy rains, hail, and high winds. These occur all over the planet, with the highest concentration over the rainforests, and are created when high levels of condensation form in a volume of unstable air. The unstable air becomes a rapid, swirling updraft of rising air currents and is often characterized by dark grey, massive thunderhead clouds. Always accompanied by lightning and can strike the ground 100 times each second, causing fires and billions of dollars' worth of damage. Because light travels faster than sound, you can determine the distance of a storm cell by the length of time between the thunder and the accompanying flash of lightning.

Tropical storm—Occurs over tropical environments and is an extremely low-pressure system moving at high speeds of approximately 40–73 miles per hour (64–117 kph).

Tornado—A particularly deadly and violent windstorm that occurs on land and often follows a severe thunderstorm. With its dark, funnel-shaped clouds, tornadoes cause billions of dollars of destruction annually and are now appearing more and more in states that rarely experienced them, such as Oregon and California, thanks to warming temperatures overall. Tornado Alley, in the middle section of the United States, remains the most active spot for tornadic activity.

Wind storm—Any storm with high winds and little or no rain that can carry debris and cause a lot of structural damage. "Derechos" are large and fast-moving thunderstorms, extending at least 240 miles (386 kilometers), with wind gusts a minimum of 58 miles per hour (93 kph).

The dangers of just about all storms (cold or heat, winds, rain, hail, etc.) can be avoided in most cases by remaining indoors when they occur. "When thunder roars, go indoors" is great advice, because not only is there the potential for lightning strikes, but also for flash floods, mudslides, hail, and even a tornado spawned by a severe storm. Storms can be predicted, thanks to radar and great advances in weather prediction systems, but even the best predictions carry the risk that a regular everyday storm can turn into a monster.

Hurricanes are particularly difficult to navigate for anyone caught outdoors, because of high winds combined with heavy downpours, causing zero visibility and flying debris. Hurricanes are easily predicted, so it is incumbent upon the individual to be ready to evacuate when told to do so, and to board up windows and take precautions to avoid flooding. Hurricanes can cover huge sections of land, unlike tornadoes, which are more localized, and create major issues when millions of people are told to evacuate quickly and get away from coastal regions.

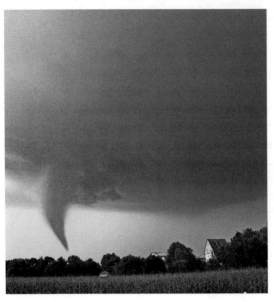

Tornados can wreak havoc over stretches of land miles long before dissipating.

Tornadoes, however, do not lose power once they hit land as hurricanes do. Tornadoes form from thunderstorms and, although they cover less territory, pack the most damaging winds should their funnel clouds reach a mile in length. Weather forecasters can easily see the formation of hurricanes over the Atlantic or Pacific and give ample warning, but being able to say exactly where and when a tornado will form out of any given thunderstorm system is a lot more difficult.

Hurricane season in the Atlantic Ocean normally runs from June 1 to November 30, with the highest activity between August and October. In the Pacific, the season can run from May to November in the northeast Pacific and November to May in the southeast Pacific. However, if the conditions are right, hurricanes and cyclones can develop any time!

Therefore it behooves you to be ready for anything when a storm occurs, even if you don't live in an area that ordinarily experiences these more severe systems and events, because they are becoming more common everywhere. If you do live in a region known for hurricanes and tornadoes, you must be prepared to either board up and shelter in place if there is no time to evacuate, or get your bug-out gear and get out of town if told to evacuate (or evacuate sooner and beat the rest of the crowd).

Tornadoes, hurricanes, and cyclones/typhoons are measured on scales of severity. For tornadoes, the Fujita Intensity Scale (F-Scale) is used, named after prominent Japanese American severe storm researcher Tetsuya Fujita of the University of Chicago in collaboration with Allen Pearson, the head of the National Severe Storms Forecast Center in 1971. The scale was updated two years later to include width and path length.

Fujita Intensity Scale

F-Scale	Description
F0	Gale tornado, 40–72 mph (64–116 kph), light damage to tree branches, signs, and brick chimneys.
F1	Moderate, 73–112 mph (117–181 kph), moderate damage, roof tiles displaced, mobile homes overturned, autos pushed from roadways.
F2	Significant, 113–157 mph (182–253 kph), considerable damage to roofs, trees uprooted, mobile homes destroyed, cars pushed over.

How Do Storms Get Their Names?

Ever wonder how a hurricane or tropical storm gets its name? The World Meteorological Organization (WMO) decided to name these storms because they are so numerous, as a way for researchers, responders, ship captains, and normal citizens to refer to them and communicate specifics of each storm.

All hurricanes and any tropical storm with sustained wind speeds of over 39 miles per hour (63 kph) gets a name, always in alphabetical order, chosen from a list of names on file at the WMO. Names can be repeated after a six-year interval, but extremely severe storms have their names retired from use. Katrina is a good example of a hurricane name that has been permanently retired.

Names were originally all female, but in 1978 male names began to be used. Female and male names are now alternated. A tropical storm that is named keeps the name if it becomes a hurricane. Outside of the Atlantic, the National Hurricane Center maintains the list of storm names. Interestingly, if there are more than twenty-one named storms in a given year, additional storms are given names based on the Greek alphabet, such as Alpha, Beta, Gamma, etc.

F-Scale	Description
F3	Severe, 158–206 mph (254–332 kph), severe damage to roofs and homes, trains and cars overturned, trees uprooted, heavy cars thrown into the air.
F4	Devastating, 207–260 mph (333–418 kph), devastating damage, homes leveled, structures blown off their foundations, cars and large vehicles thrown into the air.
F5	Incredible, 261–318 mph (419–512 kph), incredible amounts of damage, including strong frame houses lifted off their foundations and carried considerable distances, destroyed structures, automobiles turned into destructive missiles speeding through the air, trees debarked.

When it comes to tornadoes, there are a number of misconceptions and urban legends that have come into our culture. Here are some common ones.

Myth: Tornadoes don't happen near lakes, rivers, or mountains.

Fact: No place is safe when it comes to tornadoes. They can happen anywhere, even up a 10,000-foot (3,048-meter) mountainside.

Myth: Low pressure causes buildings to explode as a tornado passes overhead.

Fact: Most structural damage is caused by extreme winds and flying debris.

Myth: Open windows when a tornado is near to equalize pressure.

Fact: Keep windows closed to avoid flying debris and high winds.

Myth: If caught in the open, you can seek shelter under an overpass.

Fact: Take shelter in a sturdy building. Hiding under a bridge or overpass can get you sucked into the high winds.

Myth: While driving, if you see a tornado, drive at a right angle to it.

Fact: Seek shelter when you see a tornado. Staying on the road in your car can get you killed, and tornadoes change direction.

Try not to get your advice from storm-chasing shows on the television, which often involve irresponsible and sensationalistic behavior just for the TV cameras. You don't want to chase, outrun, or outfox a tornado or stop to take selfies with an F5 in the background. It isn't worth risking your life.

When it comes to hurricanes that form in the Atlantic and northern Pacific and threaten the United States, we use the Saffir-Simpson Hurricane Scale (SSHS) to classify them according to intensity.

Saffir-Simpson Hurricane Scale

Category	Description
Category 1	74–95 mph (119–153 kph) wind speed, the weakest category
Category 2	96–110 mph (154–177 kph) wind speed
Category 3	111–129 mph (178–208 kph) wind speed
Category 4	130–156 (209–251 kph) mph wind speed
Category 5	The strongest and most damaging, with wind speeds over 157 mph (252 kph)

All these categories can cause damage when they make landfall, but the Cat 5s are the hurricanes that go down in history as being the most destructive to both life and property. It was a Cat 4 hurricane that hit in Galveston, Texas, in 1900, killing 8,000–12,000 people and destroying thousands of homes and buildings. 2005's Hurricane Katrina was a Cat 3, but caused 1,200 deaths and an incredible amount of damage ($81 billion!) because of storm surges and flooding along the coast of Mississippi and into Louisiana, where levees protecting New Orleans failed. It has become, so far, the deadliest and most costly hurricane in U.S. history.

Other notable large hurricanes were Andrew, a Cat 4 upon landfall in 1992, which struck mainly into Louisiana and Florida, killed 65, and caused $26 billion in damage; Sandy, a Cat 3 in 2012 that caused $75 billion in damage; Ike, a 2008 Cat 4; Ivan, a Cat 5, in 2004; Camille in 1969, a Cat 5 that is considered one of the most powerful ever to hit the United States; the Great Labor Day Storm of 1935, a Cat 5 that struck Florida and caused over 400 deaths; and Dean and Felix in 2007. Hurricane Matthew in 2016 mainly hit Haiti and Cuba but also caused enough damage there and in the United States, at $15 billion, to make it one of the most costly.

Though Category 5 is the highest on the Saffir-Simpson scale, there is no upper boundary. This means that hurricanes can be absolutely monstrous, with winds high above a Cat 5, and still be called a Cat 5. Perhaps it will be necessary to add on Cat 6 and higher to accommodate the more powerful storms we are seeing. Cat 6 hurricanes might be those with wind speeds of between 176 and 196 miles per hour (283–315 kph), according to "How Strong Can a Hurricane Get?" a September 5, 2017, article for Live Science. This article was written in response to the massive Hurricane Irma, which was moving towards the mainland and already labeled one of the biggest, most powerful Atlantic storms on record.

VOLCANOES

"Roughly 450 million years ago a region that was likely the size of Europe started to stretch and tear. Deep gashes opened in Earth's crust, spewing lava that leaped into the air … although the ground eventually grew still, the damage had just begun." This excerpt is from an August 1, 2017, *Scientific American* article by Shannon Hall titled "Volcanoes May Have Triggered the Last Unexplained Mass Extinction." In the article, Hall reports on a recent research study that appeared in *Geology*, a scientific journal, that posits that the last five mass extinction events were directly tied to volcanic activity and its after-effects, which include "volcanic winters" that darken the sun for years and render many areas of the planet lifeless, on top of the initial damage done by the eruptions.

Though the earth was still being formed millions of years ago, volcanoes still present a huge threat today, and because the most active regions are found in some heavily populated areas of the planet, they affect millions of people. Not to mention all those affected by the ash that remains in the air for years to

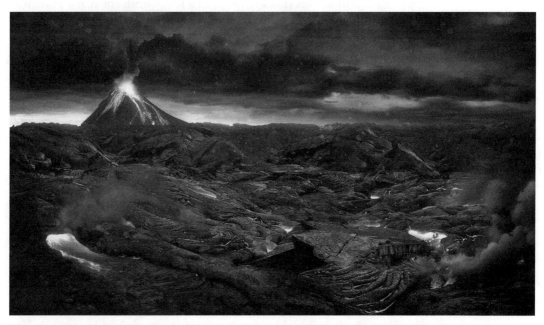

Eruptions of multiple volcanoes may have caused a mass extinction on Earth 450 million years ago.

come. Volcanoes pose a one-two punch threat because of the initial event and the longer duration of the consequences.

Over 80 percent of the earth's surface above and below sea level is of volcanic origin, and without volcanoes we wouldn't have the vital ingredients that were needed to create the oceans, the atmosphere, mountain ranges, valleys, and plains, and the fertile soils that were needed to grow food. So no matter how violent and destructive they may be, volcanoes have been instrumental to the earth's formation as well.

A volcano is a conical hill or mountain built around a vent or fissure in the earth's crust. Beneath the volcano is a reservoir of molten rock, or magma, that accumulates and eventually erupts in an explosive display of lava (magma exposed to air), ash, rock, and gases that can be ejected miles into the atmosphere and carried around the world on the winds. Ash fall can occur hundreds of miles away from the eruption location, and lava flow can continue for days, even weeks, when larger volcanoes erupt.

Tectonic plates basically float upon layers of magma beneath the surface of our moving planet. Geologists group volcanoes into four types:

Cinder Cones—The simplest and most recognizable type of volcano. Also called scoria cones, these are somewhat symmetrical cone-shaped volcanoes that eject lava fragments, or tephra, from a single vent. The cooled lava forms a crater at the summit of the volcano. These are smaller in size and can form very quickly, often in a few months or years. Parícutin in Mexico is a cinder cone volcano that, during a nine-year period of active eruptions, destroyed the town of San Juan, Mexico, and covered approximately 100 square miles (259 square kilometers) in ash.

Composite Volcanoes/Stratovolcanoes—Built upon layers of alternating lava flow, ash, and stone blocks, larger than cinder cones, and can erupt with violent energy. They can rise up to 8,000 feet (2,438 meters) and have magma chambers that, when built up to extreme pressure, release via an explosion of materials that can blow both out of the top of the crater and out the sides of the volcano. Mount St. Helens is a stratovolcano. Its eruption in May of 1980 killed 57 people, destroyed over 200 miles (322 kilometers) of forestland, and deposited ash on eleven states. Over 85 miles (137 kilometers) from the volcano, towns were thrown into darkness in the middle of the day from the ash.

Shield Volcanoes—Built of lava flows that spread in different directions from a central vent or summit, these volcanoes are more sloping cones, broad, and shaped somewhat like a shield. They can have diameters of several miles and rise up to 2,000 feet (610 meters). The Hawaiian Islands are chains of shield volcanoes, including two highly active volcanoes, Kilauea and Mauna Loa.

Lava Domes—These volcanoes start out as small masses of lava that is too thick to flow over distances and instead piles over and around a vent. A bubble or a plug of cooling rock forms over the vent or fissure. As the dome expands, the cool outer surface can explode and form lava flows known as "coulees." These can often be found as part of larger composite volcanoes, including Mount St. Helens and the Katmai Volcano in Alaska. Mount Pelée in the Lesser Antilles and California's Mono and Lassen peaks are lava dome volcanoes.

Just as there are types of volcanoes, there are different categories to describe how they erupt.

Strombolian—Huge clots of molten lava explode out of the summit and form luminous arcs in the sky overhead. Lava clots collect on the cone's sides and form fiery streams to the ground.

Vulcanian—Dense clouds of ash-laden gases are ejected from the crater and rise high, forming a white cloud of ash at the top of the cone.

Pelean—A "glowing cloud" eruption made of gas, ash, dust, and incandescent lava that explode out of, and back into, the crater and form glowing avalanches along the cone's sides.

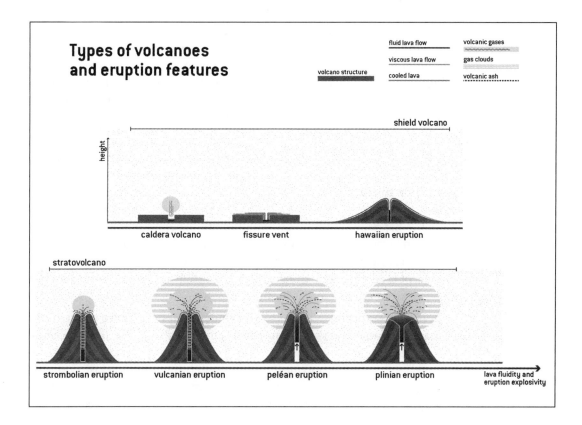

Hawaiian—These are linear vents along fractures or fissures, or one vent, and form incandescent lava that shoots into the air and also streams down the slope of the volcano itself. Can form lava lakes and feed into other lava flows.

Vesuvian—Massive quantities of ash and gas are exploded out of the crater and form a mushroom- or cauliflower-shaped cloud above the volcano. Think of the eruption of Mount Vesuvius in Italy in 79 C.E., considered one of the most powerful eruptions in history.

Phreatic—More of a steam eruption that is caused by a colder water or ground surface coming into contact with hot, flowing magma that then blast out not only rock but also new magma itself.

Plinian—The most powerful eruption category, exploding viscous lava and ash fallout over hundreds of miles. Pyroclastic flow is heavy and fast-moving, destroying anything in its path. Think of the 1980 Mount St. Helens and 1991 Pinatubo, Philippines, eruptions.

SUPERVOLCANOES

When a volcano collapses into its magma chamber, it can create a bowl-shaped depression called a "caldera." This is one of the hallmarks of a super-volcano: a massive volcano that causes eruptions thousands of times more explosive and destructive than the other types. There are approximately forty known supervolcanoes in the world today, many in the form of lakes, such as Lake Taupo in New Zealand, the result of a supervolcanic eruption approximately 28,000 years ago and the last known supereruption in geological history.

In *Supervolcano: The Catastrophic Event That Changed the Course of Human History,* my father and I wrote extensively about the Toba, Sumatra, supereruption approximately 75,000 years ago that literally may have altered the genetic history of human beings. It did so by wiping out enough of the living population to create a "population bottleneck." Think of small pebbles in a bottle that are suddenly forced into the neck of the bottle when you turn it over. That is what happened to us on an evolutionary scale, when up to 90 percent of the existing population was killed, leaving the remainder to repopulate the planet. A supervolcano today would not be able to do that, simply because there are billions of us alive, and many would survive. But it is still not an event we would hope to experience in our lifetimes.

A true supervolcano is an "explosive caldera eruption," as we wrote in the book, "namely a large-scale subsidence-resurgent caldera, where large scale implies an exceedance of a threshold volume of about 120 miles (193 kilometers) of material." So a supervolcano must eject enough pyroclastic flow, ash, gas, and debris to cover 120 square miles (310 square kilometers) and be in the shape of a caldera. But there can be calderas that are the result of massive volcanic erup-

Volcanic Ash

Volcanic ash is one of the most dangerous aspects of an eruption because of its ability to be carried on winds over long distances, cause respiratory problems, and even bury large objects.

But what is it made of? Volcanic ash is made of pulverized rock and glass that is the result of an eruption. It is deadly to those nearby, especially infants and the elderly with compromised breathing ability, and can also destroy machinery, jet and car engines, and exposed electrical equipment. It can be very abrasive, acidic, very high in mineral content, and have a gassy, sulfur smell because of the chemical compounds. Silica and oxygen are the most abundant chemicals in volcanic ash, but carbon dioxide, sulfur dioxide, hydrogen, and halogen are also found.

Ash from larger eruptions can not only travel hundreds of miles but also enter the atmosphere and literally block sunlight from reaching the surface of the earth for weeks, months, even years, resulting in a "volcanic winter" that is much like a nuclear winter created after a nuclear cloud disperses into the atmosphere.

tions such as Tambora in 1815 and the Mazama eruption over 7,000 years ago that created Crater Lake in Oregon.

In the United States, there are two supervolcanoes that must be watched and possibly more, as new research indicates there may be underwater calderas near our landmass and possibly a caldera beneath the Cascades in the Pacific Northwest. But we most have to be concerned about Yellowstone and Long Valley. Yellowstone caldera in Yellowstone National Park in Wyoming, which also stretches into Idaho and Montana, has produced three supereruptions in the last 2.1 million years, including one that created the caldera most people view at Yellowstone, which is 60 miles (97 kilometers) across. The most recent eruption was about 640,000 years ago. There are many earth scientists watching earthquake swarms and carbon release/tree kill in the area to monitor a possible coming supereruption, but because one has never occurred in the course of recorded history, we don't yet know all the factors that lead up to a supervolcano eruption along the lines of what has happened in the past.

Long Valley caldera is located in east-central California, just south of Mono Lake and close to the Nevada state line. Long Valley last erupted about 760,000 years ago and ejected over fifty times the amount of magma ejected during the 1991 Mount Pinatubo eruption in the Philippines. Ash fell as far east as Nebraska, and the entire eruption lasted for ten days. While not as big in scope as the Yellowstone caldera, what makes Long Valley so unnerving is its proximity to major fault lines such as the San Andreas. Many research studies have shown a direct correlation between major quake activity and quake swarms at or near both Yellowstone and Long Valley.

So the threat exists of a major quake triggering an eruption at either caldera—or an eruption at either caldera triggering major quake activity nearby. Long Valley is particularly worrisome because of its proximity to major urban areas such as Southern California, which would result in extensive loss of life and damage to infrastructure. The 1992 Landers earthquake caused seismic activity and deformation to the Long Valley caldera, as reported in the October 1998 issue of *Nature*. Scientists at the Carnegie Institute of Washington reported that, within a day or two of larger earthquakes they reviewed, there are more eruptions within a 460-mile (740-kilometer) range than normal. The Hector Mine quake in the Mojave Desert in 1993, which was a 7.1, was located about the same distance from both Yellowstone and Long Valley, but only triggered seismicity at Long Valley.

The question then becomes, how much of a threat is volcanic activity? If you live in other parts of the world near active volcanoes, it's a huge threat. In the United States, again the major activity is along the Ring of Fire, stretching up into Alaska, and further inland at Yellowstone—unless a supervolcano is discovered in the Atlantic or Pacific oceans, creating even more potential for disaster. The United States Geological Service (USGS) has monitoring stations at all major volcano sites, tracking activity 24/7. But it is only a matter of time before one or more erupt, and if the Big One hits the San Andreas Fault, we might be facing vent eruptions at Long Valley—maybe even a supereruption.

Some of the most violent eruptions in history include: Krakatoa, Indonesia, in 1883, which killed about 36,000 people, sent debris flying over a 50-mile (80-kilometer) swath, and caused huge tsunamis to boot; Tambora, Indonesia, in 1815, which also caused tsunamis and whirlwinds, killed over 12,000 people, and ejected four times as much material as Pinatubo; 1902's Mount Pelée on Martinique Island, killing almost every resident on the island (approx. 29,933 out of 29,937 people!); Mount Shasta in California, which erupted in 1786 and is predicted to occur every 600-plus years; and Hawaii's Kilauea and Mauna Loa, both of which erupt on a regular schedule of two to three years and have become a fixture for tourists visiting the islands.

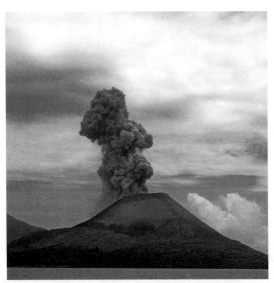

The volcano on Krakatoa is still active over a century after the 1883 eruption destroyed half the island and killed 36,000 people.

Volcanic eruptions are more predictable than earthquakes, allowing for a little more time to plan reaction and response. Even though the USGS states that the "danger zone" is only about a 20-mile (32-kilometer) radius from the volcano, the after-effects can cause damage, even death, for over 100 miles (161 kilometers) away and, in the case of supereruptions, over 500 miles (805 kilometers) away. This does not include the dangers of surviving a volcanic winter.

In the chapters on preparedness and response, we will look at what to do before, during, and after an event of this magnitude and how to focus on long-term survival, which may not be a major concern in other types of disasters.

WILDFIRES

Before 1995, the United States on average experienced one massive "megafire" per year. But between the years 2005 and 2014, that number jumped to 9.8. The federal cost of fighting these increasing megafires rose from around $300 million per year to $3 billion per year. And these massive wildfires show no signs of slowing down, thanks to climate change, increasingly hot temperatures, droughts, and drier seasons that result in more dry brush to burn.

Whether started by human hands or by a lightning strike, wildfires have become public enemy number one not just in the United States, but also in other countries experiencing drier and hotter conditions, including Canada, Greenland, and parts of Europe that may have only seen an occasional large fire before. The new norm burns hot, fast, and wide.

In the August 6, 2017, issue of *Emergency Management* magazine, an article originally published in the Boulder, Colorado, *Daily Camera* by Charlie Brennan, titled "Boulder Author Warns of More 'Megafires' on Nation's Horizon," states that we are likely to see these monster fires increase in the coming years. Michael Kodas is the author of *Megafire*, and he is also the deputy director of the Center for Environmental Journalism at the University of Colorado. Kodas writes, "The biggest and baddest of them all are still to come." In 2015, wildfires burned over more than 10 million acres in the United States, and fire scientists anticipate that rising to "12 to 15 million acres a year" and possibly even as high as 20 million. "We've got a century of climate change already built into the system," Kodas writes, and four factors play into this rising wave of megafires:

1. Wildlands-urban interface and increased development—with more populated areas built up against wildlands, forests, and hills.
2. Global climate change
3. Political and economic decision-making
4. Forest management policies

Problems in those areas could lead to more catastrophic fires, but policy and practice changes can also mitigate much of the threat about which Kodas writes.

A wildfire can be described as an uncontrolled blaze that is fueled by dry brush, hot weather, and high winds. According to *National Geographic*, humans start four out of five wildfires, but once they begin, they can consume hundreds, even thousands, of acres in minutes and burn everything in their paths. In the United States, wildfires are usually most common in the drier states, but have become an issue in all fifty states as weather conditions change. The states most affected are Montana, Idaho, Wyoming, Washington, Colorado, Oregon, and California. California especially experiences devastating fires due to the dry Santa Ana winds that blow fast and furious during the typical fire season months of October and November. Yet even in California, some parts of the state are experiencing fire season all year long!

Massive wildfires can burn for weeks before there is full containment, and if they occur in rural or mountain areas, where it is hard to get firefighters and equipment to the front lines, they can become so big they take on a life of their own and eventually spread into inhabited areas to destroy homes and infrastructure and take lives. It is not only firefighters who lose their lives to these beasts but also citizens who get caught in the fire or who refuse to evacuate and find themselves trapped when the inferno surrounds them and cuts off their escape routes.

Three things are needed for a wildfire: heat, fuel (dry brush, combustibles), and an oxidizing agent (oxygen). When those three parts of the "fire triangle" are present, wildfires occur, but at the same time, firefighters can fight a wildfire by removing one of those three things. Clearing vegetation and brush so that the fire has nothing to burn, or creating controlled "backburns" to stop the wildfire in its tracks, and dousing with water or some type of fire retardant are the methods firefighters use to control, contain, and eventually stop a wildfire.

As destructive as these beasts are, wildfires also have a positive aspect on the environment, as they reintroduce nutrients into the soil from the burned and decayed trees and brush. They also rid forest ecosystems of harmful disease-carrying insects and plants. In addition, forest fires allow for the thinning of thick treetops so that sunlight can reach the forest floor and help tree seedlings sprout and grow into new trees.

But when homes and human lives are in their paths, these benefits often seem like little comfort.

There are different types of wildfires, such as surface fires, spot fires, ground fires, dependent crown fires, and running crown fires. Surface fires are the most common and move more slowly, as they burn vegetation. Spot fires happen in smaller areas and are easy to put out but can pop up here and there as the original fire ejects burning ash that lands on dry brush or grasses. Crown fires are those spread along treetops. Ground fires start at the ground level and are usually caused by lightning strikes. The worst of these is the running crown fire, which burns extremely hot and travels over land so quickly, and changes directions even more quickly, that it is tough to get under control. Larger fires, called "conflagrations" can actually create their own weather system! When this happens, the increased flow of oxygen builds the fire up.

Smokey the Bear

Remember Smokey the Bear? His motto was "Only you can prevent forest fires." He was actually the official mascot of the U.S. Forest Service in 1985 and became iconic in his own right. In 1937, President Franklin D. Roosevelt began a fire prevention campaign that highlighted human carelessness as a major cause of forest fires. Posters of the program would include Uncle Sam, leaders of the Allied powers during the Second World War, characters from the Disney classic *Bambi*, which included a major forest fire in its storyline, and good old Smokey Bear.

Unfortunately, today four out of every five major wildfires are caused by human beings, so the program didn't seem to work for the long haul, but it did succeed in drawing attention for decades to the problem of man-made forest fires and the destruction they caused.

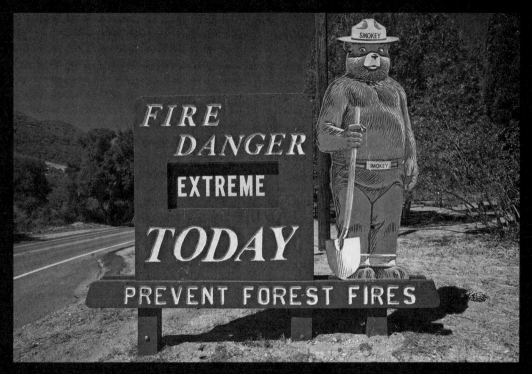

A sign put up by the U.S. Forest Service at a national park has Smokey the Bear warning visitors that dry conditions make fires likely.

Like hurricanes and tropical storms, wildfires are now named, usually after a nearby landmark such as a river, creek, mountain, or even the city most affected. Also like hurricanes, massive wildfires can generate winds of up to 120 miles per hour (193 kph). When certain conditions are present, fire tornadoes can also form, separate from or a part of the initial fire, and they can travel and cause even more damage.

Wildfires are most fatal to those fighting them and those who are trapped or remain in their direct path. In July 6, 1994, fourteen firefighters died during the Storm King Mountain fire near Glenwood Springs, Colorado. The August 2003 Boise National Forest fire saw eight firefighters die in a crash when they were returning from fighting the fire. In June of 2013, nineteen firefighters were killed fighting the Yarnell Hill fire northwest of Phoenix, Arizona. Sometimes the fire itself is the killer, and at other times it involves crashed helicopters, such as the August 2008 Buckhorn fire in Northern California, which took the lives of eight firefighters when their helicopter crashed after taking off from the fire site.

Because wildfires can be started by everything from arson to an accidentally dropped match to lightning to an explosion, it is hard to prevent them ahead of time, and firefighting efforts must then focus on containment, but one of the most important ways to make sure your home is as protected as possible is to cut brush away from your home, creating a "defensible space," which is an area of reduced or no fuel sources for a fire to spread. This space also helps firefighters fight an actual fire and defend the structure properly. The suggested minimum amount of space is 100 feet (30 meters) for homes built before 2004 and 150 feet (46 meters) for those built after, but even more space could be the difference between a standing and a charred home. Within those 100–150 feet (30–46 meters), low ground cover and drought-resistant and fire-resistant plants are best at slowing down a fire in its tracks. Having tall trees right near a home can be deadly if fire jumps from the treetops to the roofs, so it is critical to keep certain types of plants and trees far enough away so as not to aid the fire's spread.

Local fire companies will work with homeowners and communities to make sure defensible space is properly established and maintained. In addition to defensible space, it is important that access roads, alleys, driveways, and paths around homes and buildings are always kept open and clear and that the address number is prominent on the home or building so firefighters can find it when called out. Also make sure there are no combustible materials near or under the home, decks, patios, etc. Combustibles include plants, wood, cuttings, rags and gasoline, and flammable materials and products. Even firewood should be kept at least 30 feet (9 meters) away from the home or structure, and keep a clearance area of ten feet (three meters) around a propane tank.

Defensible space is like having a big, burly bouncer outside the nightclub. It protects and wards off fire, keeping it away from homes and structures. You can contact your local fire department for rules regarding how much space you need in your area, based on the fire hazard levels.

Wildfires are a problem globally, and even in Canada, record wildfire seasons are reported now more than ever. As of August 2017, there were 122 different wildfires burning in the Canadian province of British Columbia, breaking a record for the region. In the summer of 2008 alone, California was dealing with over 2,780 wildfires. Many of the most devastating wildfires in U.S. history occurred in the 1800s. A sampling of major fires of the past:

1825—The Miramichi Fire in New Brunswick, Canada, burned over 3 million acres (12,141 square kilometers) and killed 160 people.

1871—The Preshtigo Fire in Wisconsin and Michigan burned over 1.2 million acres (4,856 square kilometers) and killed over 2,500.

1894—The Hinkley Fire in Minnesota burned just 160,000 acres (648 square kilometers), but killed 418.

1902—The Cloquet Fire in Minnesota burned over 1.2 million acres (4,856 square kilometers) and killed over 450.

1933—The Griffith Park Fire in Los Angeles killed 29 firefighters.

1947—The Great Fires in Maine burned over 200,000 acres (809 square kilometers) and took the lives of 15 people.

1953—The Rattlesnake Fire in Mendocino National Forest, California, took the lives of 14 firefighters and one Forest Service employee.

1956—The Inaja Fire in the Cleveland National Forest, California, took the lives of 11 firefighters.

1970—The Laguna Fire in California destroyed over 382 homes and killed 8 people.

1994—The South Canyon Fire in Colorado took the lives of 14 firefighters.

2003—The Cedar Fires in San Diego, California, destroyed 2,280 structures and killed 14 people.

2004—The Taylor Complex Fire in Alaska burned over 1.7 million acres (6,880 square kilometers) as part of the worst fire season in Alaskan history.

2006—The Esperanza Fire in Cabazon, California, took the lives of 5 firefighters.

2008—The California Siege burned over 1.2 million acres (4,856 square kilometers)and killed 13 firefighters over the course of 2,000 fires burning in one summer season.

2011—The Wallow Fire in Arizona and New Mexico went down as the largest blaze in Arizona history.

2012—The Whitewater-Baldy Complex Fire in New Mexico went down as the largest blaze in New Mexico history.

2013—The Black Forest Fire in Colorado went down as the most destructive fire in Colorado history. It destroyed 509 homes.

2015—The Okanogan Complex Fire in Washington State went down as the largest single blaze in Washington history.

2016—The Anderson Creek Fire in Kansas and Oklahoma went down as the largest wildfire in Kansas's history.

2016—The Fort McMurray Wildfire in Alberta and Saskatchewan, Canada, went down as the largest evacuation in Alberta's history and the most costly natural disaster in Canada's history.

This list is not complete, but it does show a disturbing trend in later years, when fires broke records and became the largest in the histories of numerous states.

Mother Nature can be a cruel, cruel mistress, but the truth is, her actions are neutral. Storms, fires, quakes, and winds, unless started or exacerbated by human beings, are everyday occurrences on the planet and should not be interpreted as good or evil. They just *are*. While the gods and goddesses of olden days were assigned to natural forces and labeled positive and beneficial or negative and destructive, we now have modern science to tell us that the planet is alive in so many ways, and because of that, it will blow, explode, groan, grumble, and roar. It is our job as humans to let it, but do our best to survive when it does.

If we want our own species to outlast the dinosaurs, it behooves us to know how to survive anything nature throws our way. Or at least how to try to survive, because the honest truth is, not everyone does—even those who have a plan. At least with natural disasters we often have warning time, which we don't have with the disasters we will talk about next—those that are man-made in origin. The earth often gives us clues and time to get ourselves together and

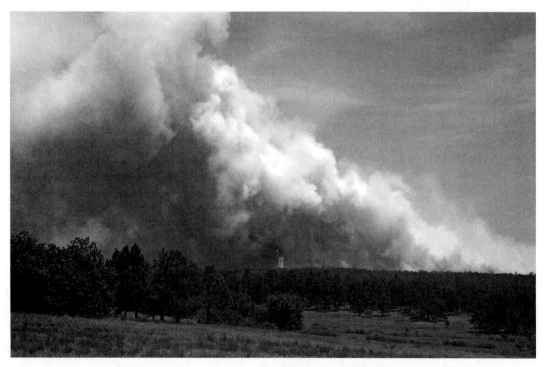

Over 500 homes were destroyed in the 2013 Black Forest Fire, the worst wildfire disaster in Colorado history.

react from a place of knowledge and power. Science advances our ability to understand what leads up to natural disasters, so we can better develop actual warning systems that will help millions of people be ready in the future.

In the chapters that follow, all different types and kinds of disasters will be covered as well as emergencies big and small and what to do before, during, and after. Hopefully, the next time there is a warning of an approaching hurricane or a nearby earthquake swarm, the disasters of the past will scare us enough to act so that we do, indeed, have a future.

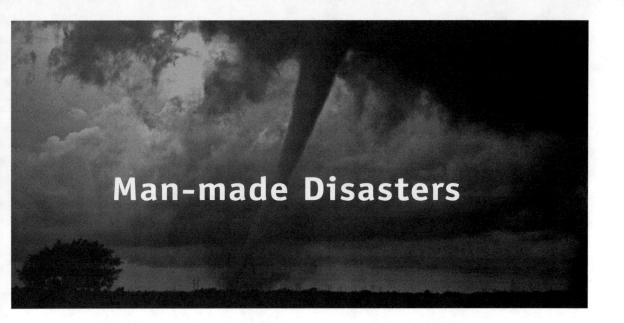

Man-made Disasters

Mother Earth may be responsible for the biggest disasters facing our world, but those due to human causes are not far behind. If we look at things like nuclear war and climate change, we can see how man-made catastrophes, especially when combined with environmental forces, might do us in much sooner. Man-made disasters add to our fear levels because unlike many natural ones, they are unpredictable and often accompany volatile social changes and geopolitical strife. Man-made disasters may be smaller in size but more powerful and horrifying in purpose and implication. Or they remind us of our capacity to make mistakes and screw up in ways that affect thousands of other people, such as a faulty mechanical inspection that might down a plane full of passengers or an overlooked valve leak that might lead to a massive gas explosion.

Humans make mistakes, and that is hard enough to deal with when they cause fatalities and injuries, but when humans commit mass acts of violence and terrorism, random or otherwise, we are rendered helpless and hopeless. Then we are forced to make sense of what happened emotionally as well as physically, and the scars these events leave behind often run deep. Global disasters take the greatest toll, leaving us feeling as if the whole world is an unsafe place.

But, just as with natural disasters, we can find ways to mitigate the threats and do our best to survive what is survivable. We can find ways to take back our power over the unknown and unplanned. It all comes down to knowing what the threats we face are, how they might play out if they actually happen, and how best to prepare for and respond to them.

According to the Disasterium website, man-made disasters are broken down into categories that include:

- Technological hazards: cyberterrorism, electromagnetic pulse, hacking, blackouts, grid outages
- Sociological hazards: terrorism, war, active shooter events, mass crime sprees
- Transportation hazards: air, roadway, railway, space, and boat disasters

Human-caused disasters are often the results of human error, human intent, or the failure of systems, including our economic infrastructure. Nuclear bombs, dirty bombs, terrorist explosions, arson fires, and plane crashes often get the most media coverage because of the fear factors involved, but we have also experienced devastating oil spills, bridge collapses, gas explosions, and the sinking of major cruise ships. Loss of life can vary from the single digits to the thousands, and often it is poorer regions and communities that pay a higher toll, simply because more expensive areas have easier and faster access to emergency response.

The frightening thing about man-made disasters is that, in the vast majority of cases, they are totally unpredictable. In the case of terrorism, they can happen anywhere at any time. At least we have some warning of a tornado outbreak or an impending volcanic eruption. However, man-made disasters can be prevented if prior actions are taken to cut down the potential for human error and provide more security in the case of acts of human intent. A solid infrastructure is a plus, but many nations of the earth, including the wealthy United States, often don't learn about weaknesses in their infrastructures until something catastrophic tests them and shows the specific points of failure. Even terrorist attacks can reveal massive holes in the security of buildings and locations, just as a cyberattack can point out the weakness of a website's protective measures.

Man-made disasters take a large toll not only on human life, but on the environment, and can often cause irreversible damage to ecosystems. The fact that we humans are building more of our homes in specific areas, such as coastal urban centers, adds to the devastation when even a moderate event takes place. If the population is dense enough, more people and structures will be affected adversely.

Even natural disasters are made worse by human actions and behaviors. Wildfires ravage homes that are built in rural areas dense with dry brush. Thick fog banks along heavily populated coastlines cause more auto crashes than along rural roads. A dirty bomb going off in an airport is much more potent than one going off in a rural grain tower.

The economic impact is often worse with man-made disasters, especially in the case of massive oil spills, toxic hazard disasters, and nuclear-related events. War is probably the biggest man-made disaster we face in terms of loss of life, environmental impact, and economic breakdown, but even a nuclear bomb or nuclear EMP set off in the atmosphere can cause billions of dollars of damage.

In 2004, the Indian Ocean earthquake and the tsunami that followed killed over 230,000 people and caused about $15 billion in damage. Yet the

2010 Deepwater Horizon oil spill in the Gulf of Mexico, which took the lives of eleven people, cost six times that much for cleanup and recovery. The 1989 *Exxon Valdez* oil spill, which resulted when the *Valdez* collided with the Bligh Reef, cost about $2.5 billion, with additional billions of dollars in damage and recovery costs. Often, with these oil spills, the environmental damage is irreversible. The *Valdez* spill alone put over 11 million gallons (41.6 million liters) of oil into the ocean, resulting in the deaths of over 250,000 birds and other wildlife near the Prince William Sound in Alaska.

TOP MAN-MADE DISASTERS

The top man-made disasters run the gamut from thick fog to oil fires to nuclear power plant explosions. While some disasters cost more in lives, others rack up massive bills for damage. In many cases, these disasters were preventable, which makes them even greater tragedies. In no particular order, some of the biggest include:

- SS *Grandcamp* disaster: Over 575 people lost their lives in April of 1947 when the SS *Grandcamp* exploded at dock in Texas City, Texas. The ship

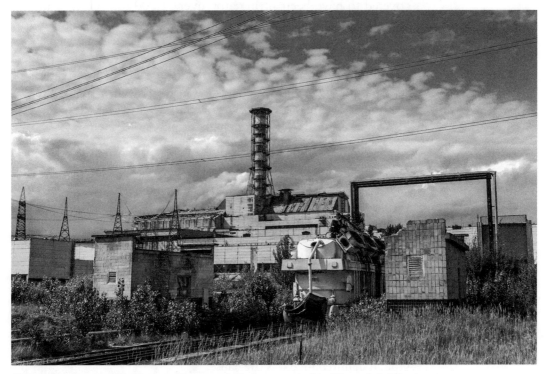

One of the worst nuclear reactor disasters of all time occurred in Chernobyl, Ukraine, in 1986, when it was still part of the U.S.S.R. The city had to be evacuated and will not be habitable by people for at least two centuries.

was filled with ammonium nitrate. When it exploded, it destroyed the entire fire department of the town of Texas City, who happened to have been fighting a fire in the ship's cargo hold. Hundreds of spectators watching along the docks were also killed. Fire spread to a nearby Monsanto chemical plant and even an oil pipeline, which added fuel to the fire and destroyed the city. Then another ship exploded hours later and finished off what was left of the town, burning hundreds of homes and structures and injuring thousands of people. This event resulted in major lawsuits and attempts to regulate laws governing the transport of toxic materials.

- The Great Smog of '52: In 1952, London was slammed with some of the heaviest combined pollution and fog in the city's history. The weather was cold, and when citizens began using fireplaces, the added smoke from burning coal created a black cloud filled with various chemicals such as sulfur dioxide and nitrogen oxide combined with auto exhaust and exhaust from nearby power plants. The toxic cloud was so thick that it enveloped the city, and over 12,000 people were killed in what became the worst air pollution crisis in European history.

- Love Canal: The Love Canal near Niagara Falls, New York, was discovered to have been sitting atop over 21,000 tons (19,051 metric tons) of industrial toxic waste that began to seep into residents' yards, leading to an epidemic of miscarriages and birth defects and a massive cleanup effort. In 1978 the seventy-acre area became one of the largest environmental disasters in history and was still oozing toxins as of 2013, according to "Love Canal Still Oozing Poison 35 Years Later," a November 2, 2013, article in the *New York Post* that reported a lawsuit by new residents in the same neighborhood.

- Three Mile Island: In 1979, Pennsylvania's Three Mile Island Nuclear Power Plant experienced a partial core meltdown at its Unit 2, causing livestock deaths, birth defects, miscarriages, and premature births and prompting an evacuation within a five-mile (eight-kilometer) radius. This would go down as the worst nuclear disaster in U.S. history and begin the downslide of public faith in the use of nuclear power.

- Flight 191 crash: One of the worst disasters in U.S. history, the ill-fated American Airlines Flight 191 crashed shortly after takeoff in May of 1979. Heading out of Chicago's O'Hare Airport, the McDonnell Douglas CD-10 crashed when the left engine broke off, sending the plane down in an open field. All 258 passengers, 13 crew, and 2 ground workers were killed. The Federal Aviation Administration found that faulty ground maintenance was the cause.

- Kansas City collapse: In July of 1981, 114 people lost their lives in Kansas City, Missouri, when a fourth-floor skywalk of the Hyatt Re-gency Hotel collapsed from the weight of over a thousand people standing and dancing on the bridge. Among the deaths were people attending a tea dance in the concourse area below. The cause was determined to be insufficient load capacity, and no criminal charges were filed against the walkway designers.

- Bhopal gas leak: In December of 1984, the Union Carbide pesticide plant in Bhopal, India, exposed over half a million people to leaks of deadly toxins such as methyl isocyanate gas. Over 15,000 died, and an additional 20,000 are said to have died later from aftereffects of the poison gas.

- Chernobyl: The "big one" of man-made disasters, the 1986 meltdown of the Chernobyl Nuclear Power Plant in the Soviet Ukraine was a catastrophe in every sense of the word. The meltdown released over 400 times more radioactive materials into the atmosphere than the Hiroshima bomb and caused thousands of fatal cancers in those near the area as well as countless thousands of babies born with birth defects. The event took place in 1986, and experts say the area will not be safe for any human activity for 200 years.

- Kuwait oil fires: The honor of the largest oil spill in history goes to the 1991 oil fires that occurred after the invasion of that year in Kuwait, when Saddam Hussein's Iraqi army blew up the oil wells. Six hundred wells were set ablaze and burned for over seven months, creating a major environmental hazard.

- Mississippi River bridge collapse: Imagine being in rush hour traffic on an eight-lane bridge over a river when a design flaw in the forty-year-old bridge causes a collapse. It's hard to imagine, but it happened in August of 2007 when the busy bridge in Minneapolis, Minnesota, collapsed, killing 13 and injuring 145. This disaster served as a catalyst for other states to increase bridge structural safety.

The above is just a sampling of the various man-made disasters that happen all over the world. We hear about them on the news and thank our lucky stars we were not there at the time and are enraged when we learn something as simple as faulty inspections were to blame for deaths and injuries. But these are the types of events that can happen to any one of us, anywhere at any time.

AIR DISASTERS

One of the most horrifying types of disasters occurs high in the air, where we already feel vulnerable. Although more people die on highways and byways all over the world because of auto accidents and crashes, the idea of being on a plane thousands of feet above the ground terrifies us, yet we continue to use this mode of transport nonetheless. While millions of flights take place each

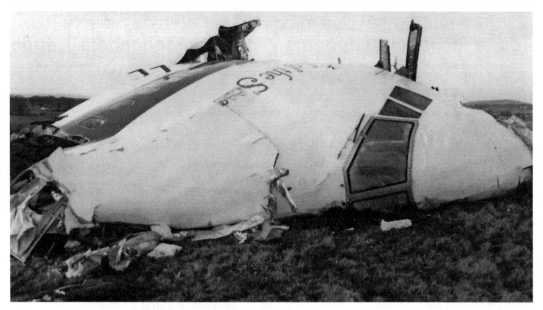

Pan Am Flight 103 was destroyed by a terrorist in 1988. The plane crashed in Lockerbie, Scotland, killing all 243 aboard.

year without incident, there are those fateful flights that result in tragedy. Whether the cause is pilot error, maintenance error, or something entirely natural, such as heavy storms and lightning strikes or blocked engines due to a flock of birds, the death tolls are always high.

- 1977—KLM and Pan Am Boeing 747 jumbo jets collide over the coast of West Africa, killing 583. Thick fog on the runway is to blame.

- 1985—Japan Airlines Flight 123 crashes in a remote area of Japan, killing 524 of the 528 on board after an explosive decompression.

- 1988—As the result of a terrorist plot, Pan Am Flight 103 exploded into three sections after taking off from Heathrow Airport in London; 243 died. Another 11 people died in Lockerbie, Scotland, when the three sections came down and a fireball burned several homes.

- 1996—TWA Flight 800 exploded near Long Island, killing 230 people aboard. The cause was later determined to be a short circuit that caused a fuel tank explosion.

- 1999—Egypt Air Flight 990, en route from L.A. to Cairo, crashed in the Atlantic Ocean, killing all 217 on board. The plane was said to have been crashed intentionally by the pilot, who was Egyptian, but the Egyptian Civil Aviation Agency determined that it was mechanical failure.

- 2001—After the terrorist attacks of 2001, American Airlines Flight 587 crashed in Queens, New York, killing all 260 on board and five people on the ground. The cause was determined to be an overused rudder mechanism.

- 2014—Malaysian Airlines Flight 370 vanished within an hour after taking off from Kuala Lumpur on its way to Beijing. It vanished somewhere over the Indian Ocean and has not been found since. It was carrying 239 people on board. No bodies or debris have been found.

- 2014—Malaysian Airlines Flight 17 was carrying 298 when it was shot down in the eastern Ukraine by a possible surface-to-air missile launched by Russian-backed separatists.

- 2015—Metrojet Flight 9268 exploded over the Sinai desert, killing all 224 on board, in a terrorist act claimed by the Islamic State.

These major air disasters all involved either mechanical issues or terrorist acts. Sadly, the disasters continue as both faulty inspections and pilot error as well as terrorist activity persist. These are not predictable, but in many ways they are preventable.

DAMS

Most of us don't think too much about dam failure unless we happen to live near a dam, yet it is the cause of major flooding and loss of both life and property, and with the increasing precipitation in many areas of the world, combined with growing populations nearby, dam failures and levee breaches are a frightening prospect.

Dam failures and levee breaches can have totally natural causes, such as heavy rains, earthquakes, and long-lasting storms, but sadly they can also be the result of poor design and maintenance practices. In the United States alone, there are over 80,000 dams, with one third considered high risk according to the National Inventory of Dams.

Dams are artificial barriers that impound massive amounts of water for storage and flow control. They can fail at any time with little warning as the result of overtopping due to heavy rains that exceed dam capacity, structural failure, settling and cracking of the concrete, earthquakes, piping and erosion within the embankments, inadequate maintenance, and even terrorist plots.

In May of 1889, the South Fork Dam near South Fork, Pennsylvania, failed due to heavy rains. The breach released over 20 million tons (18.14 metric tons) of water into communities below, killing over 2,200 people and destroying entire communities. Those who didn't perish in the initial floodwaters were left to float on debris and huddle in attics of flooded homes until help could arrive. The event would go down in history as the Johnstown Flood and South Fork Dam failure and was the first disaster that the American Red Cross, under the leadership of Clara Barton, was established to respond to and assist with.

A Sticky Situation

January 15, 1919, has gone down in history as the Great Molasses Flood. In Boston's North End, a large storage tank of molasses at the Purity Distillery Company collapsed, sending a molasses tidal wave traveling at approximately 35 miles per hour (56 kph) through the neighboring streets. Twenty-one people died, and 150 more were injured. Witnesses reported a loud roar and rumble, and the ground shook as the fifty-foot tank released over 2.3 million gallons (8.706 million liters) of molasses into the streets. Buildings were swept off their foundations, a railcar was overturned on the tracks, trucks were tossed in the air, and horses and other animals were killed in its path, unable to get out of the sticky, thick mess.

The cause was determined to be a combination of poor tank construction, insufficient testing, and rising internal pressure due to fermentation. The origin point of the stress to the tank was a manhole cover near the base of the cylindrical tank, where pressure was highest.

Cleanup went on for weeks in the immediately affected zone and months overall, with over 300 people pitching in to

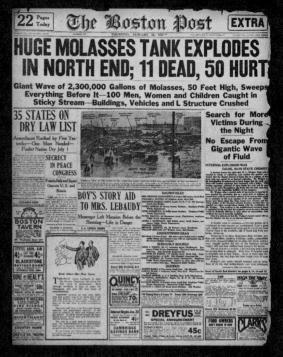

One of the more bizarre disasters in the history books is the 1919 molasses flood in Boston, Massachusetts.

remove the stickiness from the Greater Boston suburb.

More recent dam failures include the 1976 Teton Dam failure on Idaho's Teton River, which caused over one billion dollars in damage and killed 11 people. In 1977, the Kelly Barnes Dam in Georgia killed 39 people when it failed. With increasing rainfall being reported in more areas of the world, including the United States, filling levees and dams beyond their capacity, we are sure to see more of these catastrophic failures and the resulting floods.

If you live near a dam or downstream from one, you can contact your state or counter-emergency management agency or visit the National Inventory of Dams and the Association of State Dam Safety to find out if your dam is a high-hazard site. If there is a dam failure, follow all evacuation orders, and get out of the path of the water as soon as you can. Dams are structures we often just don't think about and take for granted, but they are part of the new generation of threats we face as our climate changes and storms and rainfall amounts rise each season.

According to the Insurance Information Institute, in the year 2016 alone, there were (globally) 136 man-made disasters, 4,014 deaths, and approximately $7,797,000 in insured losses. Of these disasters, which had to qualify as catastrophes in terms of loss of life and insured loss amounts, 36 were maritime disasters that included overturned ferries and ships carrying immigrants, 11 were air disasters (including space-related), 11 were rail disasters, 8 were mining accidents, 3 were bridge/building collapses, and 17 involved terrorism and social unrest. This is just a glimpse into one year and, again, only disasters with insurable losses reported.

The transportation-related disasters alone caused 2,298 deaths and over $3 billion in insured losses. Marine accidents included the horrific boat crashes near Greece and Libya, resulting in over 600 migrant deaths.

Man-made disasters could fill an entire book, but the point to be taken from these events is that they are in many cases caused by human acts and preventable. As we become more focused on regulating industries and enforcing safety codes, we still may have the occasional disastrous plane crashes, gas explosions, and dam failures, but fewer of them. Until then, it behooves us all to learn what to do before, during, and after in order to survive.

NUCLEAR DISASTER

The Fukushima Daiichi nuclear plant disaster of 2011 is considered the most significant nuclear disaster since Russia's Chernobyl event in 1986. It is also, after Chernobyl, the second nuclear disaster in history to be rated a 7 on the International Nuclear and Radiological Event Scale (INES). Though Fukushima did not result in direct deaths, it is still rated as high as Chernobyl for the potential aftereffects of the widespread radiation.

The purpose of the INES, which was created by the International Atomic Energy Agency, is to communicate to the public the danger levels of a nuclear incident or accident in terms of the ionized radiation threat. As a safety significance scale, the INES is designed to convey the critical, or not so critical, nature of an event in the same way the Richter scale signifies the size of an earthquake.

The scale is divided into two sections with seven different levels:

0—A Deviation, but with no safety significance
1—An Anomaly
2—An Incident
3—A Serious Incident
4—An Accident with Local Consequences
5—An Accident with Wider Consequences
6—A Serious Accident
7—A Major Accident

Levels zero through three are called *incidents*, with the higher levels being the more deadly *accidents*. Each level is ten times greater an event than the level before it and takes into account people and the environment, radiological barriers and control, and defense in depth. Any extremely minor event with no safety significance is rated 0. Events that don't have relevance in terms of radiation or nuclear safety at all are not even rated.

Events rated a 7 will be those that require countermeasures to protect human and other life and the environment, even if the effects haven't actually occurred.

The next time a nuclear event occurs, the media will give the rating level, which then indicates what precautions, evacuations, and other actions are necessary.

TERRORISM AND ACTS OF VIOLENCE

As the world around us becomes an increasingly violent place, new threats of terrorism, even on domestic soil, loom. Add to that the threat of war, mass shootings, and cyber attacks, and it is easy to become paranoid. While it is important to remember that we only hear about the bad news in the media and that most of our days go by without incident, it helps to be aware, alert, and prepared.

Before we can do that, we need to look at the potential threats we face. Here in the United States, the rise of mass shootings and domestic terrorism, including cyberattacks, is concerning, to say the least. As the FBI, the Department of Homeland Security, and other government agencies scramble to find new ways to stop terrorist acts in their tracks or respond to those that do happen, we must do our part to educate ourselves about what we might be facing not just abroad, but right here at home. No longer are all the headlines about countries thousands of miles away. These horrors happen everywhere, and they can happen here at any time and in any place.

Terrorism is an act of indiscriminate violence used as a tactic and a strategy to avenge or punish. It is also used to oppress a group of people by scaring them into submission and to suppress dissent. The idea behind any terrorist act is to create fear and often to achieve a specific political, social, religious, or cultural goal at the same time. Terrorist acts, by their very nature, cause extreme fear because we never know where or when they will occur, and it makes us afraid to leave our homes and live our lives in freedom. This is often exactly what terrorists, whether foreign or domestic, want. They want to control others, and their main weapon of choice is terror.

Terrorism is not just an overseas threat anymore. Domestic terrorist acts on U.S. soil happen all the time, often at the hands of white supremacist groups, antigovernment militias, and religious extremist groups (Christian and Islamic).

Sometimes the terrorist is a lone wolf acting on their own to create fear and panic. But usually it is a small cell or group that has a particular agenda they believe is achievable by killing or instilling terror in the hearts of others. Domestic terrorists can be teenagers shooting up schools with guns or a man walking into a grocery store and opening fire. Often domestic terrorism involves people who are mentally unstable, have access to vast amounts of weapons (guns and explosives), and have not committed a previous crime and therefore are not on the radar of the FBI.

When it comes to emergency situations, we know from watching headline news that a bombing or attack can occur anywhere at any time. As much as the government agencies fighting terrorism try to squash it before it happens, it is impossible to prevent all terrorist acts, especially those that are inflicted by homegrown terrorist groups and organizations.

Terrorist acts can best be classified as political, social, cultural, religious, psychological, and ideological. They may involve actual bombings, mass shootings, the intentional breakdown of infrastructure and technology

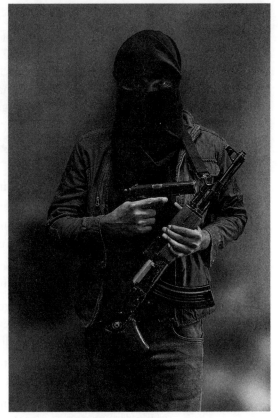

Terrorists use violence to achieve political, religious, or social goals. By attacking unpredictably, they create fear in populations, and fear keeps them from being free.

(cyberterrorism), and out-and-out warfare in more extreme cases. A school shooting is just as much a terrorist act as a bomb set off in an airport by a religious extremist group. Terror is terror, no matter what group it is inflicted upon.

It is impossible to ask people to avoid public places that can be terrorist targets, such as airports, the venues of large sporting events and concerts, subways, shopping malls, and anywhere else large groups of people gather. Even smaller locations such as a grocery store or a popular restaurant can be a target. Schools seem to be a target of choice for many shooters/terrorists, as are movie theaters. In other words, it pays to be vigilant no matter where you go nowadays and to be aware of your surroundings at all times.

Security measures since the September 11, 2001, terrorist attacks on the Twin Towers and the Pentagon, which caused close to 3,000 fatalities and over 8,700 injuries, have certainly increased public awareness of the possibilities as well as measures to protect the public. But these events will continue.

BOMBINGS

The number-one choice of terrorists, whether domestic or foreign, is explosive devices. Many bombs are improvised and easy to make with materials that are commonly found. Others are more intricate, such as the suitcase nuclear "dirty bombs." Bombs can be small, yet pack an incredible amount of deadly power. Notable terrorist bombings on U.S. soil include:

1916—Suitcase bomb—10 dead and 44 injured when a bomb in a suitcase exploded during a Preparedness Day Parade in San Francisco, California

1920—Wall Street bombing—40 dead and hundreds injured when alleged anarchists exploded a bomb on the busy New York street

1975—New York City bombing—11 dead and 75 injured when a bomb exploded in a TWA terminal locker at La Guardia Airport.

1975—Fraunces Tavern bombing—4 dead and 63 injured in the bombing of the historic tavern in New York City

1986—Hostage situation and bombing—2 dead and 79 injured during a hostage situation at an elementary school in Cokeville, Wyoming, that resulted in a bomb exploding

1993—World Trade Center bombing—6 dead and over 1,000 injured when a bomb exploded in a van in the basement garage

1995—Oklahoma City bombing—169 dead and 675 injured from a truck bomb

1996—Olympic bombing—2 dead and 110 injured when a pipe bomb exploded during a night concert in a park at the Summer Olympic Games in Atlanta, Georgia

2013—Boston Marathon bombing—3 killed and hundreds injured by two bombs thrown during the Marathon

Between 1978 and 1995, the Unabomber, otherwise known as Theodore Kaczynski, killed 3 people and injured 23 others on a nationwide bombing spree.

In many war-torn and terrorist-ridden countries of the world, bombings are a daily occurrence. Travel to such countries is often restricted, but it still behooves the traveler to beware of the dangers. On U.S. soil, many of the bombings are smaller in scope but still a clear and present danger.

Bombs are not the only weapon of choice we need to be aware of. Crashing planes into buildings has occurred more than just on the fateful day of September 11, 2001. Two hundred seventeen people lost their lives in an intentional crash of an Egypt Air flight over the Atlantic Ocean in 1999. In the past, planes were being hijacked left and right, and, as in the November 1958 Cubana Airlines crash after a plane was hijacked from Miami, some ended in disaster. Today we find many news reports of cars, trucks, and buses being driven into large crowds, killing dozens and injuring hundreds. As this book was being written—in fact, as this section was being written—a car drove into a crowd of people in Virginia protesting a White Nationalist march, killing one and injuring dozens. A few weeks later, a white van drove into a crowd in a pedestrian zone in the historic Las Ramblas section of Barcelona, Spain, and killed 13, injuring over 50 other tourists and residents, before being caught by police.

Biological terrorism and warfare is a huge concern as terrorists learn ways to weaponize deadly viral and bacterial agents. Biological agents include organisms and toxins that can kill or incapacitate people. When the agents are airborne, they are an extreme danger to heavily populated areas, where they can spread like wildfire.

There are three types of biological agents used in terrorist acts: viruses, bacteria, and toxins. Methods of dispersion include spraying them into the air, contaminating water and food systems, person-to-person contact, and infecting animals that then infect humans. The real danger of these attacks centers on the invisibility of the agents. By the time we are aware there has been an attack, the virus, bacteria, or toxin can spread exponentially, and often the first sign is a large wave of sick people showing up at urgent care centers and hospital emergency rooms.

Perhaps the most famous biological attack occurred in Japan in March of 1995 when an attack using the poisonous nerve gas Sarin occurred on a Tokyo subway. The terrorist group behind the Sarin attack was the cult called Aum Shinrikyo, a Japanese doomsday cult founded by a man named Shoko Asahara in 1984. The same group had been responsible for a smaller Sarin attack a year earlier. The followers believed in a doomsday prophecy of Asahara's that suggested instigating a third world war and bringing about a nuclear Armageddon. Twelve people died and over 4,000 were injured because of the ideology of a crazed cult combined with access to a deadly toxin. It can and will happen again so long as there are extremist groups and individuals willing to carry out such acts.

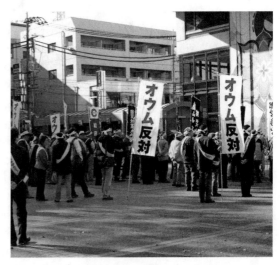

After the September 11, 2001, attacks in the United States, anthrax-laced letters were sent to numerous media outlets, congresspeople, and government officials. In September of 1984, followers of Bhagwan Shree Rajneesh in Oregon poisoned restaurants in the area with salmonella, resulting

Demonstrators protest against the Aum Shinrikyo doomsday cult, which was responsible for the 1995 Sarin attacks on a Tokyo subway.

in over 751 ill. In April of 2015, Amanda Vicinanzo, senior editor for *Homeland Security Today*, wrote in "Biological Terrorist Attack on US an 'Urgent and Serious Threat'" that a bioattack on U.S. soil could, in the words of Martha McSally (R-AZ), "cause illness and even kill hundreds of thousands of people, overwhelm our public health capabilities, and create significant economic, societal and political consequences." McSally is the subcommittee chairman of the House Committee on Emergency Preparedness. Though its main concerns are attacks courtesy of foreign terrorist groups such as ISIL and other jihadists, a threat from homegrown domestic terrorists and lone wolf "rogues" exists as well.

In an October 2014 article titled "Could US Handle Biological Attack" for The Hill, reporter Kristina Wong looked at the threat of a weaponized Ebola or other extremely virulent virus being unleashed on the country and how the virus itself is only the beginning of the problems we face: "While experts say Ebola would not make the most effective biological weapon, the problems seen in the response to the virus—from confusion over treatment protocols to a shortage of specialized medical facilities and trained workers—would be magnified if a biological agent were unleashed in the United States." This was written shortly after the United States had been dealing with the threat of three cases of Ebola and potential breakouts on our own soil.

It is very disconcerting to imagine a weaponized virus or other toxin released into the public, but even more frightening is the prospect that we may lack the proper responses to protect citizens, including ourselves, from an epidemic, or worse, a pandemic.

Mass Shootings

The biggest terrorist threat we face in the United States is the proliferation of mass shootings. Guns are the new bombs and appear to be the chosen weapon for domestic terrorists, lone wolves, and mentally unstable individuals with easy access to weapons, whether legal or illegal.

A mass shooting usually involves more than one or two victims and is often the work of someone with a distinct agenda. Often there are two or three shooters, but the vast majority of cases involve one shooter. According to "The Math of Mass Shootings," an article by Bonnie Berkowitz, Lazaro Gamio, Denise Lu, Kevin Uhrmacher, and Todd Lindeman for the June 6, 2017, *Washington Post,* mass shooting events don't even take into account gang activity, shootings that begin as another crime, such as a robbery, or family killings. We are looking at a pandemic, and it appears to be spreading.

Also called "active shooter incidents," many of these result in the deaths not only of victims, but of the shooters as well. If the shooters don't kill themselves, law enforcement usually will. Even though the majority of gun deaths in the United States continue to be suicides or one-on-one shootings, we still must be alert to the possibility that we might experience an active shooting while shopping at the local mall, attending a major concert or event, or even doing something as simple as visiting a friend at a hospital. Such incidents, like biological attacks, can happen anytime, anyplace, and anywhere and are totally unpredictable.

Everytown for Gun Safety, an advocacy group, reported some grim statistics in an NPR June 5, 2017, report titled "Most Mass Shootings Are Smaller, Domestic Tragedies."

The report states that between 2009 and 2016:

- 70% of mass shooting victims were killed during the actual incident.

- A majority of mass shootings with fewer than ten victims involve domestic violence.

- Almost a fourth of fatalities are children.

- 96% of suspects had not been subject to prior FBI terrorism investigations.

- The average shooter age is 34.5.

- 83% of shooters are male.

- 52% were *not* prohibited from possessing firearms.

- 42% were suicides.

Red flags and warning signs are possible, such as domestic abuse and violence, prior firearm offenses, mental imbalances and threats, other criminal offenses, substance abuse, and animal abuse. But often these red flags are overlooked. In the case of larger-scale mass shootings, even the FBI has difficulty pinpointing shooters ahead of time, even when they have been stockpiling weapons for months. In many cases, there is nothing to pinpoint, as with a drifter who opened fire on a Stockton, California, elementary school in January of 1989, killing five children and wounding thirty others before he killed himself. The shooter was said to have had a history of prior criminal offenses, mental illness, and drug abuse, yet he was able to buy the AK-47 and semiautomatic handgun he used in the shooting legally at the time in Oregon and California.

Despite bans on assault weapons, and security and background checks, too many of these shooters manage to get guns and use them on innocent victims. While the vast majority of gun owners are responsible and buy their guns legally, the problem persists that, at any given moment in time, the person standing next to you could open fire. Whether as an act of terror, a cry for help, or because of an extreme ideology or mental illness, the results are the same.

In the next chapters we will learn the best ways to respond in an active shooter situation, but for now we will look at some of the more recent deadliest shootings in U.S. history. Again, these don't include gang activity and normal criminal activity or shootings involving fewer than three or four victims.

- San Ysidro McDonald's, San Diego, California: July 18, 1984: A 41-year-old man opened fire in a border town McDonald's south of San Diego and killed 21 before he was killed by police.

- Luby's, Killeen, Texas, October 16, 1991: A 35-year-old man named George Hennard killed 23 people before killing himself in a Texas cafeteria.

- Columbine, Colorado, April 20, 1999: Two high school students, Eric Harris and Dylan Klebold, killed 13 people and wounded 24 others at Columbine High School before they killed themselves.

- Virginia Tech, Blacksburg, Virginia, April 16, 2007: A 23-year-old man named Seung-Hui Cho opened fire on the campus and killed 32, injuring 17 others. Then he killed himself.

- Fort Hood, Fort Hood, Texas, November 5, 2009: An Army psychiatrist named Major Nidal Malik Hasan used two handguns to kill 13 people and injure 30 others at the U.S. Army's Fort Hood Readiness Center. He was captured and sentenced to death in 2013.

- Aurora Theater, Aurora, Colorado, July 20, 2012: Twenty-five-year-old James Holmes walked into a midnight screening of *The Dark Knight* at the Aurora Theater, opened fire, and killed 12 people. Over 70 were injured. Holmes was arrested nearby shortly after the attack.

- Sandy Hook, Newtown, Connecticut, December 14, 2012: Twenty-year-old Adam Lanza walked into the Sandy Hook Elementary School and killed 26 people, including many children, before killing himself and his mother.

- Inland Regional Center, San Bernardino, California, December 2, 2015: Two men, Syed Farook (28) and Tashfeen Malik (27), killed 14 people inside a social services center before police killed them in a shootout.

- Pulse Nightclub, Orlando, Florida, June 12, 2016: A 29-year-old man named Omar Mateen committed the deadliest shooting in recent U.S. history when he killed 49 clubgoers and wounded over 50 others before police killed him.

- Route 91 Harvest music festival, Las Vegas, Nevada, October 1, 2017: 64-year-old Stephen Paddock shot over 1,100 rounds of ammunition at the country music grounds. He took the shots from the 32nd floor of the Mandalay Bay hotel, killing 58 and injuring 851. He also shot at jet fuel tanks at the adjacent McCarren International Airport, but they did not ignite. It is the worst single-person shooter incident in U.S. history. Police shot and killed Paddock; his motive is still unknown.

This is just a sampling of the mass shootings in the United States from the last thirty-plus years. They occur in offices, homes, schools, malls, even

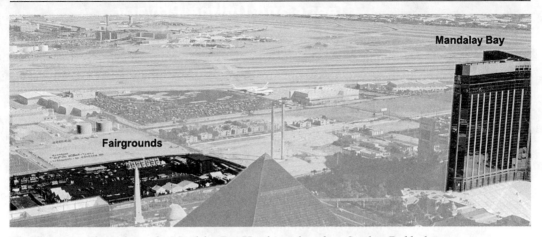

The illustration above shows the Mandalay Bay Hotel at right, where Stephen Paddock was when he shot people at the fairgrounds next to the McCarren International Airport at left. He was armed with high-powered AR-15-type assault rifles and other weapons.

churches. One of the most terrifying examples of active shooter terrorism comes in the form of sniper shootings from highway overpasses and tops of buildings. In October of 2002, Maryland and Virginia residents experienced nine different sniper attacks in eight of their communities, resulting in thirteen deaths. In July of 2016, Dallas, Texas, experienced a sniper attack that resulted in the deaths of six people, most of them police officers, before the attacker was himself killed by police.

According to the December 14, 2016, *Huffington Post,* there have been over 200 school shootings alone since Sandy Hook, and the *Los Angeles Times* in its April 11, 2017, edition stated that a gun has been fired on school grounds nearly once per week since Sandy Hook. And this is just the threat to our children and college students. We are all sitting ducks, no matter our age, gender, color, or creed.

Government and law enforcement officials have struggled to find ways to better track potential active shooter incidents before they happen, such as engaging public awareness, monitoring large gun sales, monitoring social networking sites for possible chatter, and looking for patterns of past criminal offenses, but the truth is, many of these shooters were off the radar *until* they committed their heinous crimes. This means that we have to be as proactive as possible in staying alert and aware and knowing what to do if we one day find ourselves caught in the crossfire.

CYBERTERRORISM

A new breed of terrorism lurks, feeding off our growing dependency on technology. In the first half of 2017 alone, cybercrimes were on the rise. In just

Teens and Online Privacy

Most of today's teenagers have grown up with cell phones and computers. They don't think twice about communicating openly with people all over the world in social forums and on phone apps. They friend strangers on Facebook and follow strangers on Twitter, and they send pictures and personal information without a second thought.

As parents, it is critical to sit down with teenagers and even younger children and talk to them about using common sense when leaving behind a "digital footprint." One way we can do this is ask them to think about what they are posting for the long term. Is it something they would be okay with a prospective boss seeing? Maybe a girlfriend, future husband? Will it come back to haunt them in some way? Everything they post online leaves behind a digital footprint that may be impossible to get rid of later when it counts.

Find out what their motivation is for posting. Is it to find new friends, communicate with others who have similar interests, or stay in touch with school friends after hours? Encourage them never to tell their real name or where they live to a stranger, even if it is someone they've been gaming with or chatting with for a while. Everyone is untrustworthy until they prove they can be trusted. Tell them to keep their social networking privacy settings on and not to list their age or home address and cell phone number.

When they tag each other on pictures, remind them that they are now bringing in the privacy of others. Tagging friends without permission is not cool. Have your teens set up pre-approval for others who wish to tag them so that they can keep control of the type of posts that appear on their pages.

If you suspect someone is trying to sexually engage your child or teen, get their username and report them to the website administrator. Talk to your child or teen about the dangers of being too open, even if the person they are chatting with claims to be the same age or gender. Pedophiles know exactly how to prey on young people and are adept at doing so. If your teen or child says they were asked to meet someone locally, report it to the police.

If you suspect your teen is bullying others online or being bullied, address the issue immediately before it gets out of control. If they are being bullied, help them disengage from the bullies on all online formats. Teens, like adults, use sarcasm and teasing, so help them identify real bullying from normal human behavior. Bullying is cruel and mean and is an actual

the first ninety days, cyberattacks were the highest in history, according to the security technology firm ThreatMatrix CyberCrime Reports.

The idea that terrorists can harm us via our electronics, especially our computers, is becoming more accepted as we all experience hackers getting into large corporations, banks, manufacturers, government, military, and commercial firms, threatening to expose our private and sensitive information to the world, not to mention to the hackers. Our names, addresses, phone numbers, social security numbers, bank accounts, passwords, email accounts, private photos, store

form of abuse, so report anything threatening to the local police *and* to the website administrator of the platform they are using, such as Facebook or Twitter. When bullies and threats are reported, these platforms will investigate and block them.

Even if it appears your teens are not listening to you, they are, and no doubt they want to keep themselves safe while online, too.

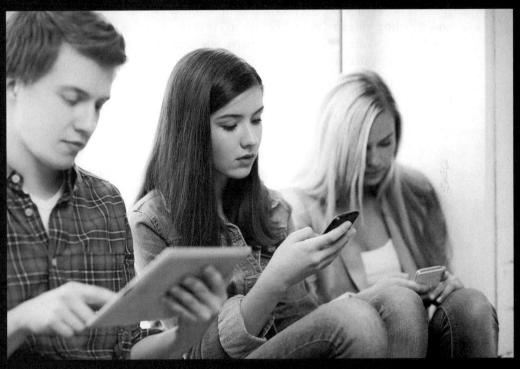

Young people are online for hours every day, accessing the Internet through phones, computers, tablets, and other devices, often talking to strangers. This can expose them to everything from credit card scams to bullying to potential sex offenders.

accounts, and everything in between can now be displayed to the public or sold on the deep Web's black market for information. Within moments, our bank accounts can be wiped out, our identities changed, and we can end up with changes to our credit reports, accounts opened in our names, crimes committed with our data, and more.

Anything that we do on our cell phones and computers is now open season for the new terrorist hackers and information thieves and traders.

Cyberterrorism, or a cyberattack, is an attack carried out via technological means, usually computer networks, by a terrorist group, individuals, organizations, criminals, or anyone else who serves to benefit from shutting down information systems and taking the data for their own agendas and motives. Malicious cyberattacks can involve the destruction of networks or the alteration of data systems, and rarely do the hackers and cyberattackers make their names known, usually choosing to remain anonymous or operating under a bizarre name. In some cyberattacks, spyware can be installed in systems without the users' knowledge—a new kind of electronic stalking.

The worst kind of cyberterrorism involves taking down infrastructures and crippling industry, as in 1999 when Amazon.com was shut down by a "denial of service" attack, exposing massive amounts of personal private data, and representing a major threat to critical systems such as air traffic control, government operations, and energy grids. Cyberterrorists play on the fears of the public, but they also play on our vulnerability, exposing to us our overdependence on technology. The individuals and groups behind these attacks can be professional hackers, lone wolves, or even groups of kids with too much time on their hands.

Although our computer use makes us vulnerable enough as individual users, a true cyberattack is one that affects a large number of people, sometimes entire nations. There are two types of attacks:

Syntactic—Malicious software that includes self-replicating virus programs that attach to other programs and files and reproduce. Often viruses are hard to find, as they can hide within the computer's memory. Worms are self-sustaining running programs that use specifically designed protocols to replicate themselves over entire networks. Think of a worm burrowing its way through an apple. Worms are fast-spreading and can infect thousands of systems in only a few hours. Trojan horses appear legitimate and are made to perform actual tasks, but hide within them unwanted and damaging activity. Trojan horses are used to introduce worms and viruses into a computer and are often embedded in free software trials found on the Internet.

Semantic—These attacks modify and disperse information, both true and false, sometimes to hide the tracks of a hacker. These attacks are often used in politically motivated cyberattacks between fighting nations eager to retrieve sensitive information or take down important systems and databases.

The FBI is the main body investigating cyberattacks in the United States, with the CIA joining in for attacks that involve foreign interests. According to the FBI website, cyber "intrusions," as they call them, are becoming more and more common, more dangerous, and more sophisticated. Both private and public sector networks are in danger of being attacked at any time with little to no warning, and unless we have the technological capability to repair or stop the damage in the first place, we remain vulnerable. Some of the ways the FBI is trying to counter this growing problem are:

- A cyber division to address cybercrime
- Specially trained cyber squads at FBI headquarters and field offices staffed with agents and analysts who are on top of the latest protection methods
- Cyber action teams that travel the world to assist in computer intrusion cases
- 93 computer crimes task forces nationwide
- Partnerships with other federal agencies, including the Department of Defense, Homeland Security, and others

Still, as we find the latest ways to stay one step ahead of the cyberattackers, we can be sure they are already two steps ahead. Prevention is absolutely critical, but so is a solid continuity plan when there is an attack.

One type of attack is called ransomware and involves the hackers demanding a ransom be paid before they will stop the attack. One such attack, called "Wanna Cry," occurred in May of 2017, involving a worldwide ransomware cryptoworm that targeted computers running the Microsoft Windows operating system. This attack alone involved over 200,000 victims and infected over 300,000 computers in over 150 countries until the worm was stopped when a 22-year-old security researcher in England found the kill switch! Which proves that for every brilliant hacker out there, there is an equally or more brilliant security researcher or anti-hacker able to find the worm and smash it in its tracks.

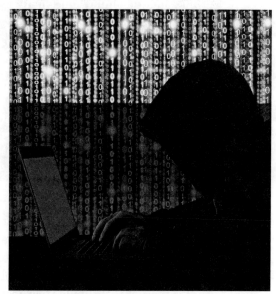

The hackers may promise federal agents a decryption key once the ransom is paid, but they don't always follow through, frustrating FBI efforts even more. Thus the need to evolve and find new ways to prevent the attacks from ever happening. Luckily, researchers are advancing methods to recover lost data from worm-infected machines. Companies are even hiring tech geniuses, often very young, to continuously come up with ways to push back against cyberattacks. It may sound like the makings of a science fiction movie, but today's terrorism involves armies of tech geeks armed with brains as sharp as razor blades.

The new battlefront is in the cyber world as people from all over the globe are stealing money and information by hacking into computers and servers at an alarming pace.

Avoiding Malicious Emails

Oh, we've all seen them. Emails that look like they come from friends, banks, financial institutions, and government agencies, yet something seems amiss when we look deeper. Unfortunately for many, you won't know it's a virus about to infect your computer until you've opened the link. Spamming and phishing is rampant and can fool the best of us.

If you get an email request for information from someone you aren't sure about, contact the company directly. Do not open the link, get the information on the actual company website. Let them know about the email. They will probably have you forward it.

Make sure your filters are on your email programs, which will help block incoming spam accounts. But when you do get spammed, try to report it so that the company is aware and can take actions to stop it.

Think about keeping your email address private, especially on social networking sites and even on your own personal website, to avoid being put on "the list" for spam and phishing attempts.

Even if an email sounds threatening and appears to come from the IRS or some powerful agency, don't fall for it. Never open the link, and do not under any circumstances give them personal information. The IRS will contact you *by mail* if there is an issue with your taxes.

One of the best ways to spot something you feel unsure about is to check the email address of the person sending it. Let's say the email appears to come from your phone company, but when you click on the address bar and see the email address, it has some strange or random name that has nothing to do with your company. There's your clue that you are being victimized. Even an email from a good friend can end up coming from a strange address. *Check before responding!*

Some of these emails can look so legitimate you are *sure* they are not malicious, so you click on the link and go to a website that *looks* like the correct site. But beware, as you may have been directed to a fake site. Check the URL and compare it to the actual company's URL. Often scammers will use a variation of the real URL, but you can still see the difference.

Mark spam as junk and get rid of it. You can also go into your email settings and block addresses that spam you often.

If you feel you have been a victim, change passwords and account numbers, contact your bank and credit reporting centers, and even consider changing your email address.

Identity theft is the biggest concern of individuals, including having their finances wiped out and financial records made available for public viewing. Identity theft is a huge priority for the FBI and other agencies, and many banks and finance institutions are implementing better protections, even insurance, for their clients should their identities be compromised. Insurance companies are also getting involved with offering identity protection for their clients. Even if this doesn't prevent the cyber intrusions from happening, it can go a long way towards helping to stabilize the potential damage to individuals who only want to live their lives and hang on to their hard-earned money.

There are some steps we can take as individuals to try to prevent major damage from cyberattacks and from smaller hackers. Having a firewall and keeping it turned on is one. A firewall will protect your computer from hackers. For individual computers that are newer, there are built-in firewalls, but firewall software can also be purchased.

Also make sure you have the most current antivirus software installed as well as anti-spyware protection, which can come in the form of a software program to download or purchase at a computer store. However, some people fall prey to fake spyware programs that can be downloaded for free on the Internet. These may actually *be* spyware or some kind of malicious code that will cause damage. Buy from trustworthy companies.

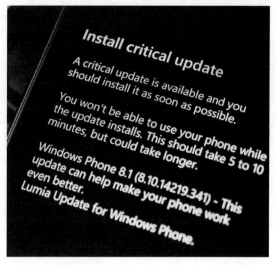

Do not ignore notices from your service providers about updating your phone or computer. Companies such as Microsoft are constantly having to upgrade operating systems to protect them from hackers.

Keep your OS, or Operating System, as up to date as possible, and watch what you download from the computer! *Never* open an email attachment or a forwarded attachment that looks strange, even if it is from someone you know. This is one of the biggest ways to spread viruses, as many poor victims have learned the hard way.

Lastly, turn off your computer when not in use. It may be a pain, but nobody can hack your computer overnight when it is not even on!

READINESS IS CRITICAL

Knowing what the threats are is the beginning of being able to develop action plans that can increase our chances of survival. We cannot begin to put together a preparedness or response plan unless we first have an idea of what the most likely emergencies and disasters we might be facing are. There will be local, regional, national, and global events, and each one will require a different method of response. Having a broad view of the potential emergencies, predictable or otherwise, allows us to face reality, as frightening as it may be, and formulate the best ways of keeping ourselves, our families, and our communities as safe as possible.

In the coming sections, we will look at detailed methods of preparing for and responding to every possible type of emergency, as well as resources for use after reading this book. Readers will begin to see patterns emerge, as many of the suggestions for surviving an earthquake can apply to living through a hurricane, with some modifications. With the advent of the Internet and social networking, there are so many new resources and educational websites that can empower the individual citizen to be ready for just about anything.

With all of the aforementioned threats we face, and many smaller emergencies that happen as a part of every day life, there is no excuse for not having solid information at our fingertips.

A personal author note here: As a single mom raising a child in earthquake and fire country, I joined Community Emergency Response Teams (CERT), coordinated through the Federal Emergency Management Agency (FEMA) and the Department of Homeland Security (DHS). CERT, which I will discuss more in the "Resources" section, allowed me to learn everything I needed to help myself, my son, my family, and my neighborhood as well as serve as a "second responder" to local emergency personnel should they need me.

My actual training in disaster preparedness and response, though, began years earlier when I was lucky enough to work at Warner Bros. Records in Burbank, California. The Warner brothers themselves were huge advocates of preparedness for their thousands of employees, especially when it came to those pesky earthquakes. I took part in free training through Warner Bros. with the Burbank Police and Fire Departments and was privileged to serve as a safety monitor at the record company, having learned everything from fire safety and disaster assessment to earthquake response, search and rescue, and triage/medical aid. It not only made me feel empowered, but it gave my fellow employees someone to turn to when they had questions.

Today, I am active with CERT in Northern San Diego County, and I have also become a licensed amateur radio operator. I continue to get training, which now includes bioterrorism, disaster psychology and trauma, fire abatement and response, toxic and chemical hazards, victim extraction, building assessment, prophylactic distribution, crowd control, and a host of other skills. I will share a lot of what I have learned in this book, but please keep in mind that I am not a superhero. Anyone can learn these skills, and anyone can do what is needed to deal with any emergency short of an alien invasion.

For that I will have to depend on my charm.

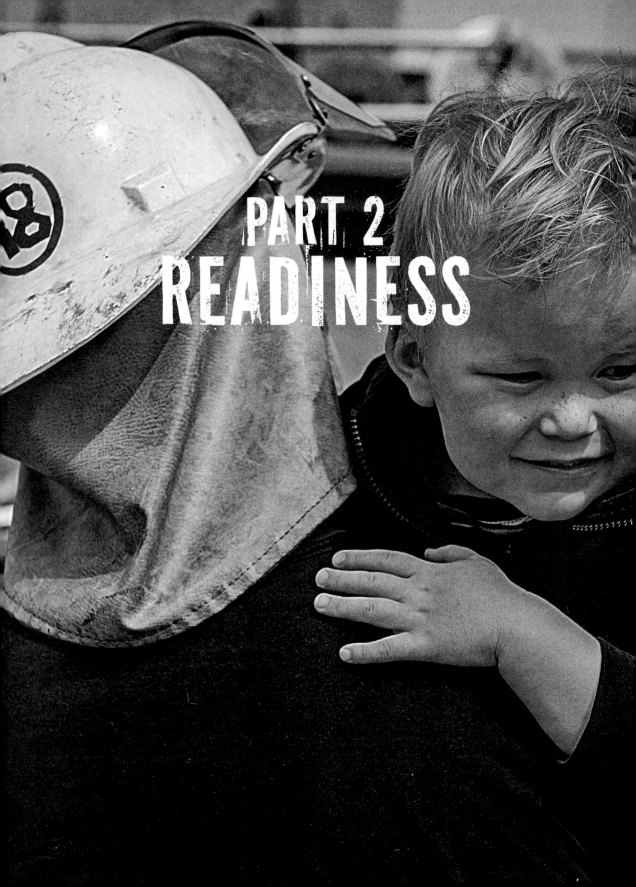

PART 2
READINESS

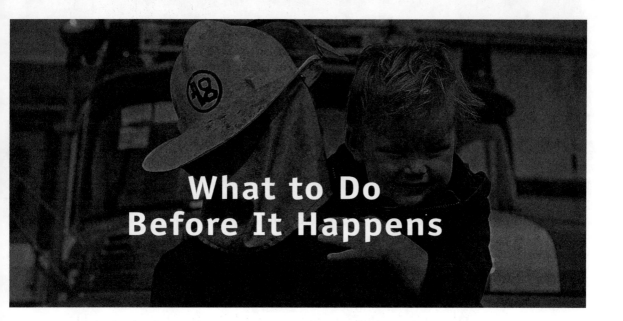

What to Do
Before It Happens

If you knew you had to give a speech in a week before 500 people, you would practice that speech until you could perform it with your eyes closed. If you knew you had a test the next day that would determine whether or not you passed a course, you would study the night before. If you knew you had to apply for a job, you would practice your interview skills, buy a nice outfit, and make sure your car had enough gas so you would have one less thing to worry about in the morning.

Why, then, would you not do what it takes to prepare for an emergency?

According to the Red Cross, "Emergencies can strike quickly and without warning. This may force you to evacuate your neighborhood or be confined to your home. What would you do if your basic services—water, gas, electricity, or communications—were shut off?" The vast majority of people are either not prepared at all or minimally prepared with a few extra bottles of water lying around the house. It's simply not enough.

In this section, the focus is on what needs to be in place before any emergency occurs, including lists of items to have in your home, office, and car, prepping ideas for everyone in every situation, a plan for yourself and your family, and a breakdown of specifics for each type of disaster we talked about in Part One.

When we were kids, our parents and teachers told us that preparation is the key to success in school and in life. It may also save our lives.

Being prepared doesn't demand a complete surrender to paranoia. Emergencies big and small will happen, and the more we are equipped to deal with them, the better we will do in responding and reacting. Not everyone will experience a mass shooting or an avalanche, but even smaller emergencies are addressed in this book, and in many cases the techniques, tips, and methods for a large event also apply to a home emergency such as a kitchen fire or a possible gas leak.

The first rule of preparedness is awareness of risk. Whatever part of the country or world you live in, there are specific natural and man-made circumstances that could lead to a major emergency or disaster in the future. Threats can be examined by categorizing them as global, national, regional, local, and individual.

- Global: nuclear war, asteroid impact, space weather event, supervolcanic eruption, war, climate change, pandemics
- National: weather events, terrorist acts, epidemics and pandemics
- Regional: weather events, flooding, earthquakes, volcanic eruptions, epidemics
- Local: weather events, flooding, disease breakouts, mass shootings

Depending on where you live, the regional and local events you will be most concerned with will vary. People who live in hurricane zones must be more prepared for those events than people who live in desert regions, yet flash flood-

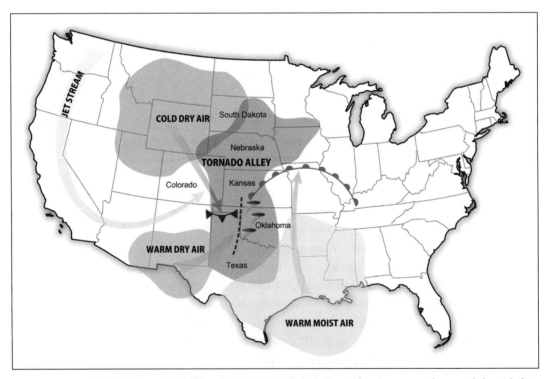

Part of being prepared for emergencies is being aware of your surroundings and the risk for certain disasters. For example, if you live in the region of the United States known as Tornado Alley, you should definitely make tornado preparedness a priority.

ing can occur in both places. Terrorist acts can affect a local neighborhood or be on such a massive scale, like the September 11, 2001, attacks that they are considered global events.

Obviously, the most imminent dangers occur with local and regional threats, and those should be addressed based on the dictates of the actual threats. It is more difficult to prepare for global events that may never happen, although we should at least take some precautions. Sometimes it's easiest to start close to home.

DETERMINE THE THREATS

Do you live in Tornado Alley? Earthquake country? Near the coastline or in a large urban center? Identify your environment and then look at the threats that are most common. A solid disaster preparation plan will include even the remote possibilities, but much of your efforts will be in learning how to survive the ones with the highest rate of occurrence.

For example, if you live in a section of the country known for hurricanes, you must be ready to board up windows and evacuate when told to, especially if you live near the coast and storm surge is a possibility. Your plan will include a before, during, and after list of what to do in the event of a hurricane specifically. Maybe your neck of the woods also experiences major wildfires during dry spells. Your plan must also include ways to create defensible space around your home, cleaning up your garage of flammables and combustibles, and knowing your evacuation routes by heart. In both cases, you will need to know how to pack a bug-out bag or shelter in place if it's too late to leave.

So, emergencies will carry with them specific ways of preparing and responding, yet many overlap, so that knowledge of surviving one carries over into another. It may seem overwhelming, but when broken down into small action steps, it can be done quickly and effectively.

SITUATION AWARENESS

Any emergency, big or small, requires a plan of action. That plan begins, though, long before the actual emergency takes place. It begins when the awareness that something can and will happen becomes reality. Just watch the news on television or on the Internet and it's easy to see how we are all targets, even if what happens is confined to our own homes or neighborhoods.

The first step is to have access to knowledge, because knowledge is power. Knowing what is going on in your environment is critical to being ready for whatever might be coming your way, from a terrorist bombing to an active shooter, from a wall of wildfire to an oncoming tornado outbreak.

"Situational awareness" is the term given to the observation of one's environment to determine potential threats and lines of defense. If you are not aware, you are not alert, and if you are not alert, you may be stuck in a situation that is difficult to extract yourself from. We have all heard of the "see something, say something" push by the government and law enforcement agencies to help identify potential terrorist attacks, shootings, and crimes in general. On a larger scale, being aware of what is normal in any given environment then allows us to have a baseline to work off of when we encounter something that feels or looks "off."

In the summer 2017 issue of *Emergency Management* magazine, Andy Alitzer writes that the baseline we should be looking for is what is normal for our community, population, a particular event, or situation. For example, what is considered normal behavior at a high school football game, versus something out of the ordinary that catches the eye and causes concern. Or think of being at a crowded beach enjoying the sun and surf, then realizing that something is amiss because things don't appear to be the norm for that particular situation. This is the kind of thing Alitzer says takes work and is different within each larger component of a community. Special events are harder still to get a baseline on, but a lot of this comes from experience, historical precedent, and often just gut instinct.

From that baseline, we then look for the possible situational issues that may arise to a disaster or emergency. A large music concert that includes fireworks has its own red flags, as does a parade of protestors in an organized march. Next, we need to look around us at the demeanor of people and notice anything out of the ordinary. Doing this may help us identify a threat such as a bombing or a shooting before it happens and possibly save our lives and the lives of others.

Man-made disasters such as auto accidents, bridge collapses, dam failures, and others require a different kind of awareness. We must know what is normal for our own environment. Walking across a bridge with ten thousand people may not be the wisest thing to do if the bridge is known to have suffered capacity load failure in the past. Driving in thick fog is a disaster waiting to happen that requires extra vigilance. Flying on a plane requires that we not only pay attention to the humans around us, but to various sounds, smells, and sights that may indicate a problem.

When it comes to natural disasters, we look around for changes in the wind, weather, smells, how we are feeling in the event of a toxic leak, the amount of water rushing down the local creek, or how high the waterline at the reservoir is. No matter what the potential emergency, being aware is the first line of defense. If we were hiking through the woods alone, we would be looking around for coyotes or wolves, mountain lions, other potentially dangerous critters like snakes, and even other potentially dangerous human beings. This same kind of vigilance, or at least a recognized awareness, is critical to being ready to respond and react.

The article "Situational Awareness: The First Line of Defense" for the March 27, 2017, *Prepper's Journal* states that situational awareness is important on a daily basis. It is a tool that must be included in any survival or emergency plan. "There is a whole world of things going on around you, some good, some not so good. You want to be able to prepare when you see the not so good. It's as close to a crystal ball as we can get." This doesn't mean you must walk around a paranoid mess, just that you must keep your eyes and ears open and trust your instincts when something, anything, in your surroundings does not fall into the usual baseline or the situational baseline that you are familiar with.

EMERGENCY ALERTS

This is a test. For the next sixty seconds, this station will conduct a test of the Emergency Broadcast System. This is only a test. If this had been an actual emergency, you would have been instructed where to tune in your area for news and official information. This concludes the test of the Emergency Broadcast System.

From 1963 to 1997, American households heard the above, or some version of it, broadcast over their televisions and radios on a regular basis. The Emergency Broadcast System was the warning system formerly used to alert citizens to a local, statewide, or national emergency situation. It was designed mainly to provide the president with a means of communicating to the public during an emergency. Between 1976 and 1996, the system was utilized to broadcast alerts for over 20,000 situations, although none of them involved a national emergency.

In 1997, the Emergency Broadcast System was replaced with the Emergency Alert System (EAS) we have today. The purpose stayed the same, and monthly and weekly tests continue to be broadcast on television and radio as well as over satellite digital audio service and direct broadcast satellite providers, cable television systems, and wireless cable systems. The EAS is designed to give the president of the United States the chance to address the nation within ten minutes of a major emergency. The new EAS has also been used in Amber Alerts of missing children as well as severe weather warnings, courtesy of National Weather Service alerts on a local and regional basis.

The Federal Communications Commission (FCC), governs the EAS along with the Federal Emergency Management Agency (FEMA) and the National Weather Service (a part of the National Oceanic and Atmospheric Administration [NOAA]) and has a number of prewritten scripts with information that would be used in a major emergency. Among the instructions in the scripts are suggestions that citizens not use phones and keep lines free, something that is a must even today with cell phones, as well as asking citizens to listen for further alerts, which might give out evacuation or shelter-in-place orders. Once official information began flowing, the sys-

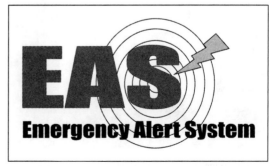

The logo of the Emergency Alert System. The EAS replaced the Emergency Broadcast System in 1997.

tem would be used for a message from the president or the next in line of command, were the president not available, as well as statewide and local emergency information.

Emergency alert tests are used to test the system at all levels so the FCC can be assured that, if needed, the system will work to disseminate proper information. It also helps the FCC identify stations that are cooperative with the system's testing schedule and those that are not. Today, weekly tests are the norm, although during potential emergencies such as severe weather, they may occur more frequently.

When a national emergency does occur, it is up to the president to activate the EAS system, and FEMA has the authority to begin the alerts.

Another mass warning system is the Integrated Public Alert and Warning System (IPAWS), which is a modernized integration of the nation's alert/warning infrastructure that combines information from federal, state, local, tribal, and territorial alerting authorities and provides the public with updated information they need during an emergency. IPAWS uses the EAS as well as Wireless Emergency Alerts (WEAs), and also broadcasts over NOAA's Weather Radio service, among others, all on a single interface. The more information that each system can contribute, the more information the public has to make the best choices during a major situation.

WEAs are a wonderful new tool for warning the public. They can be sent out at the state and local level, by the National Weather Service, the National Center for Missing and Exploited Children (Amber Alerts), and the president. These alerts come over cell phones like a text message but are accompanied by a sound or vibration to alert the user. These sounds are repeated twice. Texts are brief, including the type of emergency, the time, and any action that needs to be taken as well as the agency that is issuing the alert.

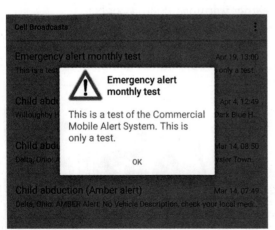

The Wireless Emergency Alert system allows government agencies such as NOAA or the police to send alerts to wireless devices such as your iPhone.

WEAs are not charged to cell phone users the way normal texts are, and they will come through even when a call or other use of the cell phone is in progress. Citizens must contact their cell phone service provider to get hooked up to the WEA system, but since nowadays most of us pay far more attention to our cell phones than to standard televisions and radios, it is critical to staying alert and up on the latest developments. This is even more important when away from home or when the power is out.

False Alarm!

It's a typical Saturday morning, around 9:33 Eastern Time, on February 20, 1971. Radio station WOWO out of Fort Wayne, Indiana, is playing a popular Partridge Family song when suddenly the broadcast is interrupted by a series of loud beeps, followed by an official message ceasing all broadcasting *immediately* for an Emergency Action Notification directed by the president. What followed on that tense morning was the first actual national emergency broadcast over the Emergency Broadcast System.

The broadcaster, Bob Sievers, sounded terrified, and rightfully so, as he went on and on for at least half an hour broadcasting a vague national emergency that he had no details of. At 10:13 a.m. Eastern Time, another message finally came through saying, "Cancel message sent at 09:33 EST, repeat cancel message," followed by a message authenticator. Turns out, the whole thing was a false alarm, a mistake caused by an accidental message sent out from the Department of Defense's base at Cheyenne Mountain in Colorado to EBS-participating stations. The teletype operator there, W. S. Eberhardt, broadcast the wrong message with an authenticator code "Hatefulness" through the entire EBS system. The message and the code ordered the broadcasters to cease whatever they were playing and announce the emergency. Shortly afterwards, around 9:59 am, a correction message was sent out, but that one contained the wrong authenticator code and didn't work! Finally at 10:13 a.m. the right cancellation message with the right code word "Impish" went out, ending the alert.

Many of the stations ignored the message, others jumped on it, as did WOWO, thinking it the real deal. But it was supposed to be only a message ordering a test, not a disaster of national proportions. President Richard Nixon never made his emergency message, the listeners and the broadcasters realized it was a mistake, and all returned to normal.

But for over a half an hour that morning, people thought the world might possibly be coming to an end. That fiasco taught the Federal Communications Commission a lot about how to fine-tune the EBS, which would later become the EAS we now have. Now we don't worry as much about mistakenly sent messages as about hackers who can break into the system to announce an alien invasion or zombie attack. The actual broadcast is available on YouTube and other sites. Simply search "WOWO false alarm of 1971."

More recently, on January 13, 2018, Hawaiians got the fright of their lives when an emergency broadcast told them to take shelter because a nuclear missile was heading their way. Given the tensions at the time between the United States and North Korea, which had been testing nuclear bombs and boasting they could now reach U.S. territory, one can understand why island residents were terrified. It turned out, however, that an employee at the Hawaii Emergency Management Agency somehow misunderstood that they were simply having a drill and instead triggered the real alarm. The employee was later fired, but an investigation led to the conclusion that insufficient protocols and safeguards, including computer software that didn't clearly distinguish between exercises and the real thing, were in place to prevent human error.

In addition to these alert systems, which can be installed on your phone with a quick visit to your state and local emergency services websites (or FEMA), apps are available that can also serve as alert and information tools for heavy cell phone users. It's as easy as visiting your provider's app store, and since most of them are free, all you need to do is install them on your phone.

The Emergency Alert System and all the additional forms of alerts are the first communication you will get of a disaster or emergency. While social networking spreads information like wildfire, it isn't always accurate. The EAS and other official warning systems will give the most updated information possible to help you know exactly what is happening, how it affects you, and what you need to do about it.

This is only a test. But one day, it could be the real thing.

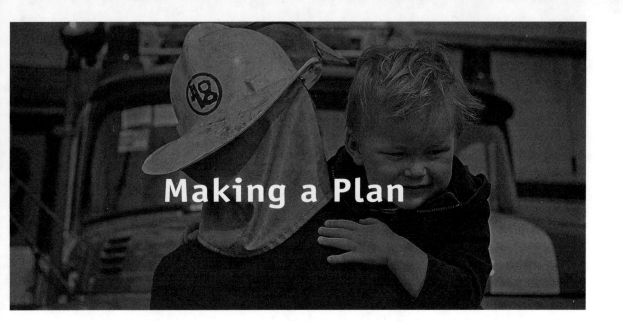

Making a Plan

Preparedness requires a plan. The Red Cross suggests putting together a plan of action for yourself and your family before doing anything else. Depending on the hazards in your area, your plan might vary a little, but the basics will always be the same. The goal of a plan is to do four things: keep you and your family fed, hydrated, safe, and sanitary.

The first order of action is to sit down with your family, if you have one, and make a disaster checklist. This list will include:

- What you need at home
- What you will do in the event of …
- How you will communicate and get news
- Where you will go if you need to leave
- What you will take
- What you will do about pets if you have them
- If you know your neighbors, get together and form a similar plan for the community

After a checklist is made, figure out how the family will communicate with each other if separated. Will there be a community meeting place chosen that everyone can attempt to get to? Will everyone try to get back home? Will you use cell phones, and if service is down, how might you get the information you need?

It is absolutely critical to make sure the identification you carry in your wallet or purse is up to date, including your current address. Pick an out-of-town relative who can be a contact person for the whole family. Did you know that after a disaster it is actually easier to make long-distance calls than local calls? Often, because disasters are regional or local, closer-to-home activity is more clogged or shut down to allow for emergency communications only.

One of the best ways to keep abreast of what is happening is to have a ham radio, but few people take the time to consider this or take the training. More on that in a bit.

Do you have a car you will need to get out of a garage? If the power is off, do you know how to open the garage door manually? If left on foot, where will you walk to get help? In some emergencies, such as an electromagnetic pulse, cars will be useless. Know where you will walk, and maybe get your neighbors involved to walk as a group to a designated shelter if needed.

If there is a home fire, do you know what to do and how to get out safely? Do you have the proper tools around the house, such as a fire extinguisher? In the coming chapters, we will go through everything that should be in your survival kit to meet any kind of emergency, big or small.

All of these questions must be answered to have a solid action plan. Remember, situational awareness! Take a look at your location and find the best escape/evacuation routes out of your home/office. Know what roads lead in and out of your community, and notice which ones tend to get bogged down the most with traffic. In some rural areas, there may be only one main road out, so look for alternative ways to get away fast, especially in the case of wildfire.

Make sure everyone in your home knows how to shut off the gas, water, and electricity if needed and who to contact afterwards to get them restored. If you turn off your gas, it will require a professional to turn it back on. Have this information written down in a place where everyone can see it, or put it in your written action plan.

What about pets? Your action plan checklist should include what to do with pets in terms of sheltering in place or evacuation. You will not be able to quickly leave animals at a local shelter in the event of an emergency. They will be overwhelmed taking care of the animals they already have!

What about an elderly or disabled family member? Will you need to have a wheelchair or walker ready should you have to leave? What about oxygen tanks and other home medical equipment that you may not be able to move? How can you improvise

Make sure you have a plan for evacuating your furry friends during an emergency, as well as a place in mind where they can be kept until things return to normal.

Family Matters

Planning for a disaster when you have a family can come down to simple things, but most of us don't take the time to address even those. Start now to put the following into place so that everyone knows what to do when disaster strikes:

- **Emergency Contact Information:** Every family member must know who the outside contact person is and how to contact them. Keep this name and phone number in a wallet as well as in the contacts on your cell phone. Make sure every family member has this information on hand. Don't just put it into your phone, because you may lose or forget your phone without having memorized the information.

- **Emergency Meeting Place:** Hopefully, you will all be together when disaster strikes, but in case you're not, have a particular place your family members can meet, preferably the designated emergency shelter closest to home. For kids who may be at school, have a family member assigned to pick up the kids and get them to the meeting place.

- **Emergency Supplies:** Make sure every family member knows where the supply kits are and what is in them. Go over how to use items such as tools, manual can openers, and shelter-in-place sheeting and tape.

Emergency Resources: Does each family member know how to dial 911? Does everyone have the same apps on their cell phones for communication and shelter location purposes? Do family members know where the closest hospital is? Fire station? Police station?

In a September 2017 article for the *Daily Independent* called "When Natural—or Any—Disaster Strikes, Being Prepared Matters," Jack Barnwell interviewed Georgianna Armstrong, the manager of Kern County (California) Emergency Services. She stated that a family communication plan was one of the basic recommended actions and that writing the contact information down is essential. Our dependency on cell phones can often make us forget that we no longer have phone numbers of important people memorized. Smaller children should know where the contact information sheet is in the home.

Armstrong's main point of urging people to have a family plan revolves around the possibility that emergency services will be crippled during a major disaster. "In a very big event, resources are going to come pouring in from other areas, but that takes time. The more strength and resilience you have to take care of yourself in the immediate after-effect of an event, the better prepared you are to withstand that event."

If preparing for an emergency comes down to *one basic thing,* it is this, in Armstrong's words: *"We are all our first line of defense."*

if asked to leave immediately or if the power goes off? Do you need to think about a small power generator?

Most people know all about having extra food and water around the house, but few think about how important it is to have critical documents such as birth and marriage certificates, social security cards, passports, deeds, insurance information, and mortgage information all in a safe place, preferably a small fireproof safe that can be easily grabbed if you have to evacuate quickly. Do this before an emergency happens, because you won't have time to search through records when it does.

SPECIAL CONSIDERATIONS

When making plans for those living in an assisted living facility, check with facility management or the resident council for a copy of the evacuation plans, meeting places within the facility, and who will assist residents in sheltering in place. These facilities should have supplies on hand for residents.

Home caregivers should also know of your emergency plans and know where supplies and important items are in the house in case they happen to be alone with a family member at the time of an emergency. If a family member requires a constant power source for a medical device, make sure everyone, caregivers included, know of the contingency plan if the power goes out, including how to find and turn on the generator.

If a family member is bed-bound, evacuation can be tricky, so be sure to have their medical supplies in case you must shelter in place. Ideally, there will be someone to help get them into an emergency vehicle or a family automobile that is equipped to handle them. Check into an emergency transport cot that can be kept with your supplies.

Know where the nearest hospitals are for anyone who must receive care as soon as possible when no ambulance service is running. Be prepared for hospitals to be overrun with people seeking aid. There also may be a shelter set up that can provide medical support in the interim.

Now that you have a written plan or checklist that covers these key points, the next big step is to get the things you need in the form of emergency survival kits. Don't just assume the things you have around the house now will suffice or that you can ask your neighbors if you run out of food or water. They may not have made any plans either.

Notice the word "kits," because the truth is, you will want to have emergency supplies for your home, your cars, and your workplace if you spend a great deal of time there.

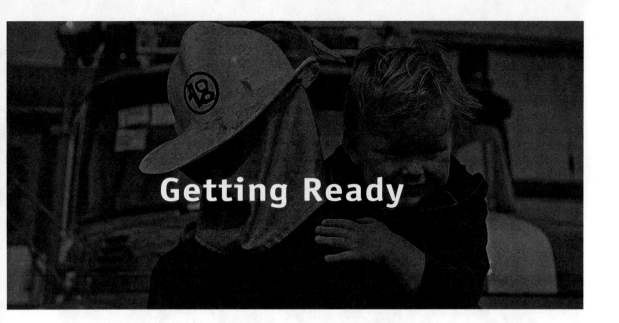

Getting Ready

Whether you call them emergency supply kits, bug-out bags, survival kits, or disaster kits, they are essential. In fact, in an emergency, these supply kits are, quite literally, your lifeline. Not having the basics, and a few other items that are specific to your location's hazards, can mean the difference between survival and helplessness. Being prepared is power, and along with the knowledge needed that is described in "What to Do before It Happens," you need things to ensure that you can get through a short- or long-duration event in case there is no help to be found.

It used to be common sense to have enough water, food, and medications for about a 72-hour period, and although that may work for a car survival kit, or a smaller bag you might send along with your college student or have at your workplace, at home it just isn't enough anymore. It is now recommended to think in terms of not being able to access food, water, and prescriptions for at least two weeks should a major event occur, regionally, nationally, or globally, that would cripple infrastructure and prevent local stores from getting supplies. Think about a massive earthquake, a volcanic eruption, or a nuclear bomb detonation. Having only three days of supplies is like putting a bandage on a hemorrhaging wound. You must have enough vital supplies on hand for at least a couple of weeks, as recent disasters have shown, because things will not get "back to normal" as quickly as you think they will. Infrastructure involves a lot of bureaucracy, red tape, and just plain good old-fashioned time, so if you aren't prepared, you will run out of time with your supplies.

It may take infrastructure even longer to get up and running, so more is always better. Can you stock nonperishables and water enough for you and your family for a month? Are you able to get an extra month's prescriptions to keep in your emergency kit? And don't forget pets. They need to eat and drink too.

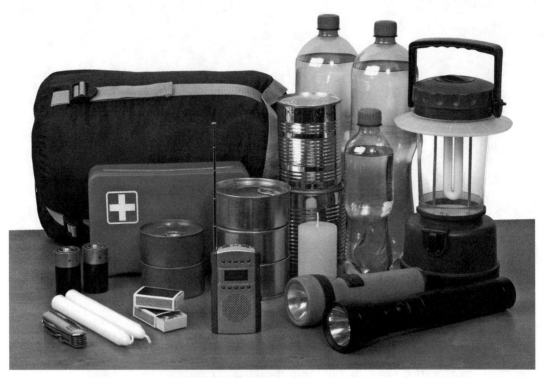

Always have emergency supplies ready for the unexpected. They should include such items as flashlights, batteries, a first aid kit, water, flares, a radio, candles, matches, toiletries, and more.

Let's start with the basics of an emergency kit that can be kept at home, in the car, or in the workplace. These items can be kept at home in a large duffel bag or a bucket with a handle that can be grabbed in case of evacuation. Or have a smaller bag such as a backpack filled with supplies, and keep the larger stock in a pantry, cupboard, or designated area in a closet or garage that everyone can get to. Where you keep your kit is important. If you live in tornado or earthquake country, think about keeping the supplies in an area that is in the center of the house. A garage can work well, but only if you can access it from the house. Otherwise you may find you are cut off from your supplies!

Ideally, have three kits. Large for home, medium for the workplace, smaller for the car.

- Water—one gallon per person per day—two weeks' worth at least for home kits, three days minimum for car and office. This is the minimum suggested amount!

- Food—nonperishables to last two weeks, and be sure to include something to open them with in the case of cans and bottles, such as a manual can and bottle opener. For a car, keep as much food as possible, although water will be the higher priority.

- Radio with batteries or a hand crank—a ham radio if you are a licensed operator (keep your charger with the radio)
- Cell phone batteries or a solar-powered charger
- Flashlights
- Flares
- First aid kit with a manual (more on this later!)
- Leather or heavy cloth work gloves
- Goggles
- Masks to cover mouth and nose
- Sanitation such as large trash bags, or you can use a bucket, toilet paper, and hand sanitizer
- Wrench, crowbar, and other tools needed to turn off gas and pry open doors
- Matches (keep in waterproof container)
- Knife—sharp, preferably a hunting knife
- Rope
- Tarp for shelter if caught outdoors
- Duct tape for sheltering in place
- Plastic sheeting for sheltering in place
- Pet food and extra water
- Medications, also for pets
- Blankets and/or sleeping bags
- Changes of clothing
- Spare contacts or eyeglasses
- Toothbrushes, deodorant, toothpaste, soap
- Baby food, formula, diapers, and some toys
- Small travel toys and games for kids
- Local maps with evacuation routes highlighted
- Utensils, washable metal dishes, small pan, and cups (not paper!)
- Cash, passports, traveler's checks, debit cards. (*Cash is king,* remember that. In an emergency, it may come down to cash-only transactions for extra food and supplies.) Cash should be in small denominations.
- Writing implements for leaving notes and taking down information
- Orange spray paint for leaving exterior information on home/building

- Triage tape
- Whistle
- An ID tag on each bag with your contact info
- Comfort items for children (blankets, dolls, toys)
- Extra set of keys
- Maps of local areas in case cell phones can't be used
- Photocopies of important personal documents
- Emergency contact information for family, friends, and local services
- Nearby keep necessary medical equipment such as walkers, wheelchairs, medical devices, oxygen tanks, etc.
- A power generator
- A grill and charcoal or some type of small cooking device that is transportable
- An emergency survival manual such as this book

The above items make the perfect home survival kit, but for work or the car you will probably want to streamline the essentials into smaller kits. Or you can actually buy premade emergency kits today over the Internet. They come in a variety of sizes, items included, and prices, and many are specifically designed for particular situations like fire, earthquake, and flood. The only problem with buying a kit, whether online or at a nearby survival goods store is that you need to do it *before* the emergency occurs. It might make sense to buy a few kits if you don't have the time or ability to get out and put your own together. You can even buy one kit per person with enough food and water for two weeks. Having plenty of kits means you will worry less about what you need once it is impossible to get out to the nearest store or get online to shop.

Either way, there is no excuse for not having at least a basic kit. Some things to remember:

- Make sure you choose a bag or a carrier with wheels that is easy to move around. You don't want your kit to be so heavy and unwieldy that you can't get it into the car if you need to evacuate.
- Label bigger equipment with your name, address, and cell phone number in case you get separated from it.
- Make sure you trade out old water, medications, and foodstuffs when they expire and go through the kit every year, if you've used anything, in order to resupply.
- Pay attention to flashlight and radio batteries, and make sure they are still usable. These too expire, and many can become corrosive inside the kit or bag.

A Battery Is a Battery Is ...

There are different kinds of batteries for different needs. We use single-use batteries for a variety of items in our homes, such as television remotes, portable radios, video game controllers, and even fire and carbon monoxide alarms. It helps to know the difference between heavy-duty, alkaline, lithium, and nickel batteries and which are good for what. We also need to keep a supply of various battery sizes, such as triple A, double A, C, and D as well as the rectangular 9-volt. You want to keep in mind the shelf life and cost of batteries first and foremost. Heavy-duty batteries have a general shelf life of a bit over two years, as opposed to alkaline, which can last for more than five years. Both are low-cost choices and do pose the risk of leaking, with alkaline being the better choice, but for basic use they are great to stock up on.

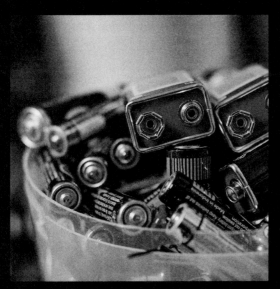
When selecting batteries for emergency purposes, buy ones with a long shelf life such as lithium batteries.

Nickel batteries and lithium batteries last a lot longer, well over six years for the nickel and ten for the lithium, and both have a much lower rate of leakage, which can be important when they are stored in unused emergency kits. Both cost a lot more money, though, and may have more limited uses, so stock up moderately on these according to what items you have that will need them. Fire and smoke alarms often use 9-volts, so keep a few extra on hand.

The most important batteries will be those used to power flashlights and lanterns if the power goes out, cell phones (exclusive to the brand of phone), and battery-operated radios. But if you are stuck inside for a length of time with power, you want to have extras of everything you normally use. Don't forget about your cell phone. If service stays on, and you can't recharge the one you have (if you lost the charger!), having an extra will be worth the cost.

Rechargeable batteries are a great choice if you want to spend a little more than usual, because they are most likely going to be used on a more daily basis. They won't last as long as traditional batteries, but they can be recharged hundreds of times while they are being used on a shorter basis. The problem with storing rechargeable batteries in an emergency kit is that they may sit around unused for so long they lose their charge.

Make an inventory of all household items and items in your emergency kit that require batteries. Note the type and size, and stock up on those, as you will actually use them, and you can cycle them out before they expire and replace them with fresh batteries.

If you keep your supplies in a cupboard, you run the risk of taking items out and forgetting to replace them. One great rule of thumb is to immediately replace anything removed. What goes out goes right back in. If the power bars you have in the cupboard are soon to expire, eat them and buy a few new boxes. Don't assume you can wait a few weeks or months to restock water you use, because you may forget. Replace it quickly. In fact, add a few more gallons while you're at it.

The month of September has been designated National Preparedness Month by the Federal Emergency Management Agency, so perhaps that can be the month you do your annual emergency kit and plan check. Things to include in the annual check will be:

- Updating and replenishing all emergency supplies

- Updating your emergency plan of action as needed, especially evacuation routes

- Updating home fire and carbon monoxide detectors with new batteries

- Reviewing how to turn utilities on and off

- Going over your insurance plan to make sure you are adequately covered for any new additions to the home

- Updating cataloged property by taking photos and an inventory in case of fire or flooding

These are some proactive measures that can ensure you and your family have the most current knowledge and information to keep safe and to protect valuable belongings.

MASKS AND RESPIRATORS

FACE MASKS

You have some choices when it comes to a face mask that will protect you from breathing in contaminants and airborne particles, even diseases. While most basic emergency kits include disposable face masks that cover the mouth and nose, these only block out larger particulate matter, splashes, sprays, and anything that can carry toxins or germs and may not protect you from everything, because of their loose fit and potential gaps between the mask and your face.

Face masks are to be used only once and only by one person. They often come in multi-packs, so you can keep some in each of your emergency kits. Once a face mask has become dirty or possibly exposed to contaminants, you can gently remove it, throw it away in a sealed bag/container, and put on a new one.

N95s

An N95 respirator is the next step up and is more protective. The N95 refers to the percentage of very small particles (95 percent of 0.3 microns) it can block, and with its closer fit to the face, it is a great choice for emergency kits in addition to the basic face masks. These respirators have straps that can be adjusted to ensure much closer coverage of the nose and mouth, unlike basic face masks. In the case of a flu pandemic or other respiratory disease breakout, these will be best for anyone with an increased risk due to age, illness, or immune system issues. But N95s should be avoided for general face protection, especially by those who have an existing lung or breathing condition or any kind of heart condition that might be affected by the mask, which can make breathing more difficult.

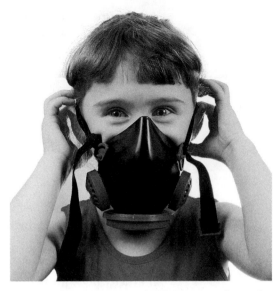

It might seem a bit paranoid to have gas masks available for your family, but if you live near a nuclear or chemical plant (or near a railway where chemicals are shipped) it might be a practical move.

Gas Masks

A gas mask protects the face from inhaling toxic gases, contaminants, and airborne pollutants by forming a tightly sealed cover over the entire face, including the eyes. Some are just protective, but other gas masks include a built-in respirator. But gas masks may not offer full protection from gases that penetrate the skin, and they usually have filters that must be changed out every twenty-four hours in a CBNR situation (chemical, biological, nuclear, radiation).

Gas masks work by filtration, chemical absorption, or by absorption and chemical reaction to neutralize a chemical. Though they are used by employees working on industrial sites, a full-on gas mask may not be something most people include in their emergency kits, but you may want to research them if you live near a nuclear or chemical plant, which increases your risk of exposure to hazardous materials. They can be pricy too, so look online or visit a survival/medical supply store, and make sure they include a filter that protects against a variety of contaminants.

PET KITS

Don't let your dogs, cats, or other beloved pets get left without the items they need should an emergency occur. They are members of your family and should be included in any plans you make. Make sure to have the following either in your larger kit or in a smaller kit that can be grabbed in case of evacuation:

- Medicines and medical records
- Leashes, harnesses, and a few toys
- Food, water, and bowls
- Sanitation items such as trash bags or small pet waste bags
- Can opener for food in cans
- Pet beds if transportable
- Pet IDs on tags if the animals are not microchipped
- Current photos of pets with their names and your contact info in case they get lost
- Pet crates if transportable (many fold down)

Sometimes you may be forced to leave pets behind, so think about leaving extra food and water. It's hard to imagine leaving your pets, but if you must, at least make sure they have plenty of water. Some people leave the toilet seats up for their pets if they evacuate quickly.

If evacuating with pets, remember that they will be panicked and anxious. Use work gloves to load them into crates or cars to avoid being bitten. Try to keep a special toy or blanket with each pet for comfort. If you live in an area that experiences numerous disaster situations, such as a tornado or hurricane zone, a floodplain, or a wildfire zone, think about asking your vet for some anxiety pills for your pets.

BUG-OUT BAGS

There is a term used by preppers, people who are passionate about preparing for any disaster. A "bug-out bag," or BOB, is a kit you can take with you in the event you need to "bug out," or get out of the area. It is also called a Get Out of Dodge Bag or GODB, a 72-hour bag, or an INCH bag (I'm Never Coming Home). As compared to a typical emergency survival kit, a BOB may have many more items included that are more oriented to longer durations away from home. These bags are equipped to be self-contained for at least seventy-two hours, usually much longer.

According to "The 7 Types of Gear You Must Have in Your Bug Out Bag" from SurvivalCache.com, you need:

- Water—One liter per day minimum as well as a purification system, which can be iodine tablets or a pot for boiling the water or water purification tablets
- Food—Three days' worth of backpack meals, energy bars, jerky, and freeze-dried meals that only require boiling water
- Clothing—Sturdy boots or shoes, long pants, a couple of pairs of socks, a couple of shirts to layer when cold, a jacket that protects against cold and rain, a hat or cap to shield the sun, and a bandana

- Shelter—A tent or ground tarp, maybe a bedroll or sleeping bag
- First aid kit—Should have plenty of bandages, ointments, bandage tape, a small pair of scissors, and aspirin. Such kits can be purchased complete if time is of the essence.
- Basic gear—Matches and other ways to make fire, ponchos or plastic rain protection, a cooking pot and small backpack stove with fuel, a couple of good flashlights, a survival knife.
- Weapons—A firearm, if legal, but keep in mind that during a major emergency, the rule of law may not exist. Pepper spray is another choice.

Other suggestions for a good BOB include utensils, bowls, cups, a manual can opener, MREs (dehydrated prepared meals), extra underwear, working gloves, a survival blanket (made of Mylar), Wet-Naps, hand sanitizer, paper towels, travel-size toiletries, a mirror for both hygiene and signaling, a multitool, glow sticks, LED lights, candles, batteries, a compass, N95 face masks, a sewing kit, sunglasses, a fishing kit, and preferably about $500 in small bills.

The bag itself is also important because it must be durable and lightweight for carrying long distances. Yet it also must be spacious enough to hold all of the items necessary. Bags with a lot of zippered compartments can help organize smaller items. The bag should be waterproof and have a place for an ID tag. Some people prefer shoulder-style bags, but they can get uncomfortable if carried for a long time, so look at a backpack-style bag that distributes weight evenly.

A BOB for a car can have just three days' worth of supplies, while a larger BOB bag will be geared towards a longer survival period, especially in cases where you are forced to go into the wild or camp out for an extended time.

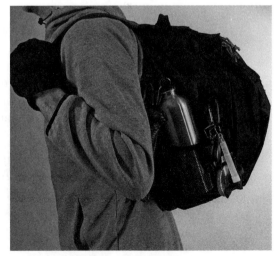

A large duffel bag is probably the last resort because of the size and unwieldiness (but it will work well for a bag meant to stay in the home). It is hard to carry a giant bag and equally hard to find what you need, because they usually don't include interior compartments.

One of the best investments you can make is some type of medical ID tag, necklace, bracelet, or ID card. But they only work if you have them with you at the time you evacuate or are found by first responders. Keep that ID on you at all times. This is especially important for seniors and children who may not be able to tell someone what

A bug out bag should be durable and lightweight so you can easily carry it for long distances.

their medical conditions are. Make sure the ID info includes any drugs, fabrics, or medications the person is allergic to.

DORM ROOMS

Smaller bags may also be ideal for college students to keep in their dorm rooms, which are so small they often don't offer much in the way of closet space. Think about having a BOB under your bed in your dorm with at least the essentials of extra food, water, flashlights, and first aid kit. Check with the dorm building manager to find out what the evacuation routes are and what happens if the power goes out, and make sure there are emergency ladders for getting out of upper-story windows safely. Walk the evacuation route out of the building to be sure there are no issues with blockage and trash.

There should also be a fire extinguisher in your dorm, or one right outside the door, but do have a crowbar in your kit so that you can get the door open in the case of an earthquake or explosion that may jam the door shut. In emergencies that involve ground movement and seismic activity, doors often sink just enough to make them impossible to open effortlessly.

Most nights on campus will be spent in the dorm, and that's when people are the most vulnerable during an emergency, so don't expect your professors and other staff to be around to help if they are cut off from the dorm building, you are cut off from the outside world, or both. If you like to take the lead, offer to put together a larger kit for your floor, and encourage other students nearby to have kits in their dorm rooms.

OFFICES

The same applies to the workspace. If you work for a large company, chances are there are emergency supplies in the building. Find out where, and what is included, because there may be missing elements that can become real issues when a disaster occurs. Are there enough water, food, and medical supplies for all of the employees? Can anyone get to the kit if they need to? Who is in charge of what is in the kit and adding to it?

If you work at a small company, chances are they do *not* have any emergency provisions on hand, other than perhaps a nearby fire extinguisher. If your boss is fine with you creating a kit, maybe take up donations from fellow employees to build one large enough for all. Think about it: you are at the workplace for hours a day, five days a week, sometimes more. Therefore, chances are good that if a disaster happens, you will be at work. Know the evacuation routes out of the building, and if your office is on an upper story, find out where the emergency fire ladders are and where the closest stairwells are should you need to leave. Remember, elevators are not ideal during any emergency, and if the power is down, you have no choice but to leave by the exit into the hallways and stairwells, or down a fire escape if that route is blocked off.

Have your own small backpack kit to keep in your workspace or in a locker if one is provided. Don't assume you will be safe at home when the you-know-what hits the fan. Be ready, encourage those around you to be ready, and have the basics you need to give you the edge on surviving and getting through an event until help arrives or you can go find help. Should you be forced to stay where you are, your fellow employees and your boss will thank you for urging them to think and plan ahead.

WATER PURIFICATION

Water purification is something you should be ready for in a variety of emergencies, both at home and outside. There are three methods of purifying water so that it is drinkable and usable for cooking:

- Heat
- Filtration
- Chemical treatment

Boiling water for ten minutes will kill any dangerous pathogens. If filtration and chemical treatment is needed, use the following guidelines:

Pathogen	Maximum Filter Pore Size
Giardia and amoeba cysts	5 microns
Enteric bacteria	0.2–0.5 microns
Cryptosporidium	3 microns
Parasitic egg and larva	20–30 microns

Chemical	Clear Water	Cloudy Water
Sodium chlorine (household bleach 5.25%)	2 drops/quart or liter (8 drops/gallon)	4 drops/quart or liter (16 drops/gallon)

Shake/stir, let stand 30 minutes before using (from the CERT Team Field Operating Guide).

THE RULE OF 3

Do you know what the Rule of 3 is? This simple set of rules is critical to remember when faced with a major disaster.

- You can survive 3 minutes without air.
- You can survive 3 hours without shelter in extreme weather conditions
- You can survive 3 days without water.
- You can survive 3 weeks without food.

The importance of having water outweighs food (although do have both) simply because we cannot live as long without water. It is absolutely essential to keep as much extra water on hand as possible. Many homeowners save rainwater in barrels, but if that isn't feasible, think about buying a couple of extra gallons each time you do a big grocery run. Before long, you will have way more water than you might ever need in an emergency, but more is more in this situation, and it can always be used for cleaning and bathing beyond what is used for actual drinking or cooking.

When it comes to food, remember to first use what is in your refrigerator if the power is going to be down for a while. If it smells bad, toss it. Great items to keep on hand are canned goods (fruits and vegetables, and if they don't have to be cooked, all the better), power bars and cereals in boxes, vacuum-packed foods, and anything that won't go bad quickly. If you have something to cook with, you can pack things like oatmeal, dehydrated foods, and any just-add-water soups and meals.

Canned goods normally have a year of shelf life, so keep them up to date, and trade out those soon to expire. Shelf-stable foods, such as noodle mixes and cereals, don't require refrigeration and are a great way to have something easy to cook or be eaten as is. If you are lucky enough to raise your own animals and grow your own fruits and vegetables, you are at an advantage when it comes to being prepared. But most people will need to stock up from their local grocery stores or box stores. See the food shelf-life list for more on how long you can keep foodstuffs.

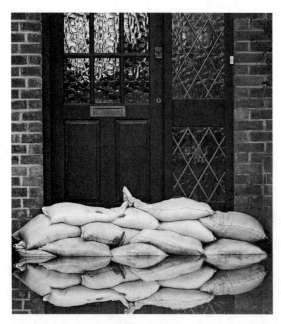

Sandbags placed around the home can keep floodwaters out, though only to a certain extent.

BEFORE THE "STORM"

Think about other items you will need before something happens. Nobody wants to stop what they are doing and think about something awful happening, but isn't it better to be more empowered when it does? Power comes from being knowledgeable and prepared. Depending on the hazards most likely to occur in your area, you may also need things like:

- Boards and planks of wood for boarding up windows and doors during hurricanes and high-wind events

- Sandbags to place around your home for periods of heavy rain and flooding

- Newer, less flammable roofing in wildfire areas (older shake-shingle roofs go up like dry tinder!)

• Garden hoses for protecting fence lines and homes during a wildfire (hosing them down long before you are asked to evacuate!)

Also think about keeping access to the garage clear from both inside and outside the home. If you live in an apartment complex with underground gated parking, ask the management what happens in the case of an emergency. Will the gates open manually, or are you better off parking out on the street? You have to weigh the risks of parking outside against what might happen during an earthquake, electromagnetic pulse, or any event that causes a long-term power outage. What would you do if you couldn't get your car on the road? You would be left to get to safety by bicycle, if you're lucky enough to have one, or on foot.

'TIS THE SEASON TO BE READY

If you celebrate Christmas (or even Halloween!), it is important to think about safety precautions so that you don't come home one night to find your home has burned to the ground. The U.S. Fire Administration reported that over the winter season of each year, there are over a half million fires, 1,900 deaths, 8,000 injuries, and upwards of $3 billion in property damage. The worst thing is, this could all be prevented.

The biggest offender is decorative candles, which can easily be knocked over, set down too close to flammable items such as curtains, and left burning overnight. Candle fires increase fourfold during the holiday season, and when children are around, the risk of burns rises. The best way to avoid candle fires is to keep them away from anything the flame can reach, make sure all candles are extinguished when going to bed or leaving the house, and never put candles on or near the Christmas tree.

Christmas trees are also a fire risk, especially live trees that get too dry and are near open flames or hot bulb lights. Make sure a live tree is watered enough so that the needles bend, but do not break. Keep the tree away from a heater vent or any other heat source and *never* place a room heater near the tree. Lighted trees should not be left on overnight or when out of the home. *Never* put electric lights on a metal or aluminum tree!

Decorative lights are another issue, because sometimes-faulty bulbs, wiring, and gaps in insulation can lead to fires. Make sure there are no frayed wires, broken or cracked light sockets, or too much wear and tear before you hang the lights and end up with a fire on your hands. Outdoor lights should be kept out of puddles, snow, and other areas of wet ground, and make sure bulb sockets face the ground so moisture cannot get inside them. Check for sparks when plugging in lights, and if you see any, buy new lights. Never leave them on overnight or when away, because you never know what could go wrong, and you won't be there to react quickly.

At Halloween, house fires are more frequent because of people leaving candles and pumpkins lit overnight. Common sense tells you to blow out all candles, no matter where they are located and what they are for. Turn off Halloween lights inside and outside as well.

Obviously, make sure smoke detectors and fire extinguishers are working and near areas where flammable items are on display. The holidays are meant to be a time of enjoyment, and a fire can ruin not only plans, but property and even people. Be ready.

GETTING CHILDREN INVOLVED

No survival plan of any kind is complete without first including your children. Children are the most fearful and vulnerable during an emergency because they are used to routines and normality. An emergency shakes up their security and threatens the normal life of home with loved ones. Unless they are too young to walk, talk, and understand what is happening around them, children can be an important part of developing a workable emergency plan. Involving children also gives them an outlet for their own fears, anxieties, and feelings of helplessness that a disaster can create. As adults, we have a responsibility to make sure our children are safe, but letting them help prepare can give them a stronger sense of security and, when the SHTF, they will be better able to process and respond to what is happening.

The family emergency plan, whether designed for fire, earthquake, tornado, or terrorist attack, must include the following:

- What roles will each person take on, including children?

- Who will be responsible for what?

- Where will the family meet if they should be separated?

People feel better and more empowered when they have an assigned role to play in the event of an emergency. What can your children do? Can one of them be in charge of gathering up the pets and pet food? Maybe another child can be given the task of making sure all the windows are closed or doors are locked. Another child can carry a clipboard and ask other family members if they have accomplished their assigned tasks. Getting kids in the middle of preparations and involved can take some of the pressure off of parents or adults who may also be attending to a dozen other tasks.

Assign each child tasks that fit their personalities. An outgoing child might be a better "leader" who can supervise the actions of other children. A child who pays attention to detail would be wonderful for making sure the bug-out bags and emergency kits are always fully stocked all year. A quiet child is often the most observant and can be critical in identifying things others might miss.

Before anything happens, children should know exactly what the plan is for home, if they are at school or away from home, and in the car. Families should review these plans a few times a year to keep them fresh in a child's memory and even give little tests or quiz challenges to see if the child is retaining what he or she learns. It can become a bit of fun, even though it is serious fun. Teach them how to open a window and use an escape ladder if they are on an upper floor and a fire breaks out. Have them practice getting beside the bed or a desk during an earthquake drill. Show them where the storm cellar is and how to lift the doors if there is a tornado and you cannot help them. And above all, make sure they know how to call 911 if phones are operational.

Everyone should know where to meet if sheltering in place is out of the question or the family is separated, and children must be able to find their way to the meeting place if on foot. A neighbor or relative who lives close by and the children know is the best bet, but if that isn't feasible, perhaps a fast food place or library that would be open during the day. Even a shopping center parking lot. Hopefully, when the SHTF, you will be with them, but there are times when that is just not possible, or if you are injured, this is how they can help you and themselves.

They should also know their address and home phone number or the number of a parent's cell phone. Nowadays we assume that our phones with all our contact information will be handy, but in a major disaster, that may not be the case. Also make children aware of how to locate the nearest shelter (this will be easy if there is Web access, harder if not) and of dangers to avoid if they have to get there on foot. Look for apps that can be loaded onto their cell phones as well. There are several emergency alert apps that work on a local and even regional basis.

The best way to prepare with children is to take a course on survival and disaster preparedness, if one is offered in your area. If not, become the teacher and do it yourself, and do it soon so that they have plenty of time for review. Take the family shopping for survival goods and equipment. Explain what each item is and how much food and water each person needs. Let kids try out high-powered flashlights and get their hands on things for a richer experience. Show them how to pop a tent out in the backyard. Engage them and they will feel like they are a contributing part of the family.

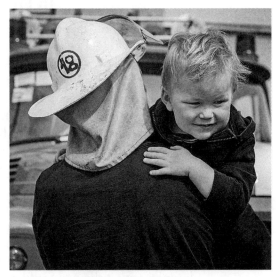

Children should be prepared for emergencies, too, of course. For example, should they get separated from the family, they should know the home telephone number, address, and how to call for help.

Be sure to find out what they will do if they are at school and something happens. Most states do have disaster plans in place for teachers and staff to carry out, and drills throughout the school year, but having your children aware and ready will help them help themselves and others. A fun class project might be having your child give a short presentation on how to be prepared for a disaster!

In addition, evacuation charts are posted throughout most schools, including colleges and universities, which have a lot more area to cover and far more students to get safely out of harm's way. But younger children, when away from parents, will tend to respond with fear and panic unless they are given structure and instructions to follow. Even children are empowered by knowledge and a good plan of action.

The key is to not create paranoia and fear but rather a sense of readiness and strength that comes with knowledge and preparation, as well as having a specific job to do to bring a sense of proactive pride and accomplishment. You will know how much your own children can handle, from teaching them how to build an earthquake kit to showing them how to make a fire outdoors to giving them instructions on boiling water and sheltering in place, even minor first aid such as treating cuts and burns. Let them dictate how much they want to learn and how much they can retain, but you'd be surprised how children have a way of stepping up to the plate when needed.

BEFORE YOU TRAVEL

Ever think about what you would do if something happened while you were abroad, traveling for work or pleasure? Aside from having a valid passport and current ID, few people think about what actions they can take if they are in another country when a major disaster or emergency occurs. It seems ironic, because being far from home should cause people to be more safety-oriented than ever, but we often feel that nothing will happen or, if it does, there will be someone to take care of us at the hotel or the local embassy. But the truth is, we are more on our own than ever once we leave U.S. shores.

Staying informed of any possible weather situations, or even potential terrorist acts, can help you determine if you should be traveling at all. Might you think about changing a vacation if a hurricane is predicted to hit the area around that time? It's hard enough to survive a natural disaster at home, let alone in a strange country without your food and water supplies. Although there is no such thing as a perfectly safe time to take that vacation or go on that business trip, if the news is filled with stories of bombings in a particular part of the country you are going to, or a looming cyclone or typhoon, it would behoove you to think about changing your plans even if it means losing your airline deposit.

If you are already on the road or at your location abroad, the first thing you should do is make sure you know the evacuation routes out of the hotel you are staying in. Know where the fire exits and extinguishers are, and ask at the front desk upon check-in if the hotel has an emergency contingency plan you should know about. Become familiar with your room location in reference to two different exits you can take if needed. If one of those exits is blocked by fire or fallen debris, you will be glad you took the extra time to stake the place out.

Find out in advance where the U.S. embassy or consulate is in the country you are visiting. Make visiting the building a part of your trip if you can, so you know exactly where it is located. That might end up being where you need to go in an emergency if asked to evacuate from the hotel or wherever you are staying. International travelers can call the Overseas Citizens Service through the Department of State to find out what to do in a variety of situations from being arrested to a natural disaster, child abduction, being the victim of a crime, or if you lose your passport.

In the United States and Canada: 1-888-407-4747

Overseas: +1-202-501-4444

Before you ever leave home, you can sign up for the STEP, or the Smart Traveler Enrollment Program, which is a free service that allows U.S. citizens who travel or live abroad to enroll with their nearest U.S. embassy or consulate. Once you enroll, which can be done online on the Department of State's STEP page, you will be alerted in the event of any situation with news and information on what to do and where to go, get help in notifying friends and family, get travel warnings and alerts in advance and as they happen, and stay connected to the nearest embassy for whatever your needs may be. STEP also provides fact sheets and country-specific information to assist travelers. The Department of State can only do so much in a crisis or emergency, so it pays to be prepared before you set foot in another country. But it can assist in certain emergences that occur overseas and affect U.S. citizens, including mass evacuations and getting citizens out of the foreign country and back on American shores safely. The Department of State uses cell phones, landlines, the Internet, and television and radio to broadcast alerts and information in major crises, and if you don't enroll in STEP, it provides constantly updated information on its website if you have access to the Internet as well as to its Facebook and Twitter accounts (see the "Resources" section).

GET TRAINED

Most people wait until after an emergency to seek out training. But wouldn't it be better to take a little time in advance to learn everything from CPR to first aid to how to shelter in place? Most cities offer training through their emergency services departments. You can also contact the Red Cross, Sal-

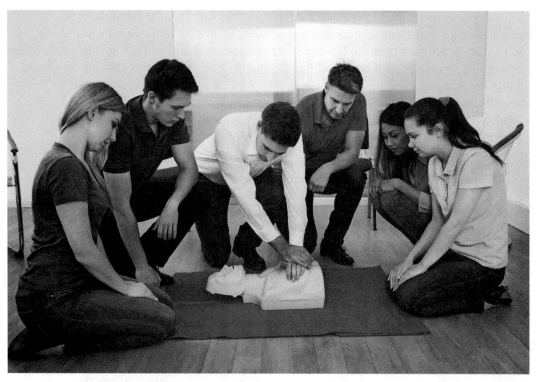

Organizations such as the American Red Cross and American Heart Association offer CPR courses across the nation and online.

vation Army, and the local police, sheriff, or fire department and ask if they offer classes for citizens who want to be ready and responsible.

The American Red Cross offers many classes, especially in CPR and first aid basics, but also trains anyone who wants to volunteer to set up and run a local emergency shelter. Volunteers are much needed, and it might be a great way to be of service during a natural or man-made disaster. The American Red Cross, in its own words, "prevents and alleviates human suffering in the face of emergencies by mobilizing the power of volunteers and the generosity of donors." You can find out about local classes at www.redcross.org or call the local Red Cross office in your area. The American Red Cross also includes a number of volunteer and training opportunities for teenagers and youth, including clubs and development classes.

Emergency shelters are usually opened by the Red Cross and operated by trained Red Cross volunteers. They often provide comfort kits with basic personal necessities such as a toothbrush, toothpaste, deodorant, and shampoo as well as hot meals and cots for those who must stay in a shelter. The Red Cross also supplies emergency items such as tarps, tents, shovels, rakes, and trash bags to assist people in the cleanup efforts after a disaster, and they can also provide health and mental health assistance to those who need it, including replacing eyeglasses, contact lenses, and prescriptions. There are trained members who can give emotional and psychological support too, because one of the most ignored issues in a disaster is dealing with shock and trauma. If people cannot get to the shelters in their areas, the Red Cross has many emergency response vehicles (ERVs) that can bring food, relief supplies, information, and water into affected neighborhoods.

But the Red Cross cannot handle every emergency without the help of volunteers willing to take the time to train and be deployed, often within a day or two, to disaster areas. Often volunteers are asked to work long hours in relentless cold or heat, dealing with the elements, trying to maintain order, and caring for victims even as they might be worried about their own families back home. Red Cross team members who do deploy must check in with their Volunteer Services Department and supervisors before they leave to ensure a strong workforce and that their whereabouts are accounted for.

In 1993, CERT (Community Emergency Response Teams) was formed as part of the U.S. government's Citizens Corps program. It is now operated under the banner of the Federal Emergency Management Agency and the Department of Homeland Security, through which all training methods and materials are coordinated. The motto of CERT is "Doing the Greatest Good for the Greatest Number of People." CERT training is found in most major cities around the country, and best of all, it is *free!* CERT volunteers receive training in disaster preparedness and response, including:

- Fire Safety
- First Aid/Triage
- Disaster Assessment
- Search and Rescue
- Terrorism and Shooter Response
- Disaster Psychology
- Shelter in Place
- Evacuation
- Epidemic/Pandemic Response

The goal of CERT is to act as "second responders" to assist first responders in a major emergency, provide disaster response services to their communities and neighborhoods, and to teach others to be prepared and how to properly respond to emergencies. CERT programs are for adults and, in some areas, teens. Training consists of weekly intensive programs, followed by quarterly training classes, drills, regional exercises, and other events throughout the year. CERT groups are active in hundreds of cities across the United States. CERT members receive a large emergency bag with all the necessary supplies as well as a smaller backpack with essentials and emergency kits for cars and motor homes. These "bug-out bags" are free for active members.

In the event of a major emergency or disaster, CERT members are activated by their local agencies, such as the fire department, working with the emergency operations command center, and are activated via cell phone, email, text, and ham radio notice. CERT members are encouraged to become amateur radio operators, and in many cities, training is offered to meet that goal.

The objective of CERT is: Save yourself first, then your family, then your neighbors, then your community. Those who take the training are able to empower themselves during times of panic and confusion and step up to help their neighborhoods with leadership skills that are needed. Even when things are quiet, CERT members can educate their families and neighbors on how to be prepared for anything and how to become proactive during emergencies rather than give in to panic and chaos.

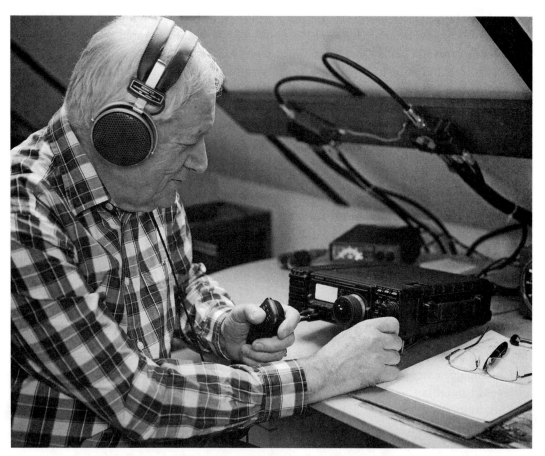

Ham radio operators are amateur broadcasters who have, at times, filled the communication gap during emergencies, informing people of news when phone service is down.

To find a local CERT group, visit the Federal Emergency Management Agency's website at www.fema.gov, and look for Community Emergency Response Teams, or call your local emergency services department or city hall. If there isn't one in your area, ask how you might get involved in starting one. Preparation and knowledge are powerful tools to have at your disposal.

THE ROLE OF AMATEUR RADIO

In the event of a major emergency, the power may be cut. Landline telephones, radios, television, and even cell phones may be down or impeded. Cell phones will experience drastic cuts in service time, due to clogged lines and high call traffic, if there is any service at all. One mode of communication reigns supreme when all else has failed, and that is amateur radio.

Amateur radio operators, also called "hams," have been a mainstay during major emergencies for decades and still prove to be the beacon of light that cuts through the communication fog. There are more than 750,000 licensed amateur radio operators in the United States and millions worldwide, providing a web of communication that can convey information within a matter of minutes. Many fire departments and law enforcement agencies are bringing ham radio into their arsenal of disaster response tools.

Whether it's during a flood, wildfire, terrorist event, earthquake, or hurricane, all of which will disrupt cell phone service, the 100-year-old technology of amateur radio will still be standing and providing a critical service during a critical time. During the 2013 Boston Marathon bombings, it was hams who provided key information when cell phone service was down due to system overload. Coordination of emergency responses depended on hams during the devastation of Hurricane Katrina in New Orleans in 2005. Local hams helped tremendously during the massive Las Conchas Fire near Los Alamos, New Mexico, in 2011. It doesn't matter what the emergency is, hams are at the ready to send and receive information, assist first responders, and help in any way they can.

Many hams volunteer with the Amateur Radio Emergency Service (ARES). ARES members are trained radio operators working in conjunction with local and county hospitals, police, sheriff, fire, Red Cross, and emergency management. Anyone with a ham license can look into joining ARES, as it has a presence in most cities across the country.

Though many people become hams for pleasure, joining any number of local and regional clubs across the country, they can do many things in an emergency that cell phone operators cannot. Amateur radio offers wider coverage when cell phones may have very little or no coverage at all, and amateur radio provides a means for all operators listening in on the same frequency to chime in with information in their area for a bigger picture of the disaster overall.

Amateur radio equipment is often usable with smartphones, tablets, computers, and the like, but it can also be used independently and does not rely on cell phone or Internet service to work. Many hams use battery-operated radios, gas generators, and even solar panels to keep their communications going and can also rely on "repeaters," which are electronic devices that can take a weaker signal and retransmit it as a stronger signal over longer distances. Many repeaters are located on tops of hills or mountains and are always within range, and enough repeaters can carry a signal over hundreds, if not thousands, of miles.

To get an amateur radio license from the Federal Communications Commission (FCC), you must take a test for an entry-level license, known as the Technician Class. It's a difficult test, but you have ample time to study, and many ham radio clubs offer the tests for free or a small fee. Once you become a Technician, you are given a call sign (you can request a vanity call sign; mine is K16YES). Then, after getting to know your equipment and what it can do, you can decide whether you want to level up to a General License, which allows you to communicate over a wider bandwidth, and eventually an Amateur Extra, which has the most privileges. The vast majority of hams in the country are Technician level—about 48.7% according to *Ham Radio for Dummies*, second edition. General Class makes up about 23%, with Amateur Extra covering the remainder.

The tests consist of between 35 and 50 questions, depending on the level, and your license will be good for ten years. Renewal does not require a new exam. Many hams who participate in emergency communications services use handheld radios that can be purchased for under $200. More advanced hams can have home base setups as well as handhelds for the car, running in the thousands of dollars. It is a fast-growing hobby, thanks to publicity received during national disasters from 9/11 to Hurricane Katrina to recent wildfire outbreaks in Southern California and Arizona.

Even though it is no longer required in order to get an amateur radio license, Morse code remains a highly entertaining and still usable method of communication. The code uses a series of on-off clicks or audible tones, even lights, that follow an international set of letters and numbers. Anyone trained in Morse code can both transmit and receive information using a unique sequence of dots and dashes to represent letters of the alphabet or numbers from 0 to 9.

Morse code was named for Samuel F. B. Morse, who is also one of the inventors of the telegraph. It is still a useful mode of communicating information when there are poor signal conditions that may hamper voice communications. Morse code is also used by aeronautical navigational aids, and most pilots and air traffic controllers do have a basic understanding. In emergency situations, Morse code can be sent by any method that mimics the dots and dashes or keying on and off. Think of the SOS distress signal that is known all over the world as three dots, three dashes, and three dots.

According to "Emergency Communications Driving Increase in Amateur Radio Operators" by James Careless for the April 11, 2017, *Emergency Management* magazine, the public's growing interest in amateur radio during emergencies "is a legacy of 9/11, when Americans saw their cellular telephone networks become overwhelmed by excess traffic and system outages." Hams were there to fill the communications gap, and hams are not just interested in their own safety during emergencies, but the safety of their communities.

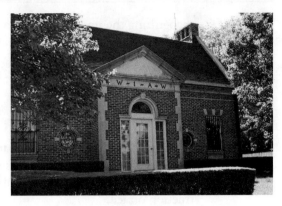

The Amateur Radio Relay League headquarters in Newington, Connecticut, is also a station that broadcasts bulletins regularly.

The Amateur Radio Relay League (ARRL) created the ARES units to assist in times of crisis. The ARRL is really considered the National Association for Amateur Radio in the United States and was founded in 1914 by Hiram Percy Maxim. Local ARES units are made up of hams who register their talents, skills, and equipment with their local ARES leadership to create a sort of database that can be put into action in an emergency. Members are all well trained to work with local emergency management and also play specific roles within the emergency operations command systems if needed. In most emergencies, it will be ARES units or teams that respond, but in times of large-scale disasters, ARRL headquarters will assist ARES teams and provide guidance, equipment, and coordination on a national scale.

Amateur radio operators also work with SKYWARN, the National Weather Service's program for providing ground-level information during severe weather events.

Interest in amateur radio peaks after large-scale events, especially when the media lets it be known that hams played a positive role in assisting with communications. According to Jack Ciaccia, ARRL Colorado Section manager, "The major capability that hams bring to emergency management is our varied modes and frequencies. We can usually make a communications path when others do not exist." That's why ham radio operators are a critical asset during any emergency, when getting and receiving information can be all that stands between life and death.

You can look for a local amateur radio club in your area, as most will have all the information you need for becoming a ham and getting tested, buying the right equipment, and getting on the airwaves. New members are always welcome. Many CERT groups around the country ask their members to get an amateur radio license as well, although it is not mandatory, but as in the case of this author's city, emergency planning agencies are increasingly recognizing the importance of having their staff, and as many civilians as possible, radio ready.

Also see the "Resources" section for information about contacting ARRL, ARES, and the FCC.

CAR READINESS

Finally, is the vehicle you may be in at the time of an emergency loaded up and ready? Do you have your emergency kit in the back? How about a spare tire, ice scraper, flares, jumper cables, and even cat litter or sand for better tire traction on ice?

Even if you are ready, make sure your car is operating well, with proper antifreeze levels, a clean battery and cables, good brakes, cleaned out fuel and air filters, a working heater and air conditioner, a working defroster, good oil and washer fluid levels, and make sure your flashing hazard lights work! Keeping to a regular maintenance schedule can ensure that your car will respond best when you need it the most.

Most people assume an emergency will happen when they are safely at home, but think about the time we all spend driving kids to school, going grocery shopping, or just commuting. Always try to have as close to a full tank of gas as possible, make sure tires are not bald, and if your car is experiencing any mechanical issues, get them attended to as soon as you can. Don't wait and end up getting stuck on the side of a road during a disaster, especially in a situation where the stability of the road, bridge, or overpass you are on is at stake, power lines are coming down from high winds, or flood waters are accumulating all around you.

If you are told to evacuate, your car is going to be your best friend, especially if you will be driving to a distant location to avoid the disaster back home. Keep it working at its best, and stock it with what you need beforehand so you don't waste time and energy looking around for your first aid kit or the extra water bottles you had in the garage.

ARE YOU READY YET?

Make it a priority now to get as ready as you can be, and make sure your family is on board too. Getting ready for the worst can often lead to the best outcome, so schedule an emergency plan check a few times a year, with one big annual overhaul of your emergency kits if supplies are approaching expiration dates. Incorporate any new information you've learned from local disasters, and make sure the information you have is up to date.

It's not rocket science, but it's a lot more important to your survival.

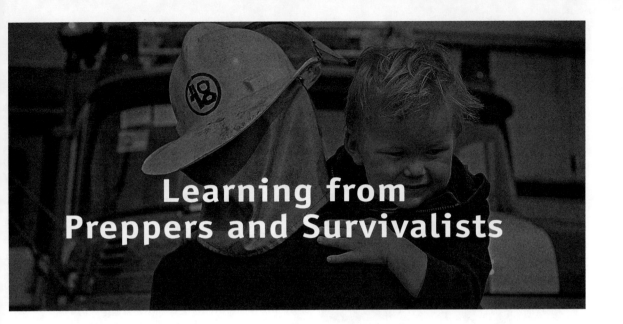

Learning from Preppers and Survivalists

If you've ever seen the plethora of reality shows about preppers and doomsday survivalists, you probably got a very negative impression of people who are committed to making disaster preparedness a high priority—maybe even too high a priority for those who think they may be anticipating the end of the world or are too paranoid to enjoy daily life.

But you can learn a lot about survival from those who have made it their lifestyle focus. These people, more than anyone else, know how to make do in situations that are less than desirable and often live their lives off the grid, functioning independently of traditional power, food, and water sources.

Long before the preppers we hear so much about today, there were survivalists. These people formed an American subculture focused on actively preparing for nuclear war, political unrest, economic meltdown, and a host of other catastrophic disasters that might happen on a local, national, or international scale. Survivalists often moved to rural areas, forming camps and retreats where members trained in self-defense, medical aid, growing food, water storage, and building shelters that would withstand the most intense disasters, such as underground bunkers.

Survivalists in America came to the forefront during the Cold War era, when citizens worried about bombs being dropped and began building fallout shelters, holding bomb drills in schools, and promoting survival tools and techniques to the general public. It was a time of great unrest, so the movement took off and made a lot of believers out of those who felt that a nuclear bomb could be dropped at any time.

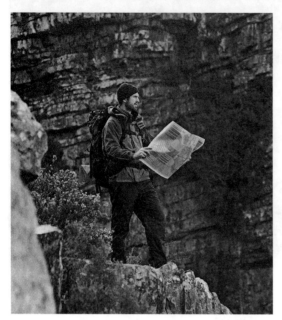

Preppers are concerned about having many skills to help them get through tough times, including how to survive in the wild.

Any time in our history, as far back as the Great Depression and the crash of 1929, when there was economic, political, and/or social unrest, the topic of survivalism entered the forefront of public perception and awareness. Over the decades, and most certainly after the September 11, 2001, terrorist attacks, the subject waxed and waned in popularity, until reality television elevated it to cult status and stardom.

The prepper movement is more recent, having come into the picture after the non-events of Y2K, but also prompted by the 9/11 attacks and the proliferation of television shows dedicated to showing preppers doing what they do best: getting prepared for the worst. The term itself seems a lot less extreme than "survivalist," but in the end, the goals are the same. In fact, we all really should be preppers and survivalists to some extent, with the myriad possible emergencies and disasters we face on a daily basis.

Preppers are concerned with all of the same things that emergency management personnel try to encourage the public to educate themselves about:

- How to survive any life-threatening situation, from a snake bite to nuclear war
- Storing food and water for long-term survival
- Finding or building appropriate shelter before disaster strikes
- Bugging out or sheltering at home
- What to have in a bug-out bag for the home, car, and on the run
- Weapons and self-defense
- Wilderness survival
- Protection from economic unrest

There are also more extreme survivalist/prepper groups that are focused on biblical end-of-the-world preparations, government takeovers, doomsday scenarios, and the like. While many of these groups take on a more cultlike appearance to outsiders, they still have a lot to show the average citizen about what to have, where to go, and what to do when the SHTF, or the "Shit Hits the Fan." One of the main goals of survivalists and preppers is to be able to live entirely independently of others, especially the government, gas, power, and water companies, and they work hard to build their own personal and communal infrastructures so they can survive without help. They pride themselves on their ability to make what they need from what they have, or rely on nature, and sustain themselves via primitive methods of hunting, fishing, and making their own medicinals and clothing.

In "Preppers Are the Modern Survivalists" for the *Prepper Journal*, Pat Henry writes, "The skills our distant relatives used to carve a home out of the wilderness are still valued and taught today." Henry recognizes that it is harder today to just up and walk away from twenty-first-century living and live off the land, but he suggests we may have gotten too far away from our self-reliant roots. He sees survivalists as more focused on total off-the-grid, long-term survival and living, while preppers may "bug out" for a while in the woods if they must, but would prefer to be safe with family and friends indoors. Survivalism can be said then to be the extreme form of preparing, with preppers in the middle. Henry states, "We might not have the same skills, but we prepare for similar reasons. We might not have the same ideology, but our goal is self-sufficiency even though our definition of what that actually is might be slightly different...."

When it comes to self-reliance, preppers see it as having a twofold benefit. Not only can you save money creating your own energy sources and stop paying the local gas and power company their ever-increasing rates, but in an emergency you are set and don't need to worry about losing power when everyone else does. If you grow some of your own food, that makes less genetically modified, pesticide-laden food you need to buy at the local supermarket. If you store your own water in rain barrels or some other type of container, that's less water you need to pay for and less pollution you contribute in the form of plastic jugs and bottles. All of it is useful during normal times and in times that require extraordinary measures to survive.

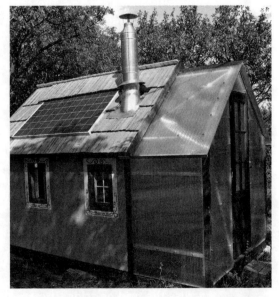

Whether you choose to be a survivalist, a prepper, or just get more prepared in general, the goal is to keep yourself and your loved ones alive and well during times of crisis. It isn't necessary to go live on a retreat and stockpile guns and ammunition for a war with the government or a foreign intruder, unless that is the direction you feel you need to go in. You don't have to start growing vegetables in every room of your house if you don't have much land to call your own, but

Compared to preppers, survivalists seek ways to live completely independently from civilization, which means generating one's own power, finding a water source, raising food, etc.

Prep Speak

The survival/prepper movement has a number of words, phrases, acronyms, and abbreviations that look like some kind of secret-club code. This handy guide helps decipher their meaning.

- ARC—American Red Cross.

- Bug Out/Bug In—In an emergency, will you "bug out," or evacuate/leave your home, or will you "bug in," or shelter in place?

- BIB—A Bug-In Bag with all the essentials you need to stay put.

- BOB—Bug-Out Bag—Should you decide to leave, you will need a Bug-Out Bag, also known as a Go Back, or a GOOD (Get Out of Dodge) Bag, which is filled with the most essential emergency survival items you can carry.

- BOL—Bug-Out Location—Where you plan to bug out during an emergency situation.

- BOV—Bug-Out Vehicle—The car, bus, van, motor home, or bike you will use to get away from the emergency, or again, Get Out of Dodge.

- CERT—Community Emergency Response Teams—Trained by FEMA and the Department of Homeland Security.

- C-Rations—Combat Rations—Survival food.

- EDC—Every Day Carry—An emergency bag or kit you should have on hand at all times.

- EMP—ElectroMagnetic Pulse—One of the catastrophes preppers are prepared for, which would wipe out all electrical and computer operations across the grid or grids. If man-made, it involves the detonation of a nuclear bomb in the atmosphere above Earth. If natural, it's the result of a massive X-class solar flare or solar storm activity.

- ESP—Extended Stay Pack—A larger bag or pack with essentials that will last over a longer period of time.

- FAK—First Aid Kit.

- Faraday cage—A homemade shield used to keep electronics from being affected by an EMP.

- FEMA—Federal Emergency Management Agency.

- GDE—Grid Down Event—Like an EMP, a large-scale shutdown of the electrical grid. Also called an Off the Grid Event (OTGE).

- Golden Horde—The masses of people who are panicked and want your supplies and are moving in on the area you are bugging out in.

- GOOD—Get Out of Dodge—Often interchanged with Bug Out.

- HAM—Ham radio operator, as in amateur radio operator. Licensed operators are the lifeblood of emergency communications and can operate even when the grid goes down and cell phones are rendered unusable.

- LTFS—Long-Term Food Storage—Usually found in a bunker-type situation or basement.

- MOLLE—Modular Lightweight Load-Carrying Equipment—Used by the armed forces as well as preppers to distribute a large bag's load weight.

- MREs—Meals Ready to Eat—Survival food that does not require cooking or preparation.

- Prepper—Someone who is dedicated to being fully prepared for a disaster or major emergency. Often interchanged with Survivalist, although preppers tend to be more focused on stockpiling food, water, and supplies.

- ROT—Rule of Three—We can generally survive three minutes with no oxygen, three hours without shelter, three days without water, and three weeks without food, depending on the circumstances.

- SIP—Shelter in Place—When you must stay where you are; often involves closing off all doors, windows, and entry points in a toxic, biological, or nuclear emergency.

- SFWF—Shelter, Fire, Water, Food—the four essentials for survival.

- SHTF—Shit Hits the Fan—A major emergency, catastrophic event, or situation where the shit has hit the fan and no one appears to be in control.

- SOP—Standard Operating Procedure—Your standard plan/needs for getting through an emergency situation.

- Survivalist—An active prepper focused on catastrophic and long-lasting scenarios that require living off the land, protection and self-defense, and other survival skills.

- TEOTWAWKI—The End of the World As We Know It—A massive disaster or catastrophe/cataclysm that alters the way survivors live afterwards.

- WROL—Without Rule of Law—A scenario when there will be no law enforcement available to uphold the law.

- YOYO—You're On Your Own—Self-explanatory.

if you can plant some fruits and vegetables, you will at least have those to sustain you when the local box store is shut down.

According to "Rise of the Preppers: America's New Survivalists" in the December 27, 2009, *Newsweek*, Jessica Bennett writes that "Some preppers fear the complete breakdown of society, while others simply want to stock up on extra granola bars and lighter fluid in case of a blackout or a storm." There is usually a rise in interest in prepping during times of social anxiety, and with today's concerns about terrorism, climate change, and political strife, the subject becomes more prevalent in the media, and more people awaken to their own lack of preparedness, which is a good thing. The last thing you want is to be fully prepared for a crisis and then be attacked by those who run out of food and water within two or three days. More on self-defense later.

Bennett also states that you don't need to own guns to be a prepper, but many do see the need to be armed, especially for long emergencies. Other people who have nothing will often come for those who have everything.

One valid point Bennett brings up is that preppers understand that government response may be limited, therefore it behooves individuals to be ready and able to fend for themselves. The Red Cross may not be able to get to you right away, if at all, and being able to take care of yourself means you won't go into a panic and become helpless because of over reliance on technology that isn't up and running, such as electricity, ATMs, and the Internet. Most people have no idea that they won't be able to access their cash in the bank, go buy more food and water, or even gas up their cars to get out of town in major events that cripple entire infrastructures.

Maybe the truth is that the preppers are not as extreme or crazy as reality television likes to make them. Maybe it's those of us who refuse to take the time to prepare at all who are truly crazy.

So what can we learn from modern-day preppers?

Food and water collection and storage, shelter, security and defense, and first aid and sanitation are the main focuses of many prepper groups. Obviously, having stockpiles of food and water is paramount, since without either you cannot survive for long.

FOOD AND FOOD STORAGE

You can divide your food stockpile into short-term and long-term. If you have a pantry where food can be kept, label the shelves, and keep foods that expire quicker in the front. Obviously, the pantry or food supply cabinet you choose will be for nonperishables only. A refrigerator that can be run by a generator should the power go down can store perishables and ice.

Start with what you can buy. Canned and bottled foods, boxed foods, power bars, cereals, and eat-as-you-go items are often fairly cheap, so either do one big emergency food shopping, or pick up items each time you visit the grocery store.

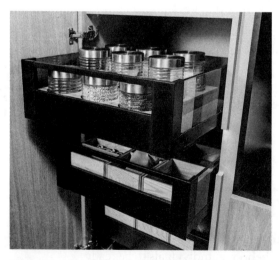

Don't keep dry foods in boxes, which can be gnawed through by rodents; rather, transfer them into glass or plastic containers.

Think about first stocking up on goods you will need for a few weeks. Once you have that, think about much longer-term needs. Preppers believe in "eating what you store and storing what you eat," meaning don't buy a ton of canned foods you and your family hate. Instead, buy extra of what you like every time you buy for present needs, and store the extra away. You may or may not wish to have bags of beans, rice, and other staples in your pantry, but remember these are foods that will need to be cooked, so make sure to keep a cooking source nearby or in your big bug-out bag.

Boxed foods are better kept in plastic containers or large pails with covers. This keeps out pesky bugs. Remember to check expiration dates and cycle foodstuffs out.

Some great items to have on hand:
- Canned fruits (jarred preserves, jellies, and fruits)
- Canned vegetables
- Jerky
- Plastic containers of fruit juices
- Pickles (great source of sodium)
- Ready Pacs of Jell-O and pudding (not all need refrigeration!)
- Juice boxes
- Power bars (energy sources!)
- Small and large cereal boxes
- Cookies and crackers (but *no breads!*)
- Instant oatmeal (the just-add-boiling-water variety)
- Boxed meals
- Cans of chili
- Vienna sausages
- Sardines
- Cans of tuna
- Soups, boxed and canned
- Bags or cans of nuts and seeds
- Peanut butter and other nut butters
- Vitamins and supplements (minerals, iron if needed)

Even though you may have a manual can-and-bottle opener in your bug-out bag, keep one near your food supply as well so you are not relying on just one of each. Keep your food area categorized and labeled so that it will be easy to find each type of item. If you are so inclined, alphabetize them! This is a great project to get kids involved in and makes them feel more empowered and proactive.

Eat refrigerated foods first, especially if you don't have an extra power source to keep the fridge running. Watch for dairy products going bad as well as meats. If you cannot cook meats at a high enough temperature, err on the side of not eating them at all.

WHAT CAN YOU MAKE OR GROW?

Maybe you had a grandmother or aunt who loved to make her own preserves and hand out jars to family members at Christmas. Maybe your brother loves to make beef jerky with his own special spices. There are food items that you can make and store that will add variety to your emergency pantry.

Jams, preserves, fruits, vegetables, and pickled foods can be stored in vacuum-sealed jars until they are ready to be consumed. Just be aware that once they are opened their shelf life diminishes. Jerky and other dried meat can provide a great protein source when food is scarce, and they last a lot longer than regular meats. Dried fruits are a wonderful source of vitamins and minerals such as potassium, and they can fit inside any size emergency kit. Whatever you can make and store that will not require refrigeration can fill in some of the gaps in your food supply and make things a little more interesting than the same power bars and water over and over again.

If you have a lot of land, grow as many different types of fruits and vegetables as you can based on the access you have to irrigation. If you have room for a chicken coop, you will have a good source of both eggs and, if needed, meat. You can also raise rabbits and ducks for food and keep goats for milk. If you live in a suburban area, you may still have room in your yard to grow some vegetables and plant a few apple or other fruit trees. The sooner you do this, the sooner you can have a harvest to use during an emergency or just enjoy your own homegrown foods. The more you grow, the less you rely on food that is laced with toxins and genetically modified.

If you live in an apartment, you can buy small tomato and pepper plants, grow your own herbs, or see about sharing a rooftop garden with other tenants. Urban gardens are flourishing in many cities, as they make the most use of the least amount of space, usually a rooftop or courtyard area. But most likely, you won't be able to sustain yourself with what you grow on your own or what comes from a small urban or apartment garden.

If you do grow your own food, be sure to look into how you will irrigate crops or larger sections of plants. Obviously, you can run them on a sprinkler system that already exists, or put in a system. Otherwise, you will have to hand-water them. If the water supply is cut off, do you have enough stored, aside from your drinking water supply? If not, think about growing foods that do not require irrigation, such as corn, sweet potatoes, watermelon, certain types of peas and artichokes, and amaranth. Ask at a local nursery for other suggestions, such as certain types of cactus and edible flowers.

You can certainly buy emergency foods in brick and mortar stores and on the Internet if doing it yourself doesn't hold appeal, but again, please remember that you must have a minimum of two weeks' worth of food for each person you are prepping for. *Minimum.*

Other great ideas for the prepper pantry that you may not have considered include:

- Distilled and seltzer waters
- Canned juices, sodas, and condensed milk
- Dehydrated powdered milk and egg products
- Protein drinks

The Power of the Bar

When it comes to compact food sources, nothing beats power, or energy, bars. They may be considered high in sugar for anyone on a diet, but your diet won't be a consideration when something big goes down and you can't cook your usual foods. Power bars are compact, lightweight sources of carbohydrates, proteins, and fats—the three macronutrients our bodies need to function. You can buy protein bars by the box, so look for those that are a blend of these three macronutrients, as they will give you the best boost for your buck.

Some bars also include vitamins and minerals. You won't necessarily need these if you've also stocked up on vitamin and mineral supplements. The most important thing about power bars is that you can buy a box or two each time you shop and end up with dozens of them to distribute among various emergency kits. Big box stores offer them at big discounts, and you can try a variety to see which your family prefers. Children will most likely go for the ones that look and taste the most like candy, but be sure they are getting some essential nutrients.

Power bars come in every flavor under the sun and include everything from chocolate chips to raisins to yogurt coatings to almond chunks, but be careful to avoid any with nuts or nut-based products for anyone who has a nut allergy.

Keep up on expiration dates, and use them in school or work lunches when the date gets close, replacing them with fresh boxes.

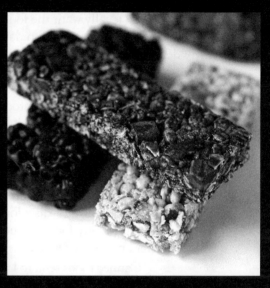

Energy (or power) bars are a great way to consume needed vitamins, minerals, and calories for energy quickly and conveniently. They're also easy to store for long periods of time.

- Raisins, dried fruits, dates, fruit strips
- Honey
- Canned hams and other meats
- Spices
- Iodized salt
- Chocolate (dark provides antioxidants)
- Instant coffee and a variety of teas
- Pet foods, canned and dry, and pet treats
- Gatorade or electrolyte waters

For longer-term survival, add things like rice, beans, baking powder, lard and butter, sugar, flour, and pasta with jars of sauce, or you can mix in butter and spices with rice, beans, and pastas. Get creative, but make sure, if you choose perishables, that you eat those first and don't buy in bulk.

FOOD STORAGE RULES

How long can you store foods? It is always a good idea to stock items by expiration date, with the soonest to expire in the front. Trade them out when they are close to expiring, and use them. First in, first out. Don't waste good food! You ideally want the food you store for an emergency to have a long shelf life, so examine expiration dates such as "use by" or "best if used by," and understand that "sell by" dates are not when a food will expire, but tell retailers how long they can display a specific product. Frozen items will have a "freeze by" date that indicates when they should be put in the freezer to extend their shelf life. Keeping all your food stock dry, cool, and tightly sealed will also go a long way toward adding to its shelf life. A good storage temperature is approximately 50–70 degrees Fahrenheit. Never leave foods in direct sunlight.

In general, watch out for any packaging that looks compromised, and don't use the food product. It may have insects, mold, or even mice! Better safe than sorry. Look at refrigerated foods first, and toss any that have any signs of mold, freezer burn, or discoloration, give off foul odors, or appear slimy. Also watch out for any food products that may be recalled, and look for the batch number on the packaging.

Canned foods tend to last a lot longer than boxed, but even canned foods will lose their taste and texture over time. Acidic foods such as tomato sauces, vinegar-based foods, and fruits will not last as long as non-acidic foods. Rusted cans should be inspected. If the rust has gotten inside the can, toss it out. Also watch for bulging cans, as they may indicate the food inside is spoiled.

Breads on average can be kept from two to four days at room temperature before mold sets in. If it can be frozen, it will last much longer, but if the power is down, use bread quickly.

Cereals (including hot cereals) have a shelf life of about six months to one year if they are unopened. Opened cereals will only last about three months.

Cheeses that are grated, such as parmesan, last up to ten months if unopened, but only two months if opened. If there is no refrigeration, they can begin to mold much sooner.

Chocolate products will vary, but most will last up to two years if kept cool and well sealed.

Coffee that is ground and unopened will last two years. If opened, two weeks at best. If there is power, refrigeration will extend shelf life. Even better, freeze coffee and remove only what you need as you need it.

Cookies can last up to two months if packaged and kept sealed. If they are homemade, they will last about three weeks if tightly sealed.

Crackers will last three months if kept tightly sealed.

Creamers (powdered) will last about nine months if unopened, six if opened.

Cornmeal can last up to a year if lightly covered, and longer if frozen.

Fish that is canned will last between three and five years.

Flour will last up to a year if kept in an airtight container. White flour will outlast whole wheat flour by a few months.

Fruit juices can last nine months, whether canned or boxed.

Gelatin products can last up to three years in their original containers.

Honey lasts up to a year if kept tightly closed. If it crystallizes, you can run warm water over it.

Mayonnaise lasts about six months if unopened. If opened, plan on about two months if refrigerated.

Milk can last up to one year if condensed and unopened. Unopened evaporated milk lasts about one year. Nonfat dry milk will last six months, and unopened refrigerated milk about three months. Always keep containers airtight.

Nuts will last about four months if shelled, up to a year if in unopened vacuum-packed cans.

Pancake mix will last fifteen months in an airtight container.

Pastas can last up to two years if kept airtight, but egg noodles will only last about six months.

Peanut butter and other nut butters can last up to six months if unopened, two to three months if opened.

Peas and beans will last about one year if dried.

Popcorn will last about two years unpopped. Microwave popcorn lasts about one year.

Potato mixes will last up to a year if kept in a sealed container.

Pudding mixes will last up to one year. Keep cool and dry.

Rice will last up to two years. Brown rice tends to last about one year. Specialty rices will last up to six months. Keep them all tightly sealed.

Sauces will last about one year if the can or jar is unopened or, in the case of a jar product, tightly sealed.

Sodas have a shelf life of about six months.

Soup mixes, if dry and unopened, can last a year.

Sugar can last two years if granulated. Brown sugar only lasts about four months, so consider keeping white granulated for longer shelf life.

Tea in bag form will last eighteen months. Instant tea and loose teas will last about two years. Keep all teas in an airtight container.

Toaster pastries will last about three months.

Veggies (fresh) last a few weeks at most, less if not refrigerated. Potatoes and onions last the longest, at about four weeks maximum.

Vegetable oils last unopened about six months, but only one to three months if opened.

Vinegar lasts a year if opened, two years if unopened.

When dealing with cold cuts, meats, eggs, poultry, deli items, breads and cakes, pastries, fish, and shellfish, without refrigeration you are looking at a maximum of four days' shelf life. Obviously, these are the foods you want to use first in a major emergency. Some hard cheeses, if coated with wax, can go two months, and processed meats and bakery products that contain preservatives can last from two weeks to two months or more. We've all heard the jokes about the eternal shelf life of Twinkies, and the preservatives and chemicals in baked and processed foods are meant to keep these foods around for long periods of time. Whether that is a good thing or not depends on whether there is an emergency.

For most fruits and veggies, if they were purchased fresh, the rule of thumb is that they can go about six months before decomposition sets in, but you might need to blanch them in ice cold water before cooking.

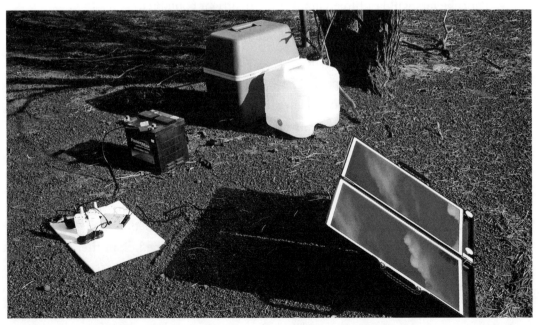

Campers sometimes use solar-powered appliances such as this ice chest for long trips; they can come in handy, too, in greater times of need.

THE DISASTER SURVIVAL GUIDE

The above list is general, and in a major disaster you won't mind eating food a little past its expiration if it means not starving to death. Always check the dates when buying your food, and buy the freshest with the longest expiration date. Having power extends all food expiration dates, as refrigeration and freezing preserve foods, but if you are without power, eat the perishables first.

Consider purchasing a quantity of airtight plastic containers of various sizes to use to keep food fresh, dry, and free of bugs. Do not use foil or plastic wrap, as they don't seal food well enough and can pose problems chemically if the food is wrapped too long.

Appliances such as blenders, food processors, toasters, bread makers, pasta makers, fryers, and mixers are great to have, but again only if you have the power source for them. The best-case scenario will be sheltering in place with the power still on!

Outdoor grills, both charcoal and propane/gas, are a must for cooking meats without having to worry about electricity. Keep grills and supplies in a shed or outdoors with covers to protect them, and keep them clean from the elements. Be sure to have the right kind of charcoal and lighter fluid, and check your propane tanks to make sure they are full ahead of time. Any meat you have in the refrigerator, or meat you acquire yourself from chickens, rabbits, squirrels, or other animals you either raise or hunt, will be an important source of protein and iron to supplement carbohydrate-heavy boxed and pantry foods.

Consider also investing in a solar-powered or propane-powered refrigerator or ice chest. They run the cost range from a hundred dollars to close to a thousand dollars, but in the case of propane, you must have the fuel on hand; think a few tanks for the grill and a few for the fridge. Solar is your best bet, but be ready to pay a little more for the convenience of not having to worry about propane or a generator.

WATER AND WATER STORAGE

Most preppers plan on storing a gallon of water per person per day. Extreme heat conditions, nursing mothers, children, and pets may increase the amount needed. Over a long period of time, that is a lot of water, which takes up a lot of space. When it comes to water, a survival staple, you can run into some big problems finding a place to keep it, especially if you live in a small home or apartment. But there are options.

Do

Store bottled waters wherever you can. Keep them away from extreme heat and cold and out of the sun, which can cause chemicals in the plastic bottles to leech into the water. Many stores carry 32-packs of bottled water, so buy one every time you go to the store. Keep in a cool, dark place.

Store gallon jugs, but again keep them out of the direct sun. Jugs should be made with BPA-free, UV-resistant plastic if possible. Gallon jugs of water are very inexpensive, often under a dollar, and you can refill them at water machines outside grocery stores for far less. Pick up a few every time you shop. Keep in a cool, dark place.

Purchase food-grade water storage containers. Clean them with dishwashing soap, and change out this water every six months. Disinfect by filling with water and one teaspoon of liquid household bleach for every quart/liter of water. Swish around to clean all surfaces, then rinse well with plain water. Choose water storage containers marked "HDPE" and "recyclable," and make sure they are marked "food grade" or "food safe" or have a knife-and-fork symbol.

Use stainless steel containers or, as a last resort, glass jars. Stainless steel containers should be prepared first by immersing them in boiling water for ten minutes. Do not use chlorine bleach to disinfect stainless steel! It can corrode the metal.

Label all containers as clean, drinkable water or gray water. Store all in a cool, dark place.

Open one container at a time when using your supply. If refrigerated, the rule of thumb is that you can use water from an opened container within 3 to 5 days. If not refrigerated, but kept in a cold area, 1 to 2 days. If kept in a warm area, opened water must be used within a few hours. After that, you must purify any remaining water in the container.

DON'T

Store water in plastic soda bottles or milk jugs. Soda bottles break down quickly and cannot be stacked. Milk jugs are often made of thin plastic that is not recommended for long-term storage of drinkable water.

Touch the rim of water bottles or containers with dirty hands, or you may contaminate the contents.

Drink from a container with a crack, hole, or leak.

Rely on iodine tablets to purify water, as they do not kill as many organisms as chlorine bleach.

Water does expire, although it usually has a five-year shelf life. Trade older water out with newer, and use the older water for home needs such as washing dishes and bathing. Or keep the older water, called "gray water," in the back of the storage pantry for cleaning and sanitation. Gray water can be kept in old milk jugs (since you won't be drinking it) that have been rinsed out well. You can also freeze some of the older water supply to use later.

Also keep bleach and water purification tablets with the water supply as well as handheld water filters if you are stuck drinking good old tap water!

Treating Water

If you do not have access to clean water sources, then you must treat the water you do have. This goes for drinking water and water used for cooking as well as brushing your teeth. Don't even make ice with water that has not been treated. You can use a coffee filter or a clean thin cloth to first filter out large particles from the water.

Boiling water for one minute is the safest treatment method. Use a large pot, or a kettle if you have one. Let the water cool before drinking.

Chlorination is a great way to treat water using household liquid bleach, which kills a variety of microorganisms. Use bleach containing 5.25% to 6.0% sodium hypochlorite, and avoid scented, color-safe, and cleaner-added bleaches. Add 16 drops or 1/8 teaspoon of bleach per gallon of water. Stir and let it stand for a half hour. The water may smell like bleach. If it doesn't, repeat the dosage and let it stand for fifteen minutes. If there's still no bleach odor, throw the water away and find another source.

An even better method is distillation, which kills all microbes and, unlike boiling and chlorination, removes contaminants. To distill, you boil the water and then collect the vapor. Fill a pot or pan halfway with water. Tie a cup to the pot lid's handle. The cup should hang right-side up when the lid is on the pot. Boil the water for twenty minutes. The water that drips off the lid into the cup is considered distilled. This is a longer process, but ensures the safest water for drinking and using.

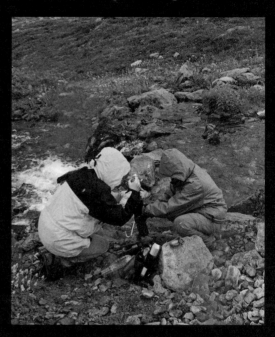

You can try chlorinating or distilling water to kill microbes and filter out impurities, or you can also try a number of commercially available filtering products designed for campers.

If you live in an area with a lot of rainfall and have room around the house outside, buy a few water storage barrels to collect rainwater. This is ideal for storing enough water for up to a year, but the water must be purified before drinking, either by bleaching or purifying.

GOING OFF THE GRID

Many preppers pride themselves on being able to survive without depending on electricity provided by their local electric company. When the commercial power grids shut down in a catastrophic emergency, those who are prepared will be those who survive and thrive. But even in a smaller situation or a more localized disaster, there are ways you can live a little or a lot "off the grid" and be ready with backup power for your basic needs.

GENERATING POWER

Few people plan ahead for power outages. We have such strong faith in our electric companies to keep the power on or get it back on quickly when something takes the grid down. Yet in the case of larger disasters, the power may be out for weeks, not just a day or two, and suddenly we are thrown back into the Stone Age, when humans had to make fire and depend on the sunlight for warmth. It can happen at any time, so a number one rule of prepping is *don't wait*. Find other sources of power, especially if you have medical devices that must keep running.

It may not be feasible to have enough smaller generators to power your home for years to come, in which case you may want to think about installing solar panels to power your home on a regular basis. Not only will this save you money over the long haul, but you will be depending on the sun and not the local utility company when things go wrong.

Wind power, if you have the land, can also be a great alternative to electrical power. But for most, the expense is too big. A Honeywell turbine, of which you might need eight or nine, can run about $8,000 to $10,000, and you have to be able to maintain them throughout the year. Preppers who rely on wind power have a large tract of land and the financial ability to build the turbines needed to bring in enough power to run their homes. You may not have that luxury.

Some preppers utilize streams or creeks on their land for hydroelectric power, building systems on their own for several thousand dollars. The great thing about the Internet is that you can buy systems and hire people to install them properly if you don't yet have the know-how.

If that is not cost-friendly, look into a generator or two. Generators can run anywhere from a couple of hundred dollars to thousands of dollars, depending on your needs and the amount of power you require. You will want to have smaller, hand-crank generators and small solar-powered battery chargers for cell phones and smaller devices. Solar power systems for use in emergencies can also be purchased or even built if you are a do-it-yourself kind of person. Though they can be complex to build, there are plenty of guides and videos online and off to help you.

Generators can run on batteries, diesel, propane, and solar power. Obviously, these will be kept outside the home, especially diesel and propane for safety purposes. Think about a whole-house generator with automatic start controls, but again this is not for long-term survival, as even larger, industrial-sized generators don't have an unlimited fuel supply (unless they are solar). And that is the caveat. A generator, while affordable, runs on fuel, so you must also remember to stay fully stocked with fuel. Yet if there is an emergency that keeps you from getting out of your house, you won't have an infinite supply.

Even a large, 500-gallon propane tank of fuel can run out after about seven days if the whole house is operating off of it. Generators should be thought of as a means, then, for powering *only* necessities, like cooking, medical devices, and a light source, when absolutely necessary.

Whether you buy a large or small generator, if it runs off a battery, that battery can die, especially during long periods of nonuse. If you use any kind of fuel, the tank can begin to corrode, starters may get stuck or break, and the elements can take a toll if the generator isn't covered. Maintenance of generators is important because, even though two years may go by before you use it, you want to be sure it will work when you do.

So what do you look for in a basic generator? You want a "standby" generator because it will automatically turn on when the power goes out and doesn't require you to do anything. The size must be proportionate to your needs (and finances!), and sizes are measured in kilowatts. A small, five-kilowatt portable generator is great for just providing power to cell phones, computers, small appliances, maybe a refrigerator, and fans. As you increase the kilowatts, you increase the amount of power you can keep going, but also the price and size of the generator.

Be sure that it is compatible with the voltage of your home's circuitry. Most are 120 volts, but check especially if you live in a much older home. Standby generators can run on existing gas or propane fuel lines, but portable generators run on gasoline, propane, or diesel and biodiesel, so be sure whatever fuel source you choose is something that is accessible and hopefully can be restocked easily in your neighborhood or city. Propane will run cleaner than gasoline, and the tanks are easy to carry and switch when they are empty. Propane also doesn't have a limited shelf life like gasoline and diesel, which can make up for the cost of the tanks.

Diesel runs longer than gasoline, and diesel-powered generators tend to run more quietly and efficiently. They can be more pricy, and the downside of diesel fuel is that, if it is stored for the long haul, it becomes susceptible to degrading algae growth.

Portable generators for appliances will need an extension cord or several, and the cords should be high quality and heavy-duty to avoid overheating and degradation that could cause a fire. You might also look into installing a "transfer switch" that is a subpanel of the home's main circuit breaker, allowing power to be used for the whole house.

Backup generators can also be used to keep power going for a business or office, although again the focus is not on long-term use.

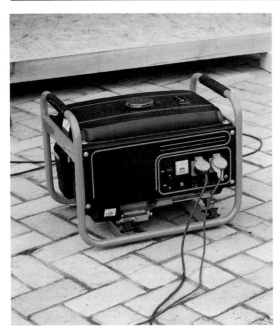

Small, gas- or diesel-powered generators such as this one can supply lighting and some appliance power for homes.

Nowadays, there are many stores that carry generators, and salespeople can help you choose the best one for your needs. While big box stores may have the cheapest offerings, it may behoove you to go to a camping or survival store to get more specific advice. You will be able to see what generators look like, how they operate, what fuel source is best for your situation, and what their limitations are. You can also research and shop online to find the best type of generator for your home's needs and actually have it shipped to you!

A cursory look online revealed over three dozen companies with dozens of types of generators priced between $150 and $5,000 and up. Obviously, you want to focus on something in your price range, but think in terms of power output needs. Some preppers say the rule of thumb is to buy something capable of giving you twice the amount of power you *think* you need.

But don't expect a generator to be the end to all your power problems during an extended outage. There are things to keep in mind, such as fuel availability. If you can stock up on fuel as much as possible before an emergency, more power to you, because once the SHTF, fuel may be as scarce as food and water. Hurricanes are a perfect example of how quickly supplies can be wiped out. After Hurricane Sandy, fuel shortages along the East Coast were fast depleted. Think about it. In a massive outage involving the entire nation, gas stations will no doubt only allow their supplies to be used for emergency vehicles. Propane tanks will sell out within hours. Diesel will dry up, and even natural gas supplies will be cut off if the supplier is no longer operational. In other words, even gasoline- and propane-powered generators rely on electricity, if only in terms of the ability to deliver these fuels to pumping stations and stores!

There won't be convoys of trucks delivering new fuel supplies for days, even weeks and months. If the average portable generator running a home goes through approximately 8 to 20 gallons (30–76 liters) of gasoline per day, and propane at a rate of about 4 to 6 or more tanks, how quickly will you run out of fuel? Unless you have somewhere to safely store massive amounts of backup, you must think of generators as more of a shorter-duration solution. Even a solar-powered generator has what is called a short load capability and cannot last forever if the battery cannot be continuously charged by good sunny weather.

For longer lengths of time, think about going solar for your home in general, or any other methods that can be used to power your home on a regular basis that free you from the electrical grid.

KEEP IT HOT, KEEP IT COLD

Yes, there are gas-, propane-, and even solar-powered refrigerators, ice chests, and freezers. These are used by RV users and operate on gas or propane as their primary source of energy. You can also find electric and solar-powered coolers as well as smaller ones that plug into your car's cigarette lighter. And think about stocking up on instant cold packs that can be shaken or hit against something to become extremely cold and usable for both first aid needs and keeping some perishable food items lasting longer. Inside these packs is water surrounding a smaller pack of ammonium nitrate fertilizer that, when released into the water upon shaking or striking, creates a heat-absorbing reaction called "endothermic" that immediately lowers the temperature of the solution to just above freezing. These packs can last for up to fifteen minutes and can even provide relief during heat waves and heat exposure.

GIMME SHELTER

An April 7, 2017, article in *Business Insider* by Melia Robinson looked at the multimillion-dollar doomsday shelter built by a man named Larry Hall in 2008 in an old missile silo. The shelter has fifteen stories, luxury living quarters for about a dozen lucky families who are rich enough to afford them, stockpiles of food, water, weapons, and even armored trucks. Hall got the idea to build the megastructure after the September 11, 2001, terrorist attacks. He purchased the silo for $300,000.

The Survival Condo Project cost $20 million to build, which seems like a lot to save only a dozen families. It is built to withstand a nuclear strike, although the jury is out as to whether it could sustain an asteroid smackdown. This is one example of the extremes many survivalists, the wealthy, and the uber-paranoid will go to. These extravagant underground vaults have all the luxuries of home, minus sunlight and nature, but promise to keep you safe (for a price) from the riffraff roaming the post-apocalyptic world above ground. In this project, there are twelve single-family homes, common areas, and operational space. Each full-floor unit is approximately 1,800 square feet (167 square meters) of living space, enough for six to ten people. It costs $3 million for the full-floor unit, half that price for a half-floor unit. Every buyer gets mandatory survival training and a five-year food supply per person (after that, they must go above ground and deal with the real world) as well as Internet access. There is also a 75-foot (23-meter) swimming pool with a slide and a gym.

Just be sure you are not claustrophobic.

You have your food, water, first aid, and other supplies. You have your generators. But do you have some place to go in or immediately outside your home if you cannot bug out and find somewhere else to survive a major crisis? Basements, cellars, panic rooms, secret rooms, cement sheds, bunkers, doomsday shelters, tarp shelters—there are many ways to set up a home shelter to protect you and your family against the elements, toxic air, and most importantly, other people, because in a major crisis, those who have will be sought out by those who have not.

Even in simple cases of natural disaster protection, you should have places to go on your home territory. In a hurricane or tornado, a storm cellar is a must, and it should be supplied with some food, water, flashlights or lanterns, and other supplies you will need for a short stay until help can get to you—or you can get to help. Storm shelters can be built within an existing cellar or basement by using plans provided by the Federal Emergency Management Agency. These free storm shelter construction plans are available on its website and offer

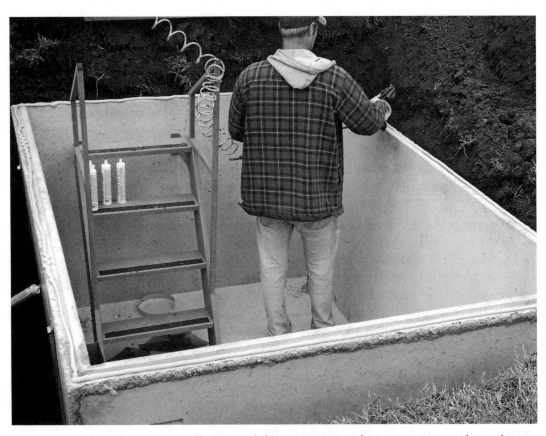

If you're going to go all-out on a shelter using concrete for construction, it is best to hire a professional contractor to do the work.

different types of shelters, some relatively inexpensive and easy to construct. From do-it-yourself "lean-to" designs that allow debris and rain to slide right off the structure to larger, more bunkerlike retrofitting, the plans include planning, framing, construction, door types, covering, costs and considerations, and advice for what style shelter is best for your home.

These shelters are usually built into the corner of a basement with at least five square feet (half a square meter) of floor space per occupant and also at least five square feet for food, water, and medical supplies. By backing the shelter into the corner, you already have two solid walls and only need to construct the inner wall. The structure will look like a long, triangular box, with the interior wall the longer wall of the triangle. This interior end wall will also have a door, which should be made of 12-gauge welded steel with welded mitered corners. The most common type of door is steel-sheathed with a honeycombed steel-reinforced core. You will also need to cover your shelter space, preferably with a "skin" of two layers of ¾-inch plywood installed over one layer of 14-gauge steel sheeting.

If all this sounds like too much, remember that the plans on FEMA's website are step-by-step guides. Or you can always hire someone to build a shelter in your basement or garage, or reinforce an existing storm cellar, perhaps even turning it into a more all-purpose bunker. If you opt for a garage shelter, there are two types: metal and concrete. You can buy these fully assembled, as the concrete storm shelter is extremely heavy and requires professional installation.

In a worst-case scenario you can make a space in your garage or even a large outdoor shed and reinforce the walls and ceiling yourself with plywood and steel sheeting to protect against strong winds, rain, and flying debris. But keep in mind that, once you have the shelter installed in the garage, you won't be able to move it or change your mind. Also remember to have adequate ventilation. FEMA shelter plans include ventilation, but if you're doing it yourself, be sure to add reinforced vents at the top of the shelter. Follow the same guidelines as the FEMA plan for square footage per person as well as additional supplies.

If one of your family members requires a wheelchair, large medical device, or medical bed, or if you have pets, you will need to add on square footage to accommodate them and also make sure the doorway or entrance allows for the large bed/devices.

Bunkers are another option. You can build your own or have one professionally built underground on your property. Before choosing an underground bunker, be sure no one in your family suffers from claustrophobia, because being in a confined space can make anyone begin to feel anxious and irritable over the course of a few days or weeks.

Some bunkers are built into existing structures underground, such as large steel drain pipes, missile silos, abandoned military bunkers, grain silos, food storage sheds, and old storage facilities. But if you aren't lucky enough to have one of these on hand, you will have to start fresh, and the best and strongest bunkers are built with concrete. If you choose to go with a steel shelter, you will have to bury it deep to get the same protection as a concrete shelter closer to the surface. Also think about excavating costs (crane or earth mover/digger, and labor) and the costs to cover the shelter with enough feet of dirt.

For example, a concrete shelter measuring 10 feet (3 meters) tall, 10 feet (3 meters) wide, and 20 feet (6 meters) long would need a 12- to 13-foot (3.7- to 4-meter) hole, with 2 to 3 feet (.6 to .9 meters) of dirt covering it overhead. This would provide about 2,000 cubic feet of space inside. You would not need a floor installed in this type of shelter.

A steel pipe shelter would require a floor, and because of its curve, would provide less interior space. Another choice is the ICF, or Insulated Concrete Form, which is made of expanded polystyrene foam blocks that fit together and connect with double rows of rebar. Once the walls are put up, concrete is poured to fill them in. A downside is that the foam blocks contain toxic chemicals that could leak. The blocks are also flammable and would require a coating of non-flammable materials.

ISBUs are Intermodal Steel Building Units. These are modified shipping containers that are often used on barges to store cargo. During Hurricane Katrina, they were used for those left homeless. They are sturdy, fire-resistant, wind- and flood-resistant, come in ready-to-use form, usually cost under $1,000, and come in a variety of sizes. The standard size is about the equivalent of an eighteen-wheeler truck and can house a family of four or five. You can even spend a little extra to customize the unit.

If you own a camper, motor home, or trailer, you can use this as your bug-out shelter with some modifications and reinforcements, such as boarding windows or adding bars, putting on stronger doors, and stocking fully with food, water, and supplies. The great thing about a mobile shelter is the ability to move it if you need to get away from home. Just remember you will need fuel, so have a few extra gallons of gas around.

Tarp and tent shelters are another possibility, although they don't hold up as well under severe weather conditions and won't protect you from nuclear radiation, volcanic ash fallout, or other human beings. These tent shelters are great, though, for traveling with and can be carried easily in a pack strapped to your back or your vehicle. Some come with detachable inner-nest linings and features to better protect against the elements, and many can be attached to your car or motor home for added space if you decide to take off, or at home in your driveway if you cannot leave.

Some people choose to build a concrete or steel shelter above ground in the backyard or reinforce a tool or storage shed. While this type of shelter may not offer the same protection as an underground bunker, it is an option if cost and space are an issue. Obviously, the stronger the materials and the more secure the door, the better. This may not work well if you want your shelter space to be a secret from neighbors and potential marauders.

Some things to remember:

- Build underground shelters as deep as possible if radiation may be a concern.
- Build as far outside of floodplains and flood zones as possible. The last thing you want or need is water leeching in from above or even below ground.
- Make sure the bunker is not too far from where the evacuees are, so they can reach it quickly. Have it marked well for anyone who will be arriving after you've gone inside.
- Build away from fuel sources, flammables, autos, hazardous materials, and fire sources.
- Don't forget to include a power source such as a generator. Solar will not work in an underground bunker, so choose the right fuel source.
- Conceal the entrance to an underground bunker, and try to conceal or camouflage the entrance to an above-ground shelter as much as possible.
- Consider adding a shelter room onto your home. It can be a multipurpose room or one specifically designed for emergencies.
- Make sure you have any necessary permits before you dig or build. Don't assume, just because it's your backyard, that you can do what you want.
- Watch out for digging near water pipes running below the ground.
- Consider a ready-made shelter or hiring professionals to build one for you.
- If you hire a contractor, look for a professional, licensed and experienced in building shelter/bunker structures.
- Err on the side of a bigger air filtration system instead of going small and cheap.
- You won't have windows, so remember to have a light source!
- If your shelter contains weapons, be sure to keep them out of the reach of your children, or have your children trained in the use of firearms.
- Show your children where the shelter is and how to get inside in the event you or any other adults are incapacitated.
- Remember to have an area for pets too and some comfort items with their food and water.
- Remember to rotate food and water out of your shelter supplies as you would your bug-out kits and in-home supply pantry.

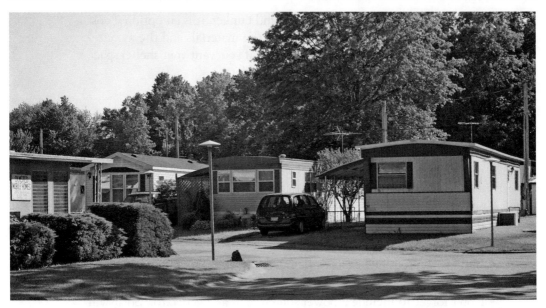

Mobile homes are very vulnerable to tornadoes, earthquakes, and other disasters, and owners of these homes are usually not allowed to build storm shelters. The best thing to do is research storm shelters in your community and flee to them in an emergency.

In the case of panic rooms, they must be stocked with food, water, and supplies, be reinforced for protection against extreme weather and attempts by criminals to break in, be easily accessible to everyone in the house/family (including anyone with a disability), and offer some of the comforts needed to survive a short-term situation. These rooms are locked off from the outside world and impossible to get into and often require a password or key that each member of the family will have to know or possess.

Also known as a "safe room," it is recommended that this room be in the center of the home, if not in the basement or cellar, and not have windows in order to ensure safety from those outside as well as from toxic gases, extreme weather, or nuclear radiation. A safe room can be built around an already existing room or as an addition, but it must be truly impenetrable from outside.

For people living in apartments, condos, and homes that have no extra room or land, not having an escape room or bunker or storm cellar may motivate you to be more ready to evacuate or bug out in the event of an emergency, unless you are told not to. But you can still identify some area where you might be safer, such as an interior closet or room that does not have many windows or doors leading outside. Many apartments have large walk-in closets that would be ideal places to keep supplies and shelter in place if needed. Even better, they tend to be connected to hallways and bathrooms that can be sealed off and included in the temporary shelter.

There truly is a shelter type for anyone in any situation. Even if all you do is have that one room inside your home with no windows, easily accessible and close to the food and supplies, you are a little better off than being fully exposed and vulnerable. In a future chapter, we will cover sheltering in place in a room inside your home, office, or anywhere else you may be when it all goes down.

PARANOIA OR PREPAREDNESS?

Watching prepper shows or seeing survivalists portrayed in movies or on the nightly news, one might get the impression these people live in a constant state of fear and paranoia. The truth is, many are simply committed to doing everything they can to survive anything the world might throw at them. Certainly, some go to extremes with paranoia and doomsday scenarios, but we can all learn something from those who are more prepared than we are. We can learn some of the tools, tips, and techniques they use to better ensure that they can survive the worst-case scenarios.

The biggest lesson preppers have to teach us, though, is to get prepared before it happens. Too many people wait until it is too late. As this chapter is being written, people on the Gulf Coast of Texas are clamoring to get away from an oncoming hurricane named Harvey. The usual images of thousands of cars on highways leading inland pepper the news channels, reminding us that it is often better to leave too soon than too late. It is often better to stock up too much than not enough. It is often better to overtrain and overlearn than to undertrain and underlearn.

Don't fear, prepare. The more you do now, the less you have to worry about doing once an emergency is underway and panic sets in.

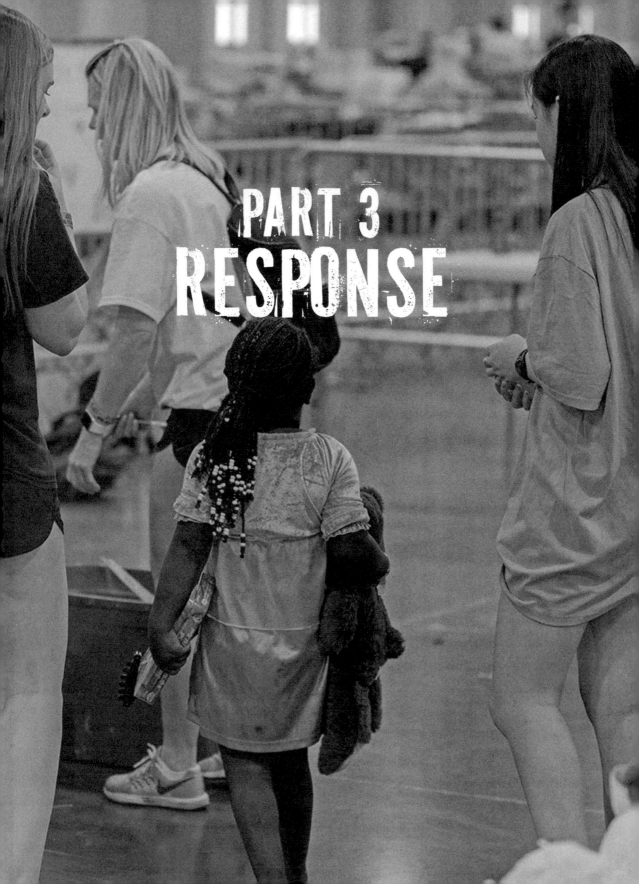

PART 3
RESPONSE

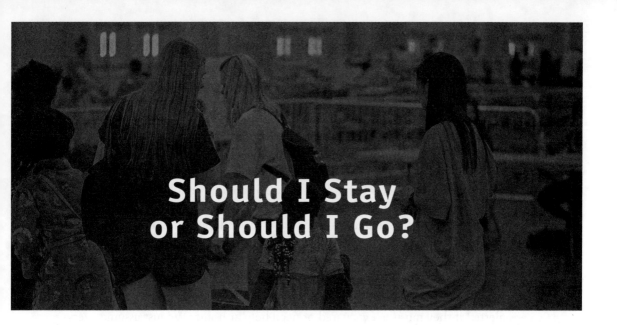

Should I Stay or Should I Go?

It happens. An emergency. A disaster. Whether it is local, regional, national, or global, the reaction is usually the same: panic and confusion. What should I do? Where should I go? How do I communicate with loved ones? Will I be okay?

Once a disaster occurs, our usual instinct is to make sure we know whether our loved ones have survived. Communication immediately following a disaster will be tricky, and in some cases, nonexistent if power is out, cell phone service is down, and those you love are not within shouting distance.

COMMUNICATE

Use whatever methods you have available to check in immediately with family members or loved ones who are not with you. This also applies to calling for help if you are injured or someone else is. 911 may be overloaded with calls within the first few hours of an emergency, and the bigger the situation, the longer the overload lasts. If you can treat your own injury or still get yourself to safety, wait to call.

Calling loved ones also blocks phone lines, preventing important emergency calls from getting through. Can you text? Email? If you are a licensed ham radio operator, perhaps you've also convinced other family members to be as well. But short of that, there are new apps for your cell phone that can be used as "walkie-talkies" if there is Wi-Fi access nearby. These apps will be available in your cell phone app store and are usually made for both Androids and iPhones. The Zello PTT Walkie Talkie is free, and you can have live conversations as long as both parties have Wi-Fi. That is the downfall, though. Without Wi-Fi, the app is useless. Another interesting app is Family Locator–GPS

Tracker, which can tell you where a family member is and if they are safe, but again GPS satellites must be functioning for it to work on both ends.

Some shelters now try to have Wi-Fi available, and during many major hurricanes this past season, many hotels that opened their doors to evacuees offered free Wi-Fi so people could get in touch with loved ones in unaffected areas. Technology is evolving so quickly that each year new apps are introduced that can do new things, extending the possible range of communication. Look in your app store and see what is available. Download a couple of good apps that have high ratings and are free, and learn how to use them properly. If you have kids with cell phones, make it a family affair around the dinner table, and download the same apps, then go over how each one operates and how it will be used in the event of an emergency.

If you have elderly neighbors who do not have cell phones, think about helping them too by getting the name and number of someone who can be alerted if they must be evacuated or need help at home. We just assume everyone has a cell phone, but that is not the case, so if you have the time to safely extend a helping hand, please do so.

Cell phone towers and antenna systems are being built more and more to withstand disasters such as high winds and floods caused by hurricanes. According to "Will My Phone Work during and after the Storm" by Nancy Dahlberg for the September 7, 2017, *Miami Herald,* major service providers such as AT&T, Verizon, and Sprint claim their towers are ready. They even have backup generators that will kick in during a power outage, and their switching centers are more prepared than ever. Some towers are being put on stilts to withstand high water levels. But is it enough?

The article discusses how the main causes of loss of service are often structural failures to the towers and damage to antennas from extreme winds. Even with shoring up, there are limits, which often revolve around getting crews up and out in the field to do the repair work in a major disaster. In a nuclear blast, massive earthquake, or supervolcanic eruption, it won't matter how retrofitted the towers are; they will go down. But it is good to know that the major cell phone providers are working overtime to try to keep open the lines of communication that so many of us have become dependent upon. Interestingly, the article recommends having a landline along with cell phones, because while strong winds can knock down telephone poles, there is actually more of a chance of loss of service to cell phones and wireless communications than the old-fashioned phones so many have given up today.

SOCIAL MEDIA

Now people have the option of using social networking sites as their check-in place to keep friends and family up to date. Facebook introduced the "check-in" feature years ago, which allows users to show their exact location. Users can also post on their personal pages that they are safe and at a local shelter or at home. Twitter is also widely used now to report in to others and let them know how you are faring.

There are also individual pages devoted to particular emergencies or disasters, such as a hurricane or large earthquake, where users can check in and leave messages and also get updated information. During 2017's Hurricane Harvey, a page was set up called "Hurricane Harvey 2017—Together We Will Make It," which featured actual maps with locations of those who needed rescuing and green marks for those who were safe. As long as there is cell phone service or Wi-Fi, social media can be a powerful communications tool because everyone is on it, and chances are that, even if you don't see a message from a loved one, someone you know will and can pass it along to you.

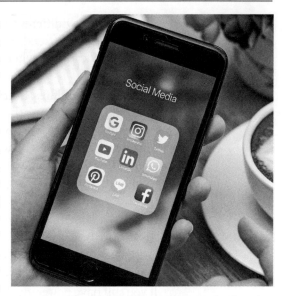

A number of social media sites such as Facebook and Twitter will set up special pages devoted to providing information about disasters such as evacuation routes and informing the Coast Guard about stranded victims.

Twitter had its own @HarveyRescue, which allowed people to tweet and ask for rescue help, boats, evacuation information, etc. This information was also reported to the Coast Guard.

Social media shouldn't be the only method of communication people plan on, simply because they rely on access to Wi-Fi or cell phone service, both of which may be down in particular situations. But they can be a valuable resource, as many people have found when they put out posts on social networking sites for others to send help, check on family members in the area, or pass on information they could not get otherwise.

Another way social media have been useful during emergencies comes after the damage is done. People are setting up GoFundMe pages to ask for financial help that they may not be getting from insurance companies or the government to rebuild their homes, buy food and water, or clean up the damage left behind.

STAY OR GO?

Do you stick it out at home and shelter in place, or do you evacuate to a designated shelter? In the event of a major emergency or disaster, you will be instructed as to which is better. If the power is out and there are no means of communication to find out what to do, you will have to use common sense.

There are many different places you can evacuate to during a disaster, including the homes of friends or family, hotels, motels, and shelters. Part of your plan must be knowing where everyone will go so that you can keep your family together.

In the case of wildfires, hurricanes, imminent storms, and weather events, the ideal would be to locate the nearest designated shelter and go there as quickly as possible. Even some toxic hazard disasters may require that you leave the area. Are you in the direct path of a major storm? Is your home close to the potential lava flow field of an active or erupting volcano? Is the local news calling for voluntary evacuations from an impending wildfire that could turn mandatory depending on how the wind blows?

Let's say you are told to *get out*, or you decide that evacuating before you are told is in your best interest. You get your family together, grab your bug-out bags and supplies, and head to a family member's home in a safe zone or to the designated shelter in your area. How do you find that shelter?

If you still have power, the local authorities will list designated shelters and even evacuation routes along with roads that are closed or impassable due to the emergency situation. If you still have cell phone service, you can do the following:

To locate the nearest designated public shelter during an emergency, text SHELTER and your zip code to 43362 (FEMA). (Example, SHELTER 90278.)

You have found a shelter to go to. Now what?

BUGGING OUT

If you can safely drive to the shelter, take your supplies with you. If you must go on foot, only do so along safe routes designated by local authorities. The last thing you want to do is get caught in a floodplain during a flash flood or be out on foot during a lightning storm—or worse.

Find out if the shelter will accept pets, as most emergency shelters for people will not allow them because of safety liabilities. The only exception to this is service animals. If not, you must make accommodations for your pets. Emergency services in many cities will provide a place for pets to go to, but you may have to transport them there yourself. Pets must be in crates or cages, and be sure to bring extra food and comfort items. Some cities set up temporary shelter trailers for local pets to stay in, and they allow their human owners to visit them if it isn't dangerous to do so.

If you have time before the disaster strikes, you can use ham radio or social media to ask for help transporting and keeping pets with others in safe zones. Call your local fire department, and ask if they offer an assistance program for evacuating horses, livestock, and other animals in rural areas. Many people just assume they can take their dogs and cats with them when they leave, but that is not the case if your destination is a shelter, unless it is designated as having a

Gassed Up

One of the most important parts of a good plan is to always have a full tank of gas. But we don't always think about the possibility that we might need to until it is too late. One of the biggest hazards to human life is being stuck on a highway or freeway in the midst of a raging hurricane or wildfire. You not only want to evacuate early to avoid congested roadways, but have enough gas to stay on the road should you get caught in that congestion. Nobody wants to have their car run out of gas while a Cat 4 hurricane is bearing down.

A good rule of thumb is to never let the tank fall below half full, which should ensure at least enough gas to get to a shelter or safe zone. As we all learned from recent hurricane news, most gas stations will run out quickly and close down, and with no open roads for gas tankers to bring in new fuel, they can stay closed for days, even weeks. If the power goes out, even gas stations with a supply on hand cannot pump it. So be prepared, and if asked to evacuate, take one car to help keep roadways less congested.

special area for pets, so check first and don't waste time later trying to find somewhere to take your furry friends.

Tragically, many pets never see their owners again, because they must be left at home to fend for themselves. Other pets escape and die out in the elements during a disaster. The best way to avoid losing a furry family member is to *plan ahead and know what to do with your pets if a disaster happens*. If you already know who can assist in transporting animals, where they can safely be taken, and what the city you live in can do to direct you to an animal-friendly shelter ahead of time, you might save the life of your pet.

Some key points to remember:

- Many disasters give you enough warning time to find out where to take your pets if you must evacuate
- Private and publicly funded rescue organizations can assist, but they cannot save every animal they are asked to rescue, so plan ahead
- Some local animal shelters will open up free cages ahead of time to those seeking emergency shelter for their pets
- Pets cannot survive on their own and will be frightened, lost, and exposed to the elements following a disaster, so don't assume you will reconnect "naturally"
- Rural areas with horses and livestock rely on trailers and trucks to get animals out, but if roads are closed, that won't happen, so get them out early
- Always have a bug-out bag filled with food and supplies for your pets if you can take them with you
- Look for hotel parking lots and campgrounds, parks, and other large open spaces that may be accommodating animals, especially livestock and horses

- Many hotels do take in cats and dogs, but they won't take in larger pets or animals
- If you live in a rural area, you must have a trailer to move larger animals, as many will not fit in the back of a flatbed or regular truck
- Mark your dogs, horses, and livestock with ink that indicates your name and phone number in case they get loose or lost. You can actually buy a livestock marking ink, but use whatever works (laundry marker) in a pinch.
- For larger animals, be sure to bring some extra hay or feed in a large bucket or plastic trash can with the bottom cut out
- If, tragically, you must leave pets at home, leave them extra water and food in bowls, and close off all doors and windows

CHOOSING A ROUTE OUT

You have your car loaded up with supplies. You've shut off all electrical appliances and televisions, leaving refrigerator and freezer plugged in (unless there is a risk of flooding in the home!), and you have shut off gas, water, and electricity to the home if instructed to by local authorities. Now it is time to *bug out!* When evacuating, you may have more than one route out of your neighborhood and into a safe zone. All routes may be clogged with people fleeing the area, and it isn't always better to choose the road you believe will be less overloaded with traffic. Think about the disaster you are escaping, and choose accordingly. If it is a massive wildfire, and the main route is a freeway only a mile from the fireline, realize how quickly a fire can burn to the road and jump the freeway, burning cars as it does. Is there a secondary route that will take you much further away from the firelines?

Hurricanes and other major flood-producing storms beg that you avoid streams, creeks, rivers, and other bodies of water that could top off and create a water hazard, as well as avoiding known floodplains and streets that are known to flood during even minor rains. Use common sense. Keep an eye out for debris in the road, downed power lines, and blocked access to roads you normally take, and know another way around or through.

The goal of evacuating is to get *away* from the hazard and *toward* safety and help. Always follow the instructions of authorities, but if there is no power or cell phone service and you are on your own, don't make your situation worse by trying to take the quicker route if it may not be the safer route.

HOW TO SHUT OFF UTILITIES

So you need to evacuate and aren't sure how to shut off power, water, or gas. If you have a family, make it a point to show everyone exactly how to do this. Keep in mind you may need to know this even for non-emergency situations.

WATER

Know where the water main is and how to turn the shutoff valve in the right direction. If you live in a warm climate, the shutoff valve will be outside, perhaps on the side of your home. Look for the point where the water pipe enters your house. This is also where your water meter is. In cold climates, it may be in your cellar or basement.

Shut off the valve that runs between the water line to the *house* and the water meter. Turn the valve in a clockwise direction until you cannot turn anymore. You don't need to shut off the valve that leads from the street to the meter unless instructed to do so.

If you do need to shut off the water at the street source, which is operated by the city you live in, look along the front boundary line of your home for the "box," which will be a metal or heavy plastic cover in the ground. You can use a screwdriver or other tool to lift off the lid. Look inside for the top valve, and turn it clockwise until it feels firm. Check a water source in the front of the house to see if the water is still running. Sometimes you have to open and close the valve a few times if it hasn't been shut off for years.

ELECTRICITY

To power down your home, look for the electrical circuit breaker box, which is usually on the side of the home. It may also be located in the cellar or basement.

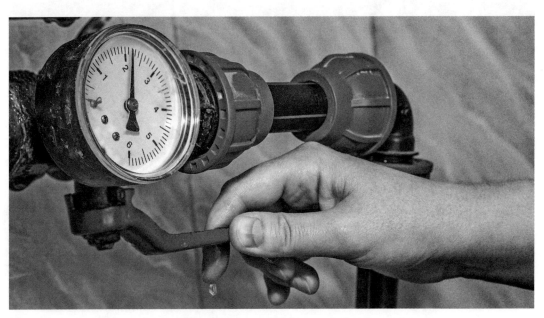

Homeowners should know how to shut off water to their houses during times when city water may be compromised by contaminants that could flow into your pipes.

Shut off *all* individual circuits before shutting off the *main* circuit breaker, which is usually at the top of the circuits. This should shut off all power to the house.

GAS

In a disaster, a natural gas leak can be more deadly than the initial disaster. Make sure you have a pipe wrench handy, preferably an adjustable one 12 inches or larger, and keep it near the gas meter and shutoff valve. The valve should be labeled, but will be running parallel with the pipe located about 6 to 8 inches above the ground. Using the adjustable wrench, turn the valve a quarter turn until the valve is crosswise to the pipe, which means it is closed.

Because home gas line configurations can be different, it is best if you contact your gas company *in advance* and ask them the steps to shutting down the gas to your home, and have those directions prominently written on the meter or nearby where any family member can find them.

EVACUATING AT WORK OR SCHOOL

If you are inside an office building, on a college campus, at school, or even in a department store or mall, there will be evacuation routes posted on the

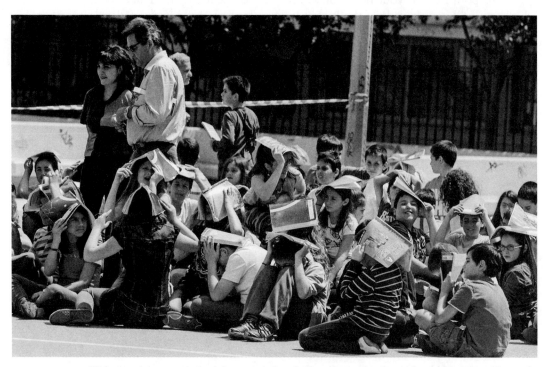

Kids practicing an earthquake evacuation drill at their school are closely supervised by teachers and administrators for their safety.

EVAC 101

The basics to evacuating safely are:

- Have your disaster kits ready to go. Load them into the car beforehand when it appears you will be needing to evacuate soon (during voluntary evacs).
- Make sure everyone in the home knows where to go and how to contact each other should anyone get separated.
- Wear long-sleeved shirts, long pants, and sturdy shoes.
- Load up your pets, but know that they may not be accepted at the local shelter. But if taking them to friends or family, or even many hotels, take them with you.
- Bring outdoor items inside the home to avoid damage from winds.
- Do not turn off natural gas unless instructed to do so by authorities.
- Do turn off propane gas service, and strap down propane tanks.
- If in a flood-prone area, put sandbags around the exterior of home.
- Have a visual record of your valuables and items in your home, whether photographs or video.
- Move objects in the home that can be damaged by any wind or water that gets in, such as computers, televisions, electronic equipment, microwave ovens, etc.
- Lock up the house after closing doors and windows.
- Make sure you have important docs with you, such as driver's license, social security cards, birth and marriage certificates, wills, deeds, insurance policies, and any stocks or financial records.

walls to show you exactly where to go in case of a fire or other emergency. Always familiarize yourself with these maps, which can also be found in hospitals, medical buildings, and doctor's offices. Take a glance at the route you would need to use to get out in an emergency. Notice where fire extinguishers and emergency axes are along walls.

Large companies should have an emergency action plan and go over it with employees at least once a year. When you are on company time, it behooves them to protect you as best they can, so the plans can be quite extensive and comprehensive—or non-existent, as in smaller companies. Office buildings and complexes will use a specific chain of command to authorize the evacuation and closure of the building and the procedures to follow in the process. This will include escape routes, where emergency supplies are located, who will be in charge of what, where employees (or students, if a school, will go), and how emergency services will be contacted. There will also be an accounting system after the evacuation to make sure all employees are out of the building. Some employees may have to remain behind to shut down equipment and secure the building.

High-rise apartment and office buildings will have several evacuation routes in case the elevators and stairwells are unusable. Fire escapes should be up to code, and some buildings are even trying out innovative techniques such as laundry-type shoots that allow people to slide down an interior or exterior cloth tunnel to ground level. Check the building you live or work in to see what the options are if the usual routes are blocked.

Schools by law have emergency plans, and teachers and staff will instruct students what to do and where to go. If the emergency requires sheltering in place, the staff will know what to do, and as we have seen in shooter-on-campus situations, will protect students and barricade rooms against the gunfire. Chemical, biological, and toxic emergencies would also require staying indoors, as would tornadoes. Each type of emergency will require specific actions to be taken by staff and students.

An Emergency Action Plan, or EAP, requires a chain of command, and usually there will be people designated for that job. However, if you are in a situation where that person or persons are incapacitated, or there is no real EAP in place, you must take action on your own behalf, and this is why not leaving your fate up to others is so critical. The more you already know, the more you can be of assistance or, at the very least, not get in the way of evacuation efforts.

Once safely outside the building or school, depending on the scope of the emergency, you may be able to re-enter after the hazard has been diffused, or you may be directed to safety elsewhere until it can be.

AT THE SHELTER

If you have never been to an emergency shelter, believe it or not, you don't just walk in, plop down on a cot, and make yourself at home. There are very specific procedures you must follow when you walk through the entrance of any designated shelter. The Red Cross, CERT, emergency services personnel, and other volunteers who set up and staff these shelters (often at a moment's notice) have a protocol to follow to ensure not only that you get the help you need, but that you are kept safe during your hopefully brief stay. Many people are intimidated by going to a shelter, but rest assured they are safe, comfortable places.

When you arrive at the shelter, you will enter the one designated main entrance (all others are closed off to keep shelter residents secure), and there will be a waiting area with chairs and tables. One by one, you will be called to the registration table to answer a number of questions for the shelter worker, who will either fill out the form for you or have you fill it out if the shelter is overwhelmed. The questions will establish your name, address, age, and any special needs you might have, such as dietary needs and medical devices you may have with you. During this intake process, you will have the chance to ask any questions about how the shelter operates. Once you have filled out the form and answered all pertinent registration questions along with any necessary for minors you may be coming in with, you will then be signed in and told where to go to find snacks, water, hot meals, and a dormitory area with cots.

Red Cross shelters provide hot meals, and you will be surprised by the quality of the food, which is donated by many local restaurants and cafes. Sometimes the shelter will have a kitchen with cooks making meals. The dormitory stations are equipped with cots, and you can bring your blankets and pillow from home, as they do not usually provide pillows because of hygiene issues (blankets can be cleaned, but pillows are tougher to keep clean and free of germs). Shelters will provide two blankets per person.

No weapons of any kind are permitted in shelters, and if you have a restraining order against a family member, the volunteers and security will not allow that person to have any contact with you if they end up at the same shelter. Many shelters have specific rules on whether or not people who are involved in custody battles or marital court–related separations can be kept in the same shelter. No animals are allowed except for service animals, and you must be able to prove that an animal is necessary for your medical or mental health.

Shelters will have an activity board with specific times for eating meals and shutting off lights in the dormitory for sleep, and how to find others who

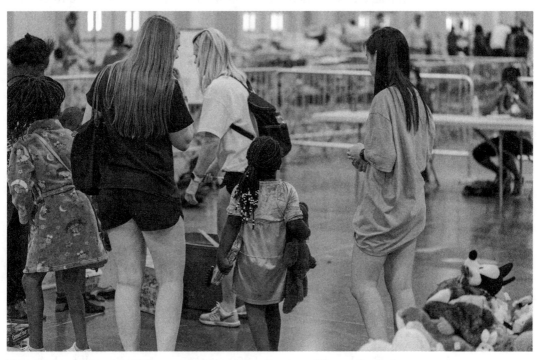

Texans take shelter at the Houston NRG Center as Hurricane Harvey floods the area in August 2017.

may be sheltering elsewhere. There may be games and activities, especially for children, as well as television broadcasting news about the disaster, but be prepared to entertain yourselves. The dormitory cots will be spaced out according to shelter rules: usually 40–60 square feet of sleeping space per person, which is about a 8 foot by 5 foot space. Bringing a ton of clutter that spills over into another person's space is unacceptable. If you have a service animal, wheelchair, or other large medical device, you will have 100 square feet of space to work with.

There will also be internal signage pointing out bathrooms, showers, staff areas, children's play zones, evacuation routes, quiet areas, snack bar and cafeteria or eating rooms, and security.

Most people fear being stuck in a shelter for long periods of time, but most shelters know that they are meant to be short-duration solutions. Yet if the emergency or disaster was to become long term, don't fear that they will run out of food and water too quickly, as they have community support as well as support from the Federal Emergency Management Agency and the Department of Homeland Security, which assist the Red Cross or CERT in making sure the shelter is well staffed and supplied. In addition to food and drink, many shelters will also have comfort kits with toothbrushes, toothpaste, and deodorant, but plan to bring your own.

All residents of a shelter are told when they enter about the rules, procedures, and mealtimes, and shelter workers will disseminate information about the disaster as they confirm it from outside sources. Being in a shelter is meant to be a calm time of knowing you have a roof over your head, food and water, and trained individuals nearby who know how to respond in a variety of circumstances. In fact, you may want to consider getting shelter operation training yourself through CERT or the Red Cross if you think you may want to volunteer to lend a helping hand during the next emergency.

HOTELS, MOTELS, PARKS, AND STADIUMS

During a major disaster, many hotels and motels will reduce room prices drastically to accommodate people forced to evacuate. There are a few hotels that will even offer free rooms, but you won't know that, unfortunately, until the disaster happens and you are looking for shelter. Parks and sports stadiums as well as some churches, preferably outside of the immediate danger zone, will often offer shelter for large numbers of evacuees who have nowhere else to go, especially if designated shelters are full.

Local news on the television or radio will provide the names and addresses of these locations, or use your cell phone's emergency app to find shelter if you are not at home. In the case of Hurricane Irma in September of 2017, the State of Florida set up a special 800 number for people to call for help getting out of their homes and safely to a shelter, including those who were too poor to afford a motel or didn't own a car to evacuate in and those who were homebound because of extreme illness.

The flow of information will be critical when you need to know where to go, so get those apps loaded onto your cell phones, have a battery-operated radio, watch television at home or wherever someone has one (many shops and stores will be broadcasting nonstop news), or get licensed to operate a ham radio, and have your handheld radio with you at all times. Sometimes even shelters have to be evacuated and relocated, should they be in the path of a hurricane, tornado, wildfire, or other threat!

STAYING PUT

If you are told point blank to shelter in place, do not attempt to leave. Obviously emergency services personnel and law enforcement individuals have determined that you expose yourself to a greater threat if you run, than if you hide out at home or work or wherever you may be.

There is an art to properly sheltering in place. For some disasters, you don't have to take every step necessary for others. Often staying put means just not going anywhere near the danger zone and not clogging up roadways needed by emergency vehicles. Sheltering in place is most important during chemical, biological, nuclear, and other hazardous or toxic emergencies, where you want to protect yourself by sealing off doors, windows, and vents to the outside and hunker down in an interior room that has no windows or as few as possible.

Look around your home or office or school right now. Locate the innermost room above ground level that you might seek shelter in, away from doors or windows. This room will be sealed off once you enter with your supplies (supplies may already be stored there), so make sure it is large enough to accommodate you and anyone else you are with. Knowing where you will go ahead of time can save you precious minutes when you need to seal off the room. Do not go into a basement, as in the case of a chemical disaster, many chemicals are heavier than air and can seep into basement areas. You can choose several interior rooms if there are a lot of people who need shelter.

Close all doors and windows to the home or office/school. Close blinds, shutters, and shades to protect against a possible explosion outside or anything that might shatter the glass and send it flying into the room. If the room has a landline telephone, this may be ideal if cell phone service goes down and you need to communicate with the outside world.

Begin sheltering in place by using duct tape and plastic sheeting to seal off all exterior windows, doors, vents, and any other possible way air could get from the outside into the room or rooms you have chosen. Make sure to tape off the area tightly and completely. Properly sealing your home/office/room can make a huge difference to survival, as it keeps the poisonous toxins or radiation outside and prevents even contaminants and airborne viruses from entering. Also turn off fans, air conditioning, and heating to avoid bringing any outside air into the area.

If anyone was outside at the time the emergency occurred, have them remove all clothing and put it in a plastic bag to avoid bringing contaminants inside. If possible, they should shower and put on fresh clothing before entering the room to be sealed.

Be sure to make a space for pets to eliminate their waste, and do not let them go outside to do so until it is safe. Have plastic poop-collecting bags, newspaper or rags, containers, and cleaning supplies handy to clean up after pets, because you may be staying with them for a few days.

Once you are in the sealed room, only use your cell phone to call 911 in an actual emergency, as phone lines will be clogged. If you have a television, radio, or cell phone in the sealed room, keep listening for news updates that will include when you can leave the sheltered area.

Once the event is over, you will be instructed that it is safe to unseal the room. Turn on fans and ventilate the room as well as the rest of the house/office. Then go outside to breathe clean air while the home/office is replacing the indoor air with fresh air.

Children and students sheltering in place will not be released to parents until the threat is over. If your child has a cell phone and there is service, they will be able to communicate with you and tell you what is happening. Do not go to the school and demand to see your child. It isn't safe for you or your child. Wait until the situation has cleared up and authorities have stated that it is safe for parents to pick up their children.

CAR TROUBLE

Yes, you can shelter in place inside a vehicle. But you must have the materials to seal off the doors and windows to make it effective. The rule of thumb is, if you are close to your home, office, or a public facility, go there immediately to take shelter. If you are not able to do so, then pull your car safely over to the side of the road. To avoid overheating, try to find a safe but shaded area to pull under, such as a bridge or large overhang of trees. Turn off the engine, and close the windows and air-conditioning vents. If you have duct tape in your car emergency kit, use it to seal off the vents. Keep the radio running so you can listen for further instructions. Stay put until help arrives or you hear that it is safe to get back out on the road again.

You can also shelter in place in a van or motor home, in which case you will need more duct tape and plastic sheeting, but a larger vehicle such as an RV or motor home can provide a much more comfortable stay for family members.

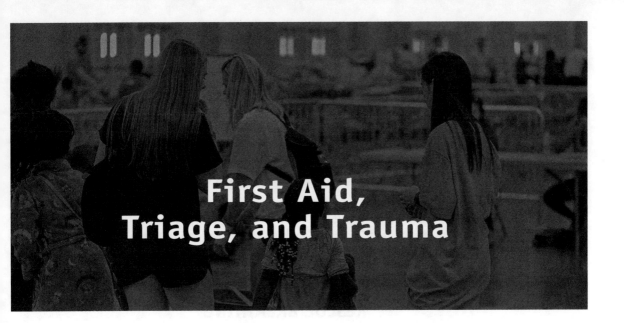

First Aid, Triage, and Trauma

People get hurt. Knowing what to do when people get hurt is the focus of this chapter, from the basics of first aid to understanding triage to dealing with trauma and psychological symptoms after a disaster or emergency. We will also cover how to deal with burns, insect bites, and stings as well as poison control. But read it all, because you never know when you might need to deal with a life-threatening medical emergency where no help is available.

Most emergency kits include the basics for first aid, such as bandages, ointments, and cleansing wipes. The best-prepared person will be sure to add as much as possible to their first aid kit, because this one kit will get used more than any other. There are a variety of first aid kits you can buy online or in many camping and sporting stores, so if you don't want to put your own together, it behooves you to order a few as soon as possible. Keep a larger kit in the home, a medium-sized kit in the car or camper, and a small kit in your purse, if you carry one. Having a small kit in every bathroom in the house could also help when you need that bandage or those tweezers in a pinch.

ABC

Any injury, big or small, needs to be assessed first and foremost for the ABCs of first aid response.

A is for Airway, B is for Breathing, C is for Circulation.

First, you must clear the airway by looking for the obstruction. You do this with the *head tilt/chin lift method.*

First shake the victim to see if they are responsive. Ask if they can hear you.

If unresponsive, put the victim on their back, kneel beside the victim, and place the palm of one hand on their forehead.

With the other hand, place two fingers under the chin, and tilt the jaw upward while the other hand tilts the head back slightly.

Put your ear over the victim's mouth, and listen for breathing. Look toward the victim's feet, and watch for the rising and falling of the chest.

Place a hand on the victim's abdominal area, and feel for a slight rise of air intake.

Sometimes just clearing the airway is enough to get the victim *breathing* again. You may find an obstruction such as a piece of food that you can remove with your fingers. If the victim is vomiting, lay them on their side so they do not choke on the vomit and clog their airway.

RESCUE BREATHING

People can stop breathing for a variety of reasons: injury, choking, drowning, overdose, severe asthma attack, etc. By breathing for them and getting air into their lungs, you raise their chances of survival until help can arrive. Brain damage can occur within three minutes from lack of oxygen, so it is imperative that rescue breathing begin immediately.

Yell for someone to call 911.

Begin rescue breathing. For an adult or child, pinch the victim's nose shut, cover their mouth with yours, and give two full, slow breaths lasting 1 to 1.5 seconds, checking the chest for rise and fall. If the victim's chest rises and falls, continue rescue breaths. If the chest does not rise and fall, check for blocked airway again.

If the victim has no pulse, administer chest compressions at a rate of thirty chest compressions, then two breaths.

Continue until the victim begins breathing or help arrives.

For infants, you will place your mouth over their nose and mouth and give two short puffs of air. If there is no response, reposition the head tilt, and continue the two short puffs. Give one puff every three seconds to an infant until help arrives or they begin breathing on their own. If you are alone, you can administer chest compressions and rescue breathing for two minutes first, *then* call 911.

If you have access to a rescue-breathing protective face mask, use that to avoid contact with a toxin or germs.

CPR OR HANDS-ONLY CPR

Check for a pulse. *Circulation* may be compromised, so a weak pulse is a concern.

Check for capillary refill by pressing on the skin. It should turn white, then return to normal color in under two seconds. This is also called the "blanch test."

Check body temperature.

If there is no pulse, begin CPR.

The proper way to do CPR has changed and now involves continuous chest compressions *without* stopping, even if the victim is not breathing. This is called *hands-only CPR* and has been proven to save more lives than CPR that takes the time out to check for a pulse or apply rescue breathing. The American Heart Association now recommends that bystanders and the general public use hands-only CPR for cardiac arrests and injuries where the victim's heart has stopped beating.

CPR stands for cardiopulmonary resuscitation and involves keeping blood moving throughout the victim's body until a medical team can arrive. The chest compressions used during CPR do this by pumping the blood in and out of the heart and moving blood to the brain to keep it alive until the heart can begin working on its own again. Hands-only CPR can keep the blood flowing continuously until help arrives or the victim recovers and increase the chances of survival because there are no short gaps for rescue breaths and checking the pulse. Any delay in compressing the chest can significantly affect the blood flow.

CPR training is a must for anyone, especially if you have children. If you do not have any training, follow these instructions: If you are alone, you may want to administer *two minutes of CPR* first to the victim, then stop to quickly call 911, then resume CPR. Shake the victim and shout at them. If they do not respond:

- Call 911 first.
- Put the victim on their back.
- Kneel on the side of the victim over their heart area.
- Put the base of one hand on top of the breastbone between the nipples. Place the other hand over this hand so that you can lean over and push down with force.
- Push hard and fast about two times per second. Be sure to release each push on the chest completely before pushing down again. Do not bounce your hands on the victim's chest, but push and compress. Lift your body weight off the victim with each compression.
- Continue these compressions until help arrives, someone can take over for you, or the victim's heart begins to beat on its own.

CPR ON A CHILD OR INFANT

Follow the same procedure, but only press down on the breastbone about *two inches* or a third of the thickness of the chest, and let the chest rise back up all the way before compressing again.

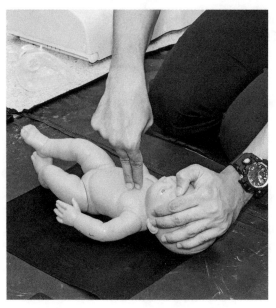

For infants under twelve months, CPR needs to be administered differently. For example, the chest should be compressed only about two inches.

You can give rescue breaths or do hands-only CPR until help arrives or the victim's heart begins to beat on its own. Ideally, you will not be alone and can have someone check the pulse while you administer breaths, and trade off tasks after you each get tired.

Even if the victim's heart begins to work again and they feel alert, call for help anyway, and let them know you administered CPR and/or rescue breathing.

We all want to do the best we can to try to save someone's life. Rescue breathing and CPR can be exhausting if you are working alone. At some point, if the victim is not breathing and has no pulse or signs of a heartbeat, you must decide if you can keep going or not. Hopefully, you will have help by then to pick up where you left off. Know that any attempt to save the life of another is brave and commendable.

ALLERGIC REACTIONS

An allergic reaction occurs when the immune system tries to fight off a foreign substance by creating antibodies. The substance may not even be harmful, but the immune system reacts anyway, and symptoms can range from mild coughing and a stuffy nose to a severe and life-threatening situation. People are allergic to a wide variety of things, from grass and pollen to animal dander and prescription drugs. An allergy can be with us from childhood or develop suddenly later in life. In any event, you must know the right way to deal with an allergic reaction to avoid making the situation much worse.

Symptoms of milder allergic reactions can include:
- Stuffy nose and runny nose
- Sneezing
- Red, itchy, or bloodshot eyes
- Skin rash
- Hives
- Digestive problems such as stomach pains
- Diarrhea
- Difficulty breathing/wheezing
- Swelling around the face

- Dizziness
- Rapid pulse

Milder allergies can be treated with over-the-counter antihistamines such as Benadryl and decongestants. The antihistamines block histamine receptors in the body so that they don't react to the presence of the allergen. Decongestants clear up stuffy noses and dry out watery eyes, especially during seasonal allergy periods. Hives and itchy skin can be treated with an over-the-counter hydrocortisone cream. If the hives and itching continue after use, you may need to get a prescription from your doctor.

These meds should only be taken for a few days, and if the allergies continue you should see your doctor and ask about a complete allergy test to pinpoint exactly what it is you are allergic to and how to treat it.

Severe allergic reactions include:

- Hives, itching, pale skin
- Wheezing and difficulty breathing
- Extreme swelling of lips, mouth, and face, with complaints of having difficulty swallowing
- Nausea
- Inability to swallow
- Swollen tongue
- Weak or quick pulse

Prescription drugs, especially if taken for the first time, can trigger what is called anaphylaxis, which can cause loss of consciousness, even cardiac arrest, if not treated quickly. Anaphylaxis is most noted for the facial swelling it provokes, especially of the mouth area. Someone who is experiencing these symptoms must be taken to the hospital as soon as possible, even if their symptoms appear to be lessening over time.

If the victim has an epinephrine auto injector or an EpiPen, help them use it or inject them if they are not able.

Call 911 and lay the victim on their back, trying to keep them calm.

Raise their feet at least a foot above heart level, and cover them with a jacket or blanket.

Watch for signs of vomiting, and get them on their side so they don't choke.

Try not to lift the victim's head, and do not administer oral meds, as this could impede breathing even further.

If the victim is not breathing and has no heart activity, you will then perform CPR at a rate of about 100 chest presses per minute until help arrives.

Again, even if they start to feel better, get them to the hospital anyway, because you need to determine what caused the reaction so that it is not repeated.

How to Inject an EpiPen

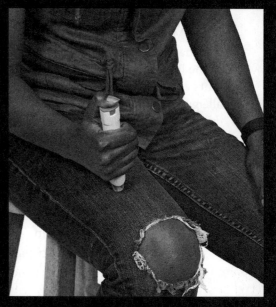

Take the pen and hold it tightly in the center, with the orange tip facing down.

- Take off the safety cap (usually blue in color).

- Place the orange tip against the victim's outer thigh. You can do this through pants if needed.

- Press the tip firmly against the thigh to release the epinephrine in the injection needle.

- Hold in place for at least 10 seconds, and make sure the entire dose is injected.

- Place the pen somewhere so you can show EMS when they arrive how much of a dose was administered.

- Gently massage the injection site for at least 10 seconds to help the epinephrine circulate.

To stave off dangerous allergic reactions to insect bites, food, or drugs, an EpiPen can be used to inject epinephrine into the leg for quick treatment.

BITES AND STINGS

The good thing about most bug bites is that they heal all by themselves, with minimal discomfort to the bitten. But there are situations that call for treatment and can even lead to distress and death, such as poisonous spiders and snakes. One of the easiest ways to avoid being bitten is to stay away from bees, wasps, snakes, and other biting critters when working in the garage or outdoors, but avoiding them altogether may be impossible. It is much better to know how to handle bites and stings if they do happen.

The range of bites runs from mildly annoying to severe and worthy of calling 911. On the mild side are bedbugs, most mosquitoes, flies, ants, fleas, chiggers, mites, lice, and some species of spiders. In the middle are bees, hornets, wasps, yellow jackets, and nonpoisonous snakes. On the more severe end of the spectrum are disease-carrying mosquitoes, scorpions, brown recluse spiders, black widow spiders, and poisonous snakes as well as ticks carrying diseases. Often it isn't the bug that is the danger, but the diseases the bug is known to be associated with, such as malaria, dengue fever, plague, Rocky Mountain spotted fever, yellow fever, West Nile virus, and Lyme disease.

Immediately after a bite or sting, the symptoms can include:

- Burning and/or itching
- Swelling at and around the bite/sting site
- Redness
- Pain

The above symptoms alone are easily treatable if that is all the victim is experiencing.

If stung by a bee or other insect with a stinger, remove the stinger with a pair of tweezers if you can see it, or by scraping it with a credit card. You can also apply tape to the stinger and quickly lift the tape. Most of the time, stingers are on the surface and should be easy to remove.

Wash the sting area with mild soap and water.

If stung on the arm or leg, keep the limb below heart level unless swelling is present. If so, elevate the limb.

Apply ice or an ice pack to the bite or sting for about fifteen minutes once an hour for six hours, but do not apply the ice directly to skin. Place a cloth between the ice and skin. If you don't have any ice packs or ice, use a package of frozen veggies or fruit!

Apply a cool, wet cloth to the area after using ice to continue to treat pain, itching, and swelling.

Elevate the area to decrease the chances of swelling.

Take an antihistamine to reduce itching. Check with your doctor before giving an antihistamine to a child.

Apply an anti-itching ointment or cream such as hydrocortisone to the affected area. Do not use hydrocortisone cream on a child under the age of two without a doctor's permission. Never use this cream on a child's rectal or vaginal area.

You can also spray with a local anesthetic to alleviate pain, but watch for any skin reactions, and stop if you see rashing or increased redness.

Cover the bite or sting to protect it against bumping and scratching.

If new symptoms arise, or current symptoms worsen, or if the victim develops a fever, call your doctor or get to an urgent care facility or hospital.

SEVERE ALLERGY SYMPTOMS

You or the victim may have an allergic reaction to a bite or sting. Symptoms include:

- Shortness of breath
- Swollen lips, mouth, tongue, throat
- Difficulty speaking and swallowing

- Dizziness and/or fainting
- Confusion
- Rapid heartbeat
- Hives, usually large in size
- Cramping, nausea, and vomiting

If the victim has an EpiPen, use it immediately and call 911. If the victim loses consciousness, turn to your ABCs.

SCORPION BITES

Scorpion stings can be very painful, but normally will not cause an allergic reaction. Symptoms include swelling, pain, and numbness at the bite site, tingling, and possibly itching. Ice can be used to reduce swelling along with an antihistamine. Hydrocortisone creams reduce itching and swelling.

If you live in the American Southwest, there are more dangerous scorpions, such as the bark scorpion. Venom from its bite can cause rapid breathing, a spike in blood pressure, weakness, and muscle twitching. If you have been bitten, get to the emergency room right away, or call 911. If it is possible to capture the bark scorpion, bag it or put it in a container or sealed bag, and bring it with you for identification. Yes, you can kill it first by dropping it into a bowl of scalding water!

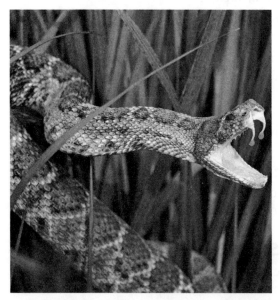

If you believe you have been bitten by a venomous snake, do not try to suck out the venom or try to dilute it with milk. These are fake remedies you see in the movies.

SNAKE BITES

Snakes are everywhere, but if you camp or hike or have property bordering woods or a canyon, you may encounter them more often. Snakes can also be found in gardens, garages, and woodsheds. Some are friend and some are foe. It helps to know ahead of time what snakes are common to the area you live in and what they look like, especially if you need to tell a first responder what bit you.

Nonpoisonous snakes tend to have pupils like a human's and more oval-shaped heads. Poisonous snakes have catlike pupils and triangular heads. If you are bitten and suspect it was a poisonous snake, call for help immediately.

If you can identify the snake as nonpoisonous, treat as a puncture wound:

Stop any bleeding from the fang marks.

Clean the bite area with soap and water for a few minutes. Pat dry and apply an antibiotic ointment, then cover with a loose dressing.

Mark the area where the swelling ends, and keep an eye on any spread of swelling that might indicate an infection.

You can make a splint to support the area if you are going to seek medical help.

Drink fluids and stay hydrated to assist the healing process.

Watch the wound! If you develop any symptoms after twenty-four hours that may indicate an allergic reaction, go to urgent care or a hospital.

VENOMOUS SNAKE BITES

In many cases, a snake will not inject enough venom to be fatal to an average-sized human being, but err on the side of caution, and seek immediate help anyway. If you can determine the type of snake, or if you killed the snake and can bring it with you to the hospital, do so. If you call 911, having the snake for first responders to identify can speed up their treatment protocol, although all emergency personnel will be knowledgeable about the snakes in your area and what their bite marks look like.

If you spot or even hear a snake you suspect is venomous, *freeze!* Snakes detect motion. Move away from the snake slowly until you are safe.

If you do get bitten, do not panic. But do get away from the snake to a safer area to treat the bite.

Keep the bite area *below* heart level to prevent venom from spreading.

Do *not* try to suck out or cut out the venom.

Do *not* use milk to try to dilute the venom.

Do *not* give the victim any type of medication unless instructed to do so when calling 911.

Remove restrictive clothing or jewelry near the bite area.

Using a cloth soaked in water, gently wipe off the bite area. If you have soap available, use soap. Do not scrub, as that can spread venom. Do not flush with water, as that too can spread venom. You may instinctively want to clean the area with vigor to "get out the venom," but this is one time you need to be gentle.

Dry the wound, and cover with a loose, sterile bandage. You may splint the area to avoid moving the bite wound until help arrives, but keep the bite below heart level at all times.

Never apply a tourniquet, as this can actually restrict blood flow too much and cause more damage to the tissue.

Never apply ice, which can cause more damage to the wound area.

Keep the victim calm and still.

Do not drink caffeine or anything that dehydrates the body or speeds up the heart rate.

Treat for shock if necessary, and apply the ABCs.

If you get to help, you will probably be given an anti-venom treatment and possibly a tetanus shot if needed.

If you do treat the bite on your own, whether at home or out camping, watch for symptoms that increase over a twenty-four-hour period. If the symptoms worsen, seek medical attention immediately.

TICK BITES

Most ticks are harmless, but they can carry deadly diseases that they pass into your bloodstream, such as Lyme disease. This is why it is important to save the ticks in a plastic container or bag once you remove them from the victim's body, as it will help health experts determine whether the victim should be tested for specific diseases.

When you see a tick on the skin, remove it with tweezers by getting the tips as close to the bottom of the tick as possible. Try not to break the tick when pulling it up and out of skin.

Pull upward firmly and evenly.

Remove any parts of the tick still in the skin with tweezers.

Bag the bug! Place the tick in a plastic bag, glass jar, or container.

Do not remove ticks with heat to the skin or anything other than a sharp pair of tweezers. Do not try to smother them with petroleum jelly, gasoline, or rubbing alcohol.

Do not try to pop or squeeze the tick.

Wash the bite area with soap and water. Dry the area, and cover with a bandage. You can apply a small layer of petroleum jelly to the bite to keep the bandage from sticking to it or pulling on it.

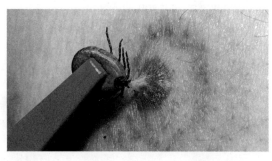

Ticks are not venomous, but they can carry illnesses such as Lyme Disease that will require medical treatment.

Wash your own hands with soap and water after removing the tick.

Apply an antibacterial cream to the bite.

If the bite area becomes infected and is warm, pussy, tender, swollen, or red, seek medical attention.

If the tick is too small to remove, get the victim to a doctor. The sooner they are removed, the less likely they are to inject diseases into the bloodstream.

If the victim experiences a rash, severe headache, or fever and joint pain, these are symptoms of tick-borne illness. Get the victim to a doctor or urgent care facility immediately.

If you live in a tick-infested area, be aware of what reported diseases ticks carry, and know the symptoms. Any time a victim experiences sudden fevers, headaches, chills, confusion, nausea, vomiting, rashes, muscle and joint pain, swollen lymph nodes, red eyes, blisters and ulcers at the bite area, and chest pain and difficulty breathing, get help immediately, as these are all symptoms of various tick-borne diseases.

Be sure to check pets and other family members for tick bites too.

Spider Bites

Most spiders are harmless, and their bites can range from imperceptible to slightly painful. For regular bites, treatment can be done at home and doesn't require medical attention, but if you aren't sure what kind of spider bit you and are anxious about it, the best option is to call your doctor anyway.

Wash the bite with cool water and soap.

Use a cool compress, such as an ice pack or ice wrapped in a cloth, to ease pain and stop swelling.

Elevate the bitten area above heart level.

Use an over-the-counter pain reliever if needed.

Monitor the bite area for twenty-four hours. If symptoms worsen, call your doctor or poison control. A bite bigger than a quarter in diameter or showing stripy marks in the skin should be attended to by your doctor or an urgent care facility.

If the following symptoms appear after a bite, seek medical help immediately:

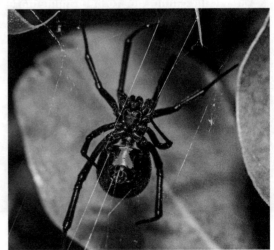

- Difficulty breathing
- Muscle spasms
- Faintness and weakness
- Profuse sweating
- Nausea and vomiting
- Difficulty swallowing, swollen throat area

Dangerous Spiders

In the United States, there are two main spiders that can cause harm: the black widow and the brown recluse.

The black widow spider is easily identified by the red, hourglass marking on its abdomen.

When People and Animals Bite!

Treating animal and human bites is all about keeping away infection. These bites must be treated quickly if the bite breaks the skin to avoid the spread of germs and bacteria. Seek medical attention immediately!

Call 911 or get the victim to an urgent care or hospital.

Clean the bite area immediately by flushing under warm water for a few minutes. To be safe, do this even if the skin is intact.

If there is anything embedded in the bite area, such as teeth, hair, or dirt, remove the objects and encourage the wound to bleed just a little to purge debris. Squeeze the bite area gently until it is bleeding on its own.

If bleeding is heavy, put a sterile pad over the bite area and apply pressure.

Dry the area, and cover with a sterile dressing.

If there is pain, the victim can take over-the-counter pain meds.

Watch for signs of infection if the victim cannot get to help immediately, and treat for shock. Symptoms can include redness and swelling, pus or other discharge from the wound, increased warmth and pain around the wound, fever, swollen glands, and red streaks coming outward from the wound site.

Once help arrives or you get the victim to the hospital, be ready to tell responders what bit the victim and whether the victim has any medical issues of concern, such as high blood pressure, diabetes, heart disease, or autoimmune diseases.

Most animal bites occur to a child's face, especially dog bites, and damage can be more severe. The risk of infection rises the deeper the bite wound, so get help immediately, and treat it as an open wound until help arrives. Apply pressure with a clean sterile cloth to stop bleeding, cover the area with a sterile dressing, and keep the child calm, watching for signs of shock.

With animal bites, rabies may be a concern (as may tetanus), especially if the animal was wild. The more information you can give responders about the type of animal and where it was when the victim was bitten, the better chance there is of the animal being caught or observed to determine if rabies is a factor. Most animal bites are from household pets. If the pet has not had a rabies vaccine, let responders know. Bats also carry rabies, so if the bite is from a bat, let responders know. It isn't just frothing-mouthed dogs and wild-eyed cats that carry rabies!

Human bites can spread a variety of diseases, including hepatitis B, hepatitis C, and even HIV, so get them treated immediately at a medical facility, even if the bite mark looks innocuous. Blood-borne viruses are transmissible through broken skin, and even though the risk is small, because viruses are not transmitted via saliva, if there is blood present in the person's mouth when they bite, it is a possibility.

The black widow is a large black spider with a red hourglass shape on its belly. They are found throughout the country and often make their homes in wood piles, sheds, gardens, closets, and garages. When a black widow bites, it will feel like a pinprick, but it will soon become red and swollen. Within a few hours, there will be severe pain and even stiffness around the bite area, followed by stomach pain, nausea, vomiting, rapid pulse, chills, and fever.

If you suspect a black widow bite and have two tiny "fang marks" on your skin, call 911 or get to a hospital immediately. The bite is rarely fatal, and there is a vaccine, but if not treated soon, it can result in a systemic reaction that may end in the loss of fingers or limbs, depending on where the bite was located.

Brown recluses come in various brown shades and are mostly found in the southeastern United States, but they have a violin-shaped mark on their backs. They have longer, spindly legs and are also found in dark places such as garages, sheds, closets, and wood piles. When they bite, it stings! A bite will be pale or bluish-purple in color and can be red around the periphery. However, if the bite is red in the center, it is probably not a brown recluse. The bite will be dry and flat or sunken in the center. Over the next eight hours, pain sets in. Fever, rash, and nausea may occur. After about a week, the bite area can ulcerate and become infected if not treated quickly. Antibiotics may be prescribed, and if the bite has spread over time, surgery might be required.

The rule of thumb is that, unless you saw a spider actually bite you, most bites can be attributed to something else, such as mosquitoes. But if you do see either a black widow or brown recluse either on or near you, do not hesitate to get help.

BLEEDING

Some injuries have minimal bleeding that can be taken care of with cleaning and bandaging to put pressure on the cut or wound. Bleeding will usually subside and cease after a while. But in the event of a more severe injury, you may be dealing with uncontrolled bleeding.

There are three types of bleeding, determined by how fast blood is flowing:

Arterial bleeding—Blood is transported via arteries under high pressure, so bleeding from an artery will cause blood to spurt.

Venous bleeding—Veins transport blood under low pressure, and this appears as flowing bleeding.

Capillary bleeding—Capillaries carry blood under low pressure, and bleeding will be oozing bleeding.

Bleeding injuries require direct pressure, elevation, and pressure on pressure points.

Place direct pressure over the wound. Use a clean dressing or a clean cloth if needed over the wound. Apply pressure firmly and evenly.

Wrap the wound tightly with a dressing that continues direct pressure, and tie in a bow so that it can be removed and replaced with a clean bandage wrap.

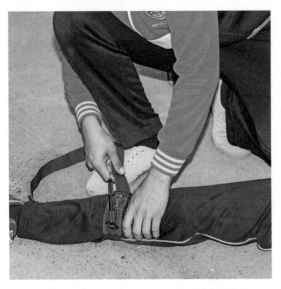

Generally speaking, a tourniquet should only be applied by a professional to stop bleeding. If you don't know what you're doing, you can cause more harm than good to an injured person.

Elevate the injured area above heart level.

Apply pressure on the nearest *pressure points* to the wound/injury. This will slow blood flow to the area. For bleeding in the arms, apply pressure to the brachial point just above the elbow.

For bleeding in the legs, apply pressure to the femoral point on the upper thigh.

Never apply a tourniquet except as a last resort or if you are instructed to by emergency personnel.

It can take between five and seven minutes for blood flow to stop when using direct pressure and elevation.

Nose bleeds: Pinch the nose at the nostril area and lean over. Do *not* lean your head back, as blood can enter the airway and go into the lungs. You can also put pressure on the upper lip just under the nose. If the blood loss is severe, treat for possible shock. If a lot of blood has been swallowed, there may be nausea and vomiting. Keep the airway clear!

BROKEN BONES AND FRACTURES

Splinting a broken bone may be necessary before you can get yourself or the injured person to the hospital.

Find any solid object that can serve as a splint, such as a board of wood, layers of cardboard, particle board, a sturdy stick, a thick blanket, even a book or anything solid that will keep the area immobilized above and below the break. You can also use pillows, folded magazines or newspapers, and even metal strips. Splints can also be used any time an injury needs to be immobilized.

Cut to a smaller size if you have the means to do so.

Remove clothing, jewelry, and anything else from the affected area.

Align the splint with the affected area so there is equal coverage above and below the break, including joints.

If you can, splint the injury in the position it is in so you do not have to move the area and cause more damage.

Never try to realign the joint and bone.

Wrap the splint in a cloth bandage, and secure the ends.

Check the area above the wrapping for warmth, feeling, and color. You can gently press down on the skin to see if it turns white, then regains color quickly. If it does not, loosen the wrap.

Keep the entire area immobilized until help can arrive. If you have to get the person to a hospital, try to get help lifting them so the broken bone can stay immobilized, and make sure, during transport, that the area is supported, lying flat, and not bouncing around.

Closed fractures only require splinting. These are fractures where the bone has not broken through the skin.

Open fractures are those where the bone protrudes through the skin. These are more dangerous because of bleeding and infection risks.

Do not wash out an open fracture, and never try to push the bone back inside the tissue.

Treat the wound area of an open fracture first, then cover the wound with a dressing, and splint without disturbing the wound area.

Use a moist dressing approximately four inches by four inches over the bone so it does not dry out.

Call for help.

DISLOCATIONS

A dislocated shoulder is excruciatingly painful. Dislocations are common in major emergencies and separate the bone from its joint. Dislocation should be treated just like a fracture, and you should *not* try to relocate the bone to the joint. Keep it immobilized until help arrives.

Sprains and strains can be immobilized and kept elevated to reduce swelling and usually don't require much more than splinting, as if it were a fracture.

Things to remember:

- Before splinting an area, remove rings, watches, and any other jewelry that can constrict blood flow.
- If you splint using a blanket or pillow, tie it at various points to ensure that the splint stays around the limb and keeps it immobilized.
- If you use a large towel, roll up the towel, wrap it around the limb in question, then tie into place.

EYE INJURIES

If you got something in your eye, what would be the first thing you would do? Too many people rub their eyes, which can cause whatever is in the eye to become even more embedded. If you get a foreign object in your eye, you need to first wash your hands with soap and water to make sure they are clean and free of germs.

First try to locate the object and remove it gently without damage to the surface of the eye. Use the flat part of your index finger to gently press on the object and lift it up. If that doesn't work, or you are afraid of scratching your eye, flush the eye with clean, warm water. You can put your face under the stream of water in a sink or shower, but make sure the stream is gentle so it doesn't cause the object to stick into the eye.

Hold your eyelid open while you flush the eye. If you wear contact lenses, remove them *first* before flushing the eye.

If the object is located over the dark center, or pupil, of the eye, flush it with water. If it doesn't budge, put on dark sunglasses and seek medical help. Try not to put any pressure on the affected eye.

If the object is located over the white part of the eye, the sclera, or inside the lower lid, you can wet a cotton swab and touch it to the end of the object to lift it off. Use a twisted, damp piece of toilet tissue if you don't have swabs handy. There may be some irritation, but hopefully the object will cling to the tissue.

If this irrigation method does not remove the object, seek medical help immediately.

Do not use tweezers or any kind of sharp object to try to lift the object out of the eye.

Do not rub the eye, even if it itches. You could scratch the delicate cornea.

If a large object is stuck in the eye, get medical help and let the professionals remove it properly, or you can do more damage to the eye.

Know that, even after the object is removed, it is natural to feel some pain and experience redness and the feeling of something in the eye for a while. It will go back to normal soon.

BURNS

Burns will be treated depending on the severity, or degree. Not all burns should be treated the same, and what works on one may be damaging to another. Burns can be caused by fire, chemicals, poisons, electrical currents, and exposure to radiation.

There are three layers of the skin:

Epidermis—the outer layer, containing nerve endings and hair

Dermis—the middle layer, containing blood vessels, oil glands, hair follicles, and sweat glands

Subcutaneous—the inner layer, containing blood vessels and covering muscle and skin cells

The most severe burns can affect all three layers. Burns are categorized as:

First Degree—Epidermal, resulting in reddened skin, pain, and swelling, such as with sunburn.

Second Degree—Epidermal, partial destruction of dermis layer, resulting in red, blistering skin with a wet appearance, pain, and swelling.

Third Degree—Complete destruction of epidermis and dermis and some subcutaneous damage—can affect all skin layers as well as underlying muscle and skin cells. The skin appears waxy and white, charred brown, or black and leathery and can either be very painful or numb and painless.

If you or someone else is burned, get away from the source of the burn immediately.

Cool the skin or clothing on the skin if still hot. Immerse in cool water for one minute, or cover with clean compresses that have been wrung out in cool water.

Treat severe burn victims (third degree) for shock immediately.

Elevate burned areas above the heart level.

Never use ice! Ice causes vessel constriction.

Never apply ointments, gels, alcohol, butter, antiseptics, or creams.

Do not remove clothing that has been seared into the skin.

Do not break blisters.

Cool burns by running cool or cold water over the area for several minutes.

Dress less severe burns in a wet dressing.

Dress more severe burns in a dry dressing (so that it won't stick to the skin and pull on it, causing more damage.)

Chemical burns: If the chemical was a liquid, wash the area with copious amounts of water. If the chemical was a powder, brush off the powder, but do *not* wash or rinse with water to avoid spreading. Cover the burned area.

Be careful of possible hypothermia when cooling a burn victim's body if the victim is a child, elderly person, or an infant. Victims with severe burns can be more susceptible. Do not cool more than 15 percent of the affected body surface area at a time.

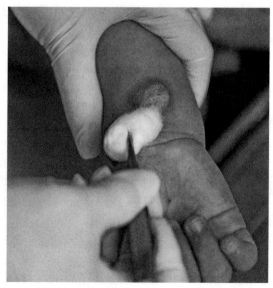

It is important to treat burns quickly because they leave the skin vulnerable to infection.

CHOKING

Choking occurs when the airway is obstructed by an object or liquid. When someone is choking, they usually put their hands to their throat. They will clearly have difficulty breathing, and their skin and lips may take on a bluish tone. If they don't get their airway clear, they may faint. If someone can talk, cough, or make sounds, let them continue until they are able to breathe clearly or dislodge the object blocking their airway. The Red Cross suggests taking on what they call a "live and let live" approach, which consists of allowing a victim to try to dislodge the object, but also taking action as follows to assist:

Give five back blows: Use the heel of your hand to give five blows to the back between the shoulder blades.

Give five abdominal thrusts, also known as the Heimlich maneuver. See below.

Alternate between five back blows and five abdominal thrusts until the object is dislodged and the victim can breathe.

Be sure to have someone call 911 first. If you are alone with the victim, call 911 *after* administering back blows and abdominal thrusts.

If the victim has no heart activity, administer CPR and keep checking the airway to see if you can find what needs to be dislodged. Continue CPR and dislodge the object when it becomes visible.

Abdominal thrusts, or the Heimlich maneuver, can also be given to yourself if you are choking as well as to infants, children, and even pets.

THE HEIMLICH MANEUVER

An American thoracic surgeon by the name of Henry Judah Heimlich created a procedure consisting of abdominal thrusts designed to stop choking which was included in *Emergency Medicine* in 1974 and has become the main technique used today to assist a choking victim. To perform the Heimlich maneuver on someone else:

Stand directly behind the victim, and wrap your arms around their waist. Have the victim lean forward slightly.

Take one hand and position it above the navel, and grasp the fist of that hand with your other hand, forming a ball shape.

Thrust hard upward with both hands gripped together. Use quick upward thrusts that almost feel like you are trying to lift the victim up.

Do five thrusts, check the airway to see if the object is dislodged, then repeat the five thrusts. Do this until the object is dislodged from the victim's mouth or help arrives.

If at any time the victim becomes unconscious, begin CPR with chest compressions and rescue breathing.

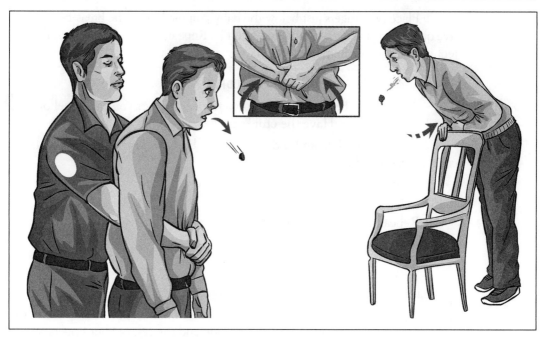

At left, a person assists a choking victim by administering the Heimlich Maneuver. If no one is around to help you and you are choking, you can perform the maneuver yourself with the help of the back of a chair or countertop (right).

If the person is pregnant or obese, place your hands a little higher, at the base of the breastbone, and press inward with quick thrusts.

IF YOU ARE CHOKING

You can perform the Heimlich on yourself by positioning your hands in the same fashion slightly above your navel and thrusting inward and upward. You can also bend over a hard object such as the back of a chair or a countertop and push your body into the chair back and upward in thrusts.

INFANTS

For a baby under the age of one year, you will hold the baby face down on your forearm and rest them on your thigh. The baby's head should be lower than their chest. Support the head with the palm of your hand.

Using the heel of your free hand, give up to five back slaps between the shoulder blades.

Turn the baby to check the airway, and if the object can be dislodged, do so.

If the baby is still choking, place the baby face up on your thigh with their head lower than the body.

Place two fingers just below the baby's nipple line at the breastbone. Give five quick thrusts just as you would in CPR. Repeat the procedure until the object is dislodged or help has arrived.

CHILDREN

A child can be set face down on a firm surface, or you can kneel or hold the child in your lap. Have the child's back to you.

Place the middle and index fingers of both hands below the child's rib cage, just above the navel.

Press into the abdomen with quick, upward thrusts, but be gentle. Do not push hard on the rib cage.

Repeat until the object is dislodged or help has arrived.

PETS

Dogs and cats can also choke, and you can administer the Heimlich to a pet that is not coughing out the lodged object on its own.

Open the pet's mouth and look for the object. Place one hand on the pet's upper jaw, with your thumb on one side and the rest of your fingers on the other side.

With your free hand, push down on the lower jaw, and sweep the mouth with your index finger to seek the lodged object.

If you can see the object, remove it.

If you cannot see the object or reach it, and your pet is small, you can hold it down with the tail toward your face and arms around its lower abdomen area for thirty seconds and gently sway the body.

If the object is still lodged, place the pet on its side on a hard surface where you can tilt its head down and rear quarters upward. You can put something under the rear quarters to lift the area above the head level.

Place one hand on the back of a smaller pet to steady it, and the other under the center of the rib cage, and press in and upward with a thrusting motion four times.

If the pet is larger, like some breeds of dog, place both hands behind the rib cage and press in, thrusting upward, four to five times.

Do this until the object is dislodged or help has arrived, but beware, because a pet can bite you out of fear once they stop choking.

DIABETIC EMERGENCY

A diabetic can have an emergency if they have too much or too little insulin in their bodies. Too much will cause low blood sugar, or hypoglycemia, and can result in an insulin shock. Too little insulin causes high sugar levels, or hyperglycemia, and can lead to a diabetic coma. Symptoms will include loss of consciousness, blue and numb hands and feet, swelling of extremities, stomach pain, seizures, slurred speech and confusion, intense fatigue, muscle weakness, and a fruit odor to the breath.

Call 911.

Have the victim sit. In the event of a low blood sugar/hypoglycemic emergency, give the victim juice, jelly, sugary candies, or anything with a high sugar content. Have them continue to eat or drink, and monitor their glucose levels until they feel better.

If they are not conscious, put them in the recovery position, laying them on the left side with the right leg out.

Elevate feet and legs and check for signs of shock.

Keep dry and warm until help arrives.

If they have their medication or insulin with them, help them take the medication or administer the shot, or do it for them.

DROWNING

Whether it be a pool, lake, river, or ocean, helping save someone from drowning is a matter of time. If you see someone struggling, or if someone calls out that they are drowning, you must act fast, but first you must assess the situation to see if it is safe for you to rescue the victim.

Active drowning victims will wave their arms, bob in and out of the water, and appear distressed *even if* they are not yelling for help. They may not be able to yell. Once it is determined that a person is in trouble, you must first get them out of the water and onto shore or ground.

Call 911 as quickly as possible, or yell for a bystander to do so.

Do a reach assist if the drowning person is within arm's length. Reach out and grab their hand or arm, and help them out of the water. Do this while you are on your stomach face down, because if you are standing or kneeling, there is a possibility that the victim will drag you into the water.

Use your dominant hand to pull them out.

Use a throwing assist if there is an emergency float or life jacket nearby, or if there is something you can use, like rope or a line of cord, to pull them in with.

Use a swimming assist only if your own swimming skills are above par and you are strong enough to withstand the water and the weight of the victim.

Once the victim is on solid ground, do your ABCs. Check airway, breathing, and circulation. If they are conscious, they may vomit water, so help them lie on their side to do so.

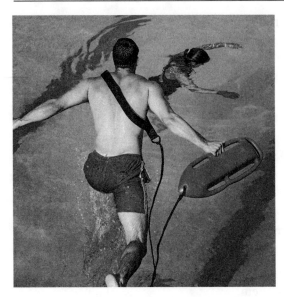

Lifeguards are equipped with a swimming or throwing assist to help them rescue people who are drowning, but if you don't have these, a rope may help you retrieve them from the water.

If they are unconscious, but have heart activity, begin rescue breathing. Again, watch for the expulsion of water from their lungs, and be ready to roll them on their side so they don't reswallow the water.

If they are not breathing and have no pulse or heart activity, begin CPR with breaths and continue until help arrives or they regain consciousness.

If you are drowning, try to take deep breaths and get on your back to float. If you can, call out for help, or swim closer to shore. Be prepared to vomit up water.

If you cannot swim, do not try to save someone out in the ocean or a river, or you will risk your own life. Ocean currents and moving waters of rivers can easily overtake you and make you the next victim. Call for help!

If you can swim, be prepared to use your body as a flotation device to get both of you out of the water.

In oceans and rivers, the water may be very cold, so watch for signs of hypothermia once you are back on shore.

If a person is injured and drowning, you must get them out of the water *first*, then treat the injury as best you can. This also applies to a heart attack or seizure. Get them *out* first, then treat on the ground.

If there are downed power lines or electric lines in the water, *stay out.* The victim will most likely have already died, and you risk your own life entering the water to find out.

GUNSHOT WOUNDS

Gunshot wounds can cause major damage to tissues and organs. The severity of a gunshot wound is determined by the penetration point, size, and speed of the bullet. It is actually the speed of the bullet that can determine the extent of the damage. A large gun can cause more damage than a small gun. The trauma created by a gunshot can be:

Penetration—destruction of flesh and tissue by the projectile (bullet)

Cavitation—damage to the body from the bullet's shock wave

Fragmentation—damage to the body caused by fragments of the bullet

If you or someone you are with is shot, call 911 immediately. If the wound has penetrated a vital organ, you may only have about ten minutes to get treated.

Until help arrives, do not move the victim or yourself, *unless* there is the possibility of more gunfire.

Assess the wound and look for an exit wound. Also look for additional bullet wounds.

Follow your basic first aid ABCs. Airway. Breathing. Circulation. Administer rescue breathing and CPR if needed until help arrives.

Control bleeding, and if you can see the bullet has exited the body, apply pressure and dressing to the wound on both sides.

Seal up a gunshot wound on the chest or abdomen with plastic sheeting or plastic wrap to keep air out of the wound.

Never apply a tourniquet unless it is the last resort and the bleeding is uncontrollable and severe. You will wrap a bandage or something that can serve as a bandage or belt tightly around the limb between the actual wound and the heart. Get as close to the wound area as you can. Wrap around several times and tie a tight knot, leaving some fabric to tie around a stick or board. Then you will twist the stick or board to tighten the bandage/belt and cut off all blood supply.

Bullet wounds are not the cause of death. It is the damage they do that you must treat. Do not wash out a wound or apply any kind of antiseptic, antibiotic, or ointment to the wound.

Treat the victim for shock if needed, but do *not* elevate the victim's legs if the gunshot wound is located above the waist or is near the spine, as that will drive more blood to the wound. If the wound is in the arm, you can elevate the legs.

Keep the victim in a comfortable position, but do not give them food or any liquids until help arrives.

If the victim was shot in the arm or leg, elevate the limb, and apply direct pressure to stop bleeding.

Chest Wounds

Special consideration must be taken for bullet wounds to the chest area, especially if you cannot find the exit wound. Because of a bullet's potential to do damage to the heart and lungs, do not move the victim if you can. There may be a sucking sound coming from the chest, and the victim may cough up blood or gasp for breath. This can indicate that the bullet has penetrated or collapsed a lung. A sucking chest wound victim must be placed in the recovery position so that blood doesn't fill the other lung.

HEAD INJURIES

The face and scalp are home to many blood vessels close to the skin's surface. Even a minor cut or wound to the head can create heavy bleeding that may look worse than the injury actually is.

MINOR HEAD INJURIES

Make sure you have clean hands by washing with soap and water. If you have access to latex gloves, use them.

If you do not have latex gloves, find some plastic bags or cloth you can put between your hands and the victim's wound. Bare hands should be a last resort.

Help the victim lie down.

Clear the wound of visible objects, but do not clean the wound.

Press down on the wound with gauze or whatever dressing you have available. In the event the wound contains an object that you are not sure can be removed, leave it, and press down on the wound around it.

Apply steady pressure for fifteen minutes, alternating with someone else if you get tired.

Replace the cloth if blood soaks through.

Keep applying pressure until help arrives or the bleeding has slowed or ceased. The wound may still ooze a little blood for up to an hour afterwards, but as long as blood is not flowing, you can treat the victim for any other injuries, including shock, or keep them calm and still until help arrives.

WHEN TO CALL 911 OR GO TO THE HOSPITAL

Even if there is no wound or bleeding, the victim may have a concussion. Are they displaying dizziness, confusion, slurred speech, or loss of consciousness? Can they talk at all, and are they aware of what day it is or where they are? Someone who has struck their head on the ground or another object needs emergency attention even if at the moment they appear fine. Call 911, or take the victim to the hospital and explain what happened.

When a child suffers a head wound of any kind, get help or get them to a hospital. Look for the following symptoms of a head injury:

- Younger than age one
- Neck pain
- Crying incessantly
- Gaping wound that needs stitches
- Blurred vision
- Vomiting
- Bad headache
- Loss of memory
- Fall from a height greater than three feet
- Head was struck by an object

The above applies to adults with a head injury as well, and anytime confusion, dizziness, vomiting, blurry vision, severe headache, or memory loss occurs, it can indicate a major head trauma that needs to be examined immediately in a hospital setting.

Other adult symptoms include abnormal behavior, sleepiness, inability to move arms and/or legs, unequal pupil size, a severe headache, and stiffness around neck.

Some major head injuries will involve bleeding within the brain tissue and the layers around the brain. This kind of hemorrhage and hematoma can be deadly, so call 911 or get to a hospital immediately.

Fracturing of the skull and spinal cord damage can occur in severe accidents, falls, and automobile crashes. Traumatic brain injuries are more severe than concussions. If you suspect the victim has broken their neck or back or damaged their spine, keep them still until help arrives and treat any bleeding issues that you can while you wait.

Do not wash the area around a deep head wound or apply pressure to a wound if you suspect a skull fracture beneath it. Do not remove any debris in the wound, as it may have penetrated the skull. Simply cover the wound with sterile gauze dressing.

Do not pick up a child that you suspect may have a head injury.

Never remove a helmet of someone you suspect has a head injury.

Only ever move a victim if they would be in more danger staying put, as in the case of a car fire or potential explosion.

If an object has impaled an eye, do not try to remove it. Treat any surrounding bleeding and wait for help. Treat the victim for shock.

Apply CPR if the victim is unconscious.

The best hope for severe head injuries of any kind is getting the victim to help. In the meantime, you can monitor them and do what you can to stop bleeding or treat for shock, but because of the delicate nature of head and spine injuries, you must be careful not to do anything that makes a bad situation worse.

Head injury symptoms may show up right away, but they also may not show up for days. If you or anyone else has been in an accident, crash, or other situation where the head was involved, get to a doctor immediately even if you feel fine and have no external issues.

INTERNAL INJURIES

In a traumatic injury or emergency, internal bleeding is the most serious consequence, but not always the most obvious one. There are internal bleeding emergencies that must be treated immediately with surgery in a hospital, and there are those that make themselves known over time or that stop on their own.

Concussions

A concussion is a traumatic brain injury that can occur from any type of blow to the head. It can result from a car accident, a fall, a sports injury, a playground accident, a fight injury, or any kind of injury that bumps or shakes the head area. When someone has a concussion, they may or may not pass out, but there will be symptoms such as disorientation, forgetfulness, dizziness, and more. During a concussion, the brain, which is normally protected by fluid, bangs or smashes into the skull. Symptoms can include:

- Confusion
- Lack of short-term memory
- Headache
- Ringing in the ears
- Vertigo
- Nausea and vomiting
- Fuzzy, blurred vision
- Problems with balance and walking
- Sensitivity to light and loud noises
- Slow reflexes

If the person was knocked unconscious, it is a good indicator that a concussion has occurred.

Over the days that follow, sleep disturbances may occur (sleeping more or less than usual) as well as mood changes and high anxiety or extreme fits of anger. Children may display additional symptoms such as:

- Excessive crying
- Sadness they cannot explain
- Temper tantrums
- Changes in behavior and eating and sleeping patterns

- Loss of balance and of the ability to walk
- Mumbling and stumbling
- Unequal pupil size
- Seizures
- Slurred speech
- Loss of skills such as toilet training or using utensils
- Loss of memory and lack of attention

When dealing with seniors, we often pass off some of the symptoms of concussion as aging, so if a head injury is suspected, or there is a visible sign of a bruise, take them to their doctor right away. Do the same if you suffer from a head injury and begin displaying any symptoms. Call your own doctor or go to urgent care right away.

Once a concussion is diagnosed, usually involving CT scans or MRIs to image the brain, you will be treated and given a plan for healing, which usually involves a lot of rest and avoiding demanding activities that can further jar the brain and cause additional injury. Don't try to "treat" a possible concussion yourself. Do not drive or even ride on a bike or motorcycle until you are cleared by your doctor, because sometimes symptoms don't pop up right away, and they can last for weeks before you feel any relief at all.

If you are the parent of a teen who plays football or other sports at school, be aware of changes in their behavior and complaints of symptoms. Concussions from sports activities happen all the time and often go unrecognized and untreated. You want to make sure you get help as soon as possible after the injury occurred.

The best ways to avoid concussions are to use seat belts when in a vehicle, wear a helmet when riding any kind of bike or participating in sports activities, and avoiding potential hazards that can lead to a fall.

Do not ever underestimate the damage a concussion can cause. Often a bonk on the head doesn't seem like much, and we joke about having a "hard head," but to the brain inside the skull, there can be invisible stress and injury that reveals themselves via symptoms that people might pass off as just not feeling well in general. It is also a fact that once you have one concussion, it is easier to suffer from another one later. People who play football for a living know this too well, being susceptible to multiple concussions. The same goes for hockey players, soccer players, even rodeo riders. Any situation that can result in the head meeting another solid object, or an impact from an explosion or movement as in a car accident, is a risky situation.

When it comes to concussions, use your head—pun intended—and get medical help immediately, even if you are the victim.

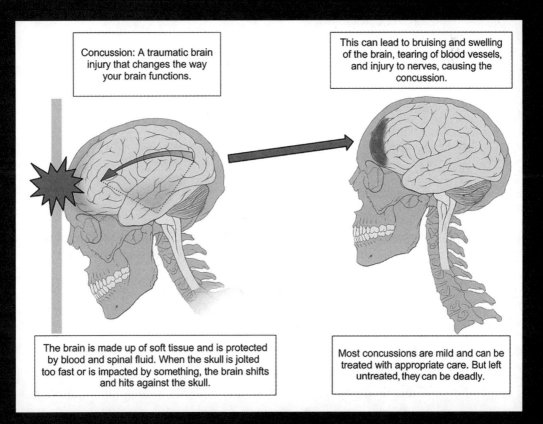

Concussion: A traumatic brain injury that changes the way your brain functions.

This can lead to bruising and swelling of the brain, tearing of blood vessels, and injury to nerves, causing the concussion.

The brain is made up of soft tissue and is protected by blood and spinal fluid. When the skull is jolted too fast or is impacted by something, the brain shifts and hits against the skull.

Most concussions are mild and can be treated with appropriate care. But left untreated, they can be deadly.

What happens when someone gets a concussion.

Trauma can be from many sources. Blunt force trauma occurs when the body, or some part of the body, crashes or collides into a solid object at high speed, causing extreme injury to skin, muscle, tissue, and even bone. It can also occur when the body is struck by a blunt object, such as in an assault or a workplace accident or vehicle crash. Penetrating traumas occur when a foreign object penetrates the body, as in a gunshot wound or stab wound or impaling by a sharp object.

Internal bleeding from any kind of trauma can occur inside the head (intracranial hemorrhage), the heart, lungs, large blood vessels, and vital organs in the abdominal area. All are deadly if not treated quickly and correctly. General symptoms might include:

Pain and swelling in the abdominal area

Severe headache

Lightheadedness and dizziness

Loss of consciousness

High blood pressure

Low blood pressure

Severe weakness

Numb areas on body

Nausea and vomiting

Diarrhea

Sweaty skin

Severe bleeding from a deep wound

Swelling and pain in an affected limb

If you are a victim of some type of trauma, or you are trying to treat a victim, call 911 immediately or get to a hospital and let the staff know the type of injury that occurred.

If you cannot call for help, remember the ABCs and make sure the airway is clear and breathing and circulation are normal. If not, administer rescue breathing and CPR immediately.

Do not move the victim.

Treat for bleeding.

Treat for shock.

Sadly, there is not a lot in the way of emergency first aid you can do for someone who has severe internal bleeding except try to get them to a hospital as soon as you can. The treatment they need will usually involve scans and surgery, so keep them still, watching the ABCs, keeping them comfortable, stopping any bleeding, and avoiding shock.

Internal Bleeding Symptoms

Symptoms of internal bleeding in the head include:

- Weakness and/or numbness on one side of the body
- Severe headache that comes on suddenly
- Difficulty speaking and writing
- Difficulty swallowing
- Unresponsiveness
- Blurred vision
- Poor hearing
- Tingling and numbness in the extremities
- Stupor
- Loss of consciousness

Symptoms of internal bleeding in the chest and abdominal area include:

- Pain in the chest or abdomen
- Shortness of breath
- Dizziness and vertigo upon sitting up or standing
- Nausea and vomiting
- Bruising around the navel and the sides of the abdomen
- Bloody urine and/or stool
- Black, tarry stool
- Bleeding from mouth, nose, eyes, ears, or anus

LOSS OF CONSCIOUSNESS

A conscious person, even if groggy and disoriented, should be asked their name, where they are, and the date. If they answer correctly, keep them warm, dry, and treat for potential shock until help arrives.

If they are in shock or fading in and out of consciousness, put them in the recovery position, and start triage for three areas:

Respiration—Are they breathing? If not, check to make sure their airway is clear.

Perfusion—Press on the skin, and it should go white, then return to color after two seconds. If not, it means capillaries are not refilling.

Mentation—Cannot answer questions once conscious, which can mean head injury, internal injury, and severe disorientation.

POISON EXPOSURE

Treating poison emergencies comes down to identifying what the poison substance was. From household cleaning agents and chemicals to overdoses of prescription drugs to ingestion of toxic berries and mushrooms to a child swallowing a button battery, poisonings account for thousands of hospitalizations every year. Timing is key, because the quicker the victim can get the ingested substance out of the body, the better for their overall recovery and survival. Symptoms of poisoning include:

- Burns around the mouth
- Stains or discoloration around the mouth
- Vomiting
- Dizziness
- Confusion
- Chemical odor to the breath
- Drowsiness
- Difficulty breathing
- Loss of consciousness

If you or someone else suspects poisoning of any type, call 911 immediately, or call the Poison Control Hotline (open twenty-four hours a day) at 800-222-1222.

Try to locate the poison. Look for berries, food items, pill bottles, open bottles of cleaning or chemical agents, sources of fumes, mouth burns (suggesting chemical poisoning), breath odors, and empty battery packages. Often the bottle or container will include instructions on what to do if the contents are ingested. Follow those instructions while waiting for help to arrive. If you are not alone, you can have another person bag the poisonous substance for emergency personnel. If you suspect a child or someone has ingested poisonous berries or plants from outdoors, see if that person can bag some of the berries or plants for expert identification when help arrives.

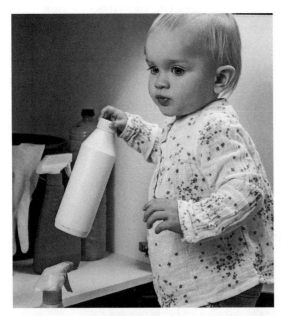

According to the Centers for Disease Control, in the United States each day three hundred children under nineteen end up in the emergency room because of poisoning, and two of those children will die.

Check the ABCs. Airway. Breathing. Circulation.

If the victim is vomiting, monitor their breathing to make sure the airway does not become obstructed. If the victim is on their back, turn them on their side. Do *not* use anything to induce vomiting unless you are instructed to do so by emergency personnel or poison control. Expert organizations no longer suggest using syrup of ipecac to induce vomiting, so throw any bottles you have in the trash!

If the victim is breathing and conscious, ask what they ingested, and be sure to alert emergency personnel when they arrive or on the phone with poison control.

Keep the person comfortable until help arrives, and monitor the ABCs.

Be ready for the victim to experience convulsions or seizures. Treat for seizure (see "Seizures" below) until help arrives.

If the victim is unconscious, administer rescue breathing and/or CPR as needed, but be careful, if the victim has mouth burns, that you do not expose your own mouth to the toxic substance during rescue breaths. You may only be able to do CPR until help arrives. Never put your own life in danger.

If the victim came into contact with something poisonous to the skin or eyes, call Poison Control and they will talk you through the process. If the actual poison has been identified, have it with you when you call.

Remove any traces of the toxic substance by removing clothing from the affected area of the body and discarding it.

Flush the affected area with lukewarm, room-temperature water, including the eyes, for at least fifteen minutes. If the victim states that their eyes are burning, continue flushing with water until help arrives.

Have the victim blink repeatedly if a toxic substance has entered the eye. Do not let them rub the eye area!

Continue to monitor the victim's breathing and pulse until help arrives.

FOOD POISONING

Almost everyone has experienced a good bout of food poisoning. Bad seafood, mushrooms, salads—there are many culprits. Nausea and vomiting are the usual symptoms, along with stomach pains and diarrhea. Severe dehydration is the biggest danger during food poisoning, so the victim must drink clear fluids, starting out with small sips to avoid vomiting and graduating to more as the symptoms subside.

Do not give a victim solid foods until vomiting has ceased, and then start with bland foods free of heavy grease, spices, sugars, and oils. Saltine crackers, bread, plain rice, and even bananas are a good start until the victim can tolerate more.

Ask the victim's doctor about administering any anti-nausea/diarrhea medications, because some can increase the risk of diarrhea and lead to more dehydration.

If symptoms persist or get worse, see a doctor after three days, especially if there is fever, bloody or dark stools, prolonged or bloody vomiting, increased heart rate, breathing difficulties, cessation of urination, or severe stomach pain.

SEIZURES

According to the Centers for Disease Control and Prevention, one out of ten people have had a seizure in their lifetime. Most of us think of seizures as something only epileptics during a grand mal experience, but many situations can cause seizures. Always call 911 in the following circumstances:

- The victim has never had a previous seizure.
- The victim is injured during the seizure.
- The victim experiences more than one seizure.
- The victim is in water at the time.
- The victim is pregnant, diabetic, or has a known heart condition.
- The seizure lasts beyond five minutes.

If you cannot call for help, do the following:

- Lay the person on their side on the floor to assist breathing.
- Clear the area around them of anything sharp or blunt, including furniture, to prevent injury.
- Protect them under their head with a soft blanket, jacket, or pillow.
- Take off their eyeglasses.
- Loosen tight clothing that might inhibit breathing.
- Time the seizure.

If you cannot get the victim on their back during the seizure, watch for vomiting and excess saliva, and use your fingers to gently clear the mouth.

Stay with the victim until the seizure ends, and ask them what happened when they can talk. Comfort the victim, and ask about medical issues that may have caused the seizure. They may also be wearing or carrying a medical emergency ID. If they have meds on them, help administer the meds. The victim may be sleepy, but be sure they are aware of their surroundings and fully conscious.

If you have transport, get the victim to a hospital to be checked out.

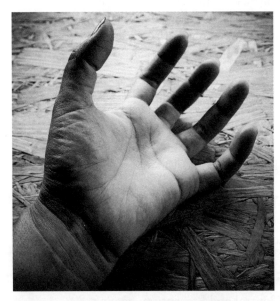

Watching someone have a seizure can be frightening, but you can help them get through it by calling for help and protecting them from injuring themselves until help arrives.

Things *Not* to Do

- Do not hold or restrict the victim during the seizure.
- Do not place *anything* in the victim's mouth. They will *not* swallow their tongue as so many falsely believe.
- Do not administer rescue breathing, as they will be able to breathe on their own afterwards.
- Do not give the victim food or drink until you know they are fully alert or are told to do so by emergency personnel.

- *Do not put anything in the mouth to keep the tongue down.* Use your fingers if you need to help.

Lay them on their left side, with their right leg out in the recovery position.

Protect the victim, and be sure to help keep their airway open, especially if their tongue is getting in the way.

SHOCK

In the event of an injury, a victim may begin to go into shock. They may appear pale, disoriented, and confused. Along with keeping a victim breathing and conscious, shock is absolutely critical because it indicates ineffective blood circulation. If a victim is in shock for too long, they will experience death of cells, tissues, and eventually entire organs. Signs of shock are:

- Shallow, rapid breathing
- Capillary refill greater than two seconds
- Inability to respond to or follow simple commands
- Pale skin or changes in skin color

To treat shock:

- Lay the victim on their back.
- Elevate their feet 6 to 60 inches (15–150 centimeters) above heart level.
- Maintain an open airway.
- Control bleeding if necessary.
- Keep the victim warm and dry by laying them on a blanket and covering them with a blanket.
- Try not to move until help arrives. If you must, move as gently as possible.

WOUND CARE

Whether it's a small cut or scrape or a gaping wound, it must be taken care of to avoid infection and control bleeding. A wound should be cleaned with water or flushed with a mild mix of soap and water, then rinsed with plain water. Never scrub a wound. You can irrigate the wound with a turkey baster or syringe if there is no running water to hold it under.

After the wound is cleaned, it must be covered with a dressing and bandage. The dressing is what covers the wound itself, and the bandages cover the dressing to keep it in place.

If the wound is bleeding, apply the bandage tighter over the dressing to add pressure and control bleeding.

If there is no bleeding, you can remove the dressing and flush the wound with water every four to six hours. Check for signs of swelling and infection. Signs of infection:

- Swelling around the wound
- Discoloration: darkening color
- Pus and discharge from the wound
- Red striations from the wound
- Foul odor from the wound
- Fever

If infection is present, you must treat the infection. Wash the wound with soap and water. Use a tiny amount of antibiotic ointment. Cover the wound with a dressing or gauze. Keep the wound clean and dry for twenty-four hours, then change the dressing while wearing sterile medical gloves to avoid spreading infection.

In the case of a severely infected wound, call 911 or go to the hospital. This also applies to amputations, such as fingers cut off by machinery or impaled objects in the body. Do not attempt to treat these yourself.

For amputations, try to save the tissue part by wrapping it in a clean material and putting it into a plastic bag. Keep the tissue part cool and with the victim. Get them to the hospital.

For impaled objects, immobilize the impaled body area.

Do not remove the object unless it obstructs the airway and prevents breathing.

Control bleeding at the wound site, but try not to put pressure on the impaled object.

Clean and dress the wound as best you can, and wrap dressings around the impaled object to keep it immobilized until help arrives or you can get to the hospital.

BASIC TRIAGE

Triage is simply the act of initially assessing victims and sorting them into treatment groups, based on the severity of their injuries. Once triage assessment is over, you begin treating the victims you can or transporting them to a treatment area for when first responders arrive. This also includes moving dead bodies to a designated "morgue" area. In major disasters, you may find yourself performing triage just to save your own family and friends.

If you come upon a group of people injured after a disaster, or your entire family is injured, even if you are not professionally trained in triage, you can still help. The first thing you can do, if you yourself are fine and not injured, is call 911, then perform a quick visual assessment of the situation and the victims.

Look around for any potential hazards that still exist after the disaster, such as crumbling buildings, loose chimneys, broken glass, sharp objects and debris, and downed electrical lines.

How many victims are there, and what are the stages of injury? Are there any victims out of sight, perhaps trapped under debris? Treat the worst-affected victims first, but try to keep an eye on other victims, as their situations may worsen.

If anyone is ambulatory and can help you, get them involved in treating others.

If someone is trapped beneath debris, but able to talk, tell them *not to move* until help arrives. You may need to treat others before coming back to try to help them, but do

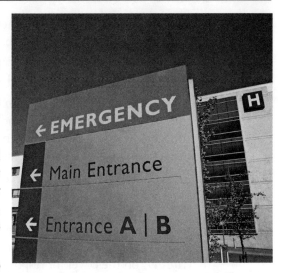

Triage is the process of evaluating a patient's illness or injury and prioritizing which patients are helped first based on need. This is done all the time in hospital emergency rooms, but you might find yourself having to assess the injured on your own after a disaster.

not attempt to move debris without help, as it may end up caving in on the victim and causing grievous injury, even death. If they can move without causing more debris to fall, talk them through helping to stop their bleeding or using their own clothing to treat and dress a wound.

Treat victims systematically, starting with those who need the ABCs and may be in shock, moving to the least injured. Do a quick head-to-toe assessment, and treat the most pressing injury on a victim first, such as breathing and bleeding.

A head-to-toe assessment will look like this:

- Airway obstruction
- Excessive bleeding
- Signs of shock
- Severe pain
- Disfigurement
- Bruising
- Swelling

The goal is to determine the type of injury, the extent of injury, and what treatment is needed.

Those who need rescue breathing or CPR come first, then treat the heavily wounded and bleeding, then those who have fractures and lighter bleeding.

If you are alone and there are a number of victims, use your judgment. Clearly someone who is not conscious, but has a pulse, should be attended to before someone with a broken leg.

Try to get the least injured to treat themselves.

Be aware of the mental status of some victims, as they may look fine physically but may have suffered a head injury or be going into shock. Often victims will demand attention even when their injuries are slight, and you have to be strong in telling them that you must attend first to the most severe cases.

The last thing anyone ever wants is to come across a dead victim. But it may happen in a major disaster. Do not stop to move or cover the dead if it means valuable lost time when you could be treating the living. But once the situation has stabilized, move the dead body out of sight of the living victims, cover it with a jacket or sheet, and if you have something you can mark with, write "D" on the cover for responders when they arrive.

Triage is meant for the trained, but even the above tasks can help you help others until trained personnel are on site. Never put yourself in any kind of danger, though, to help others. You will become another victim that first responders will need to deal with if you do. You are *not* selfish if you cannot help everyone who needs you. Help yourself first, then reach out to others if you can.

MOVING VICTIMS

In any emergency, big or small, you may be called upon to move victims away from dangerous locations or hazards. If the victim is ambulatory and can move themselves, you should assist them, because they may not be aware of their own injuries and weakness. Depending on the situation and whether or not you have help, you may need to carry a victim out of a danger zone.

The one-person arm carry is the most basic. Bending at the knees, you will reach around the victim's back and under their knees. Supporting the victim, raise yourself up with your legs so the victim's back stays straight. Keep in mind the size and weight of the victim and how far you need to move them.

The one-person pack-strap carry is another method. This time, you stand with your back to the victim. Place the victim's arms around your shoulders so you can grab their hands at your chest level. Hoist the victim up, and bend forward so that the victim's feet clear the floor.

You can also drag the victim to safety even if you are alone. Wrap the victim in a blanket. Squat down and grab an edge of the blanket, dragging the victim to safety. If you have help, you can each take a corner of the blanket, with the victim lying in the center.

Sometimes there won't be blankets around, so you can drag a victim by grasping them under the arms or by the ankles and pulling them to safety. Be careful of dragging the victim over rough ground or debris, and only use this method if none other is available.

If there are others around, you can have the victim sit in a chair, then have one of you carry by holding the front chair legs, and the other holding the chair back. Or do a two-person carry where one of you squats at the victim's head and grasps them behind their midsection, and the other stands between the victim's knees and supports them outside each knee.

Obviously, it is easier to move a human body with help, but it can be done alone. Just be sure never to put yourself in harm's way to move a victim, and if you suspect they have a head injury or internal injuries and it is not a hazardous situation, wait for emergency help to arrive.

RESCUING A TRAPPED VICTIM

If you come across a victim trapped beneath debris that cannot be easily lifted off, such as concrete blocks or stone slabs, you can help. Leveraging and cribbing are techniques that can move and stabilize even heavy debris enough to retrieve the victim. It helps if you have a few people to help, as you will want a couple of people to work on leverage, while the others crib beneath the debris.

Leveraging involves using some object such as a metal pole or rod to wedge beneath the debris, with a stationary object beneath it to act as a fulcrum. When you lean down on the lever, it is forced down over the fulcrum, and the far end of the lever lifts the object. The cribber than places pieces of wood as a framework beneath the object, preferably in a box shape. There are different cribbing patterns, but the idea is to create a stable base that can be added to each time the lever lifts the object higher, until it is high enough for the rescuers to reach the victim and drag them out. There are many cribbing videos online that show the patterns of setting the wood pieces in. Basically, you move slowly and lift an inch, crib an inch, rather than try to lift the object too high and risk it crashing down onto the victim if the levers break.

But you do not just walk away once the victim is free. You must then reverse the whole process and lower the object back to the ground so that it doesn't present an additional hazard.

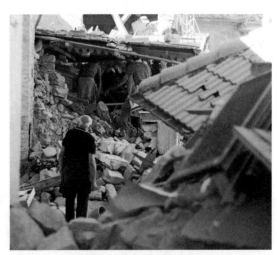

Rescue teams dig through rubble with their bare hands in this photo from the 2016 Amatrice, Italy, earthquake. Victims often survive collapsed buildings by being fortunate to find a sturdy doorway or interior room.

SANITATION AND HYGIENE

When handling another person's blood or body fluids, use protective sterile gloves and a face mask. Try to avoid letting bodily fluids touch your skin, mouth, nose, or eyes.

Always dispose of used bandages, cloths, and dressings safely in a plastic bag, trash bag, or sealed container.

Be sure to dispose of used gloves and face masks properly, as they may be infected with contaminants.

In a major disaster or emergency, be aware that frightened people may evacuate their bowels or urinate uncontrollably. If you are able to help them find water, soap, and clean clothing, do so. Dispose of their soiled clothing in a plastic bag or trash bag.

If there are no toilets available, you can make one with a bucket and a trash bag. Be sure to dispose of the bag, once full, by tying off and sealing it and placing it in an area away from people and animals. If you have something to mark with, mark the bags as "medical waste."

Never expose yourself to possible disease-spreading germs, such as in a biohazard situation. Do not risk your own life!

PSYCHOLOGICAL TRAUMA

A disaster or emergency does more than cause physical harm. It can also cause psychological trauma and even PTSD, post-traumatic stress disorder. PTSD can occur after exposure to a stressful, frightening, or dangerous situation, including a traumatic accident, act of war or terrorism, violent crime, or natural disaster. According to the U.S. Substance Abuse and Mental Health Services Administration (SAMHSA), mental health can be affected not just during the event, but long after it, causing an acute stress reaction and an inability to cope with everyday life. Children will respond quite differently than adults and often hide or suppress their fearful emotions by means of misbehavior and acting out.

Psychological first aid goes beyond just keeping yourself or a victim calm. Often signs of psychological trauma don't show up until weeks or months after the disaster took place, and then it may appear as symptoms that might be misconstrued as something else, such as general anxiety or irritability. It might be easy to pass this off as just plain old stress, but that would be a mistake and a disservice to the victim.

Following a disaster, there will be feelings of panic, terror, fear, paranoia, anxiety, sadness, grief, depression, even suicidal thoughts from survivor's guilt or the shame of not being able to save a loved one. Any kind of loss, whether it be a home or treasured material items, a beloved pet, or a loved one, will cause damage that goes far beyond the physical. Feelings of helplessness and power-lessness can turn into everything from extreme rage to complete withdrawal.

If there is an ongoing threat, such as in war, the pressure may become so overwhelming that people will not be able to cope and may turn to drugs or alcohol. Physical illness will show up as well as symptoms of mental illness. Obviously, the quicker you or any victim can get professional help via therapy or counseling, the better the chances of offsetting some of the severity of the trauma. Professionals can provide you or your loved ones with coping techniques and mechanisms that directly address the event, nightmares and flashbacks, psychosomatic illness, and the inability to carry on a normal life after the disaster. This is especially critical for children, who are deeply affected by traumatic situations but often incapable of expressing their feelings and fears.

Whether the emergency or disaster is massive, such as war or nuclear attack, or a regional earthquake or hurricane, or a home accident that injures or kills a loved one, there are steps you can take to cope:

Talk about it! Talk openly about what happened and how you feel about it. Express your anger, fears, and feelings of helplessness. Vent when you must, but in a healthy way.

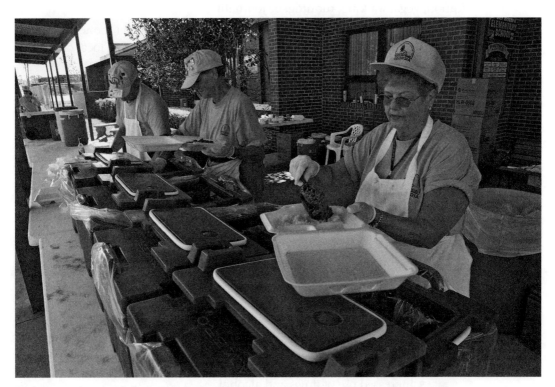

Red Cross volunteers help provide food to Florida hurricane victims. Volunteering your time and services to a charity can help you overcome your own personal traumas by helping others.

Avoid numbing your feelings with food, drugs, alcohol, prescription pills, etc. Self-medicating can be harmful.

Get help from a professional. If the family was affected, seek family counseling so you can all talk about your fears and express your needs, then put a plan into action.

If your workplace offers grief or trauma counseling, take it! Often we let shame get in the way of seeking help, only to find that we are not alone in needing help. The author of this book can attest to this. After the Northridge Earthquake, my company, Warner Bros. Records, offered trauma counseling in the huge meeting room. I was embarrassed to go but thought it might help. Imagine my surprise to find the room packed, including higher-level executives, all seeking to talk and express their feelings of fear, grief, and suffering. There were many tears shed that day. *Get help if you need it.* This is not a time to care about "saving face."

Stay away from news of the disaster to avoid adding more stress and anxiety. Keep children from watching news, and try to distract them from seeking out news on their cell phones and gadgets. An adult can keep up on any developments in the news that might affect the family unit.

Employ any relaxation technique that works for you, such as prayer, meditation, yoga, walking, running, or journaling.

Volunteer! One of the best ways to get over a trauma sooner is to help others who are in immediate need. Contact the Red Cross or a local crisis center, donate blood, or work at a shelter or soup kitchen.

Refrain from projecting anger and fears onto cultural and ethnic groups. This does no one any good and often leads to a cycle of violence and hatred that is like a runaway train. Even terrorist acts are not indicative of the beliefs of an entire culture, and all nations are capable of terrorist attacks on others, including war. Focus instead on the common humanity we share. This is important if you have children who were affected by the disaster or emergency, because they learn from adults how to react and respond to their environment and fellow humans. Keep in mind, too, that with children, some of the trauma will show up later in behaviors such as learning disabilities, developmental delays, bullying, self-harm, and suicide.

Reach out to others you suspect may be suffering. Symptoms to watch for include:

- Withdrawal
- Oversleeping
- Self-medicating
- Lack of impulse control
- Increased use of drugs and alcohol
- Anger and rage

- Irritability
- Depression
- Survivor guilt
- Feelings of helplessness
- Fatigue and weakness
- Nightmares, especially with children
- Excessive crying and mood swings
- Hypervigilance
- Denial
- Loss of concentration
- Insomnia
- Relationship discord
- Numbness
- Self-blame
- Cutting and self-harm

Right after a disaster, people, including yourself, may have a tendency to shut down in order to internally process what has happened. But if that period of being closed off goes on too long, they run the risk of being paralyzed by their own fears and developing post-traumatic stress disorder. Even though you or your loved ones may not want to "get back to normal" that soon, getting out and exercising, getting back into family or personal routines, and finding positive things to do and look forward to can go a long way toward recovery. Eating healthy foods, staying hydrated, and communicating with loved ones and friends are good medicine and cost you nothing, but they can pay off in huge dividends by helping to overcome debilitating trauma and fear.

Watch carefully for PTSD to flare up among our veterans. If you have a loved one who is a veteran, a disaster or emergency will trigger them, as will loud noises and traumatic scenes of injuries and death. Be extra observant of their behaviors and responses, and help them get help if needed. Veterans are often the first to respond and step up bravely during a disaster but often the last to recover from it. The same also applies if you have a loved one who is a first responder such as a firefighter, police officer, EMS, hospital worker, nurse, triage nurse, or doctor who may be on the scene and totally immersed in helping others. Once the disaster has abated, these people are at high risk of developing PTSD, even with their extensive training, if they are not able to properly process and deal with what they've experienced.

Be extra patient and understanding. Not everyone responds and processes trauma the same way and in the same time frame, and pressuring someone to "get over it" more quickly than they are able only adds to their existing difficulties.

Also be ready for these symptoms to pop up again later if triggered by a new situation. For example, people who experience massive earthquakes find themselves still reacting out of panic and the original trauma's effects a year later when a small aftershock occurs. If you have ever been a victim of a crime such as an assault, you know that it is possible to have nightmares years later, even after you feel you have accepted and dealt with the original event. The author of this book can attest to feeling PTSD symptoms over a year after living through a major Los Angeles earthquake, and even being triggered into a state of hypervigilance years later whenever a large truck would drive by or a high wind would rattle the windows.

The mind holds on to trauma and it also gets "stuck" in the body in the form of tension, aches, tightness, and even digestive and breathing problems.

Some things *not* to do:

- Never minimize the pain and suffering of any survivor or victim.
- Never say that you "understand" what they are going through, as you cannot possibly understand their personal perspective.
- Never tell a victim not to cry or express anger.
- Never tell a victim, "Don't feel bad, things could be worse," as that is cruel and heartless and implies the victim is in some way lucky to have suffered.
- Never *ever* tell a victim that a death or disaster is "God's will," as this can result in more grief, anger, and sadness and does not help someone with different beliefs.

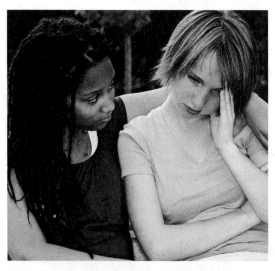

When consoling a friend or loved one who has endured a trauma, the best thing you can do is simply offer sympathy and tell them you are there for them.

The above statements will always elicit a negative reaction and add insult to injury. A simple "I am so sorry" will suffice. People grieve in different ways and according to different time frames, and never should be judged or guilted into doing otherwise, or it can impede their overall healing.

The most difficult part of psychological trauma comes when you must tell a victim that their loved one has died. If you are ever in that sad situation, remove the person from noisy surroundings, sit them down, and tell them directly. "I am so sorry to tell you that so-and-so has died." Let them react and grieve, and be there for support if they need you, but be kind, be calm, and be understanding without being offensive and insulting. They may not know what to do, so help

THE DISASTER SURVIVAL GUIDE

them find the answers and resources they need, but expect them to be in a deep state of grief and despair.

Disaster and trauma psychology is something first responders and other emergency service personnel will be trained in, so once help arrives you can ask them to take over the situation. You have done all you can.

The physical and emotional toll of disasters can show up years later, especially if you or the victim is a master at suppressing feelings and trying to "power through" grief. Many people think it is a sign of strength to suppress their feelings or be there for others, but not for themselves. Take the time to feel, process, grieve, and mourn, even if you have not lost a loved one. What you have lost is a sense of safety and security and trust that the world around you is a safe place, and that takes a long time to deal with, process, and ultimately cope with so that you can one day wake up feeling ready for living life to the fullest again.

DEATH

Yes, we will all have to face death—our own and the death of those we love. It can be especially traumatic when a disaster takes a life away, possibly right in front of our eyes. We then must deal with not only the loss of the person and the natural grief that follows but also the potential guilt and shame that we were not able to save them or help them. Survivor guilt can eat away at people and turn into full-on PTSD with nightmares and anxiety, even psychosomatic illnesses. It is important to understand that we cannot save everyone from a major disaster and that often the best we can do may not be enough. Even emergency services personnel, firefighters, police, and EMS cannot always avoid losing someone or not getting there in time to save someone.

If you find yourself in the position of helping others through the death of someone they loved, treat yourself gently. You are not a professional therapist, but you can do some small things to help, such as provide creature comforts to the person until help arrives, let them cry on your shoulder, and let them talk if they feel the need. Some people go quiet and need to be observed for shock. Often just being there makes someone feel less alone, but don't beat yourself up if you cannot stop the person's grief. You shouldn't even try. Grief is necessary.

Try to avoid all religious-oriented talk, unless the person asks to pray or asks you to sit with them in prayer. You don't want to offend someone by suggesting something that they may not believe in or accept as their religious tradition, so let them lead in this respect. Be humble, even if your beliefs are different. This person has just lost someone important to them. You can set aside your personal beliefs for a few minutes to help them grieve.

Do not leave someone alone, especially a child, with a trauma such as witnessing a death. Wait for help to arrive if you possibly can. Children will be particularly affected by a death and may completely withdraw or scream uncontrollably. Do not yell or scold them. Have compassion and empathy.

If the dead person is in the room with the mourners, ask if they would like you to cover the body or possibly carry it to another room. Sometimes the presence of a dead loved one offers comfort, but at other times it can add to the trauma. Ask for help if you need to move the body. Do so gently and respectfully. Think of how you would want your own loved ones treated in such a situation.

You can ask a family member if there is something special you can place on the body. But if the other members look too distraught to approach, leave them alone with their thoughts. This is one situation where you can do only so much and no more. Death is final, and you cannot say or do anything that will alleviate their pain, so don't try. Just be kind, see what you *can* do to help, and leave quietly when help arrives.

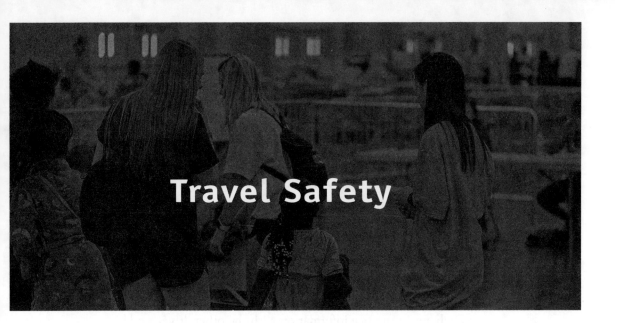

Travel Safety

We spend so much time out in the world, it is important to know what to do if there is an emergency when we are far from the comforts of home. Whether we are on a road trip, taking a train across the country, flying to another country, or relaxing on a cruise ship, things can happen, and the more we are prepared in advance, the better chances we have of surviving.

AUTOMOBILES

Imagine how many people are out on the roadways on any given day or night—it is mind-boggling. Although most of our trips pass without incident, now and then there is an accident or mechanical issue that can send us into a panic if we don't know how to react and respond.

IF YOUR CAR BREAKS DOWN

Before you hit the road, especially for longer trips, make sure your vehicle is in good operating condition by checking all fluid levels, lights, signal lights, belts, hoses, and windshield wipers.

Fill tires to the correct level as dictated in your car's operations manual.

Have a full tank of gas.

Keep a spare tire in the rear or trunk of the vehicle.

Make sure seat belts are in good working order.

Make sure the registration and insurance information is in the glove compartment, along with a number to call for roadside service in an emergency.

If you have a breakdown and you cannot get the car running again, get the car over to the side of the road safely, and put on your hazard lights.

Call roadside service for help. Many highways and freeways have call boxes if you don't have a cell phone. Be sure to give them as exact a location as you can.

Do not get out of the car and stand outside waiting if you are on the highway or freeway, as this is how many people are killed by passing cars. Do not assume people are paying attention!

IN A MINOR ACCIDENT

Do not leave the scene of the accident, as most state laws require you to stop. You can be charged with hit-and-run if someone you hit is injured, and even in an accident where you are not at fault.

Make sure everyone involved is fine, and move the cars off the roadway. Turn on hazard lights on both cars.

Be civil. Everyone makes mistakes.

Exchange insurance information with the other driver, and be civil.

Take photos with cell phone cameras of damage to both cars to document the damage at the time of the accident.

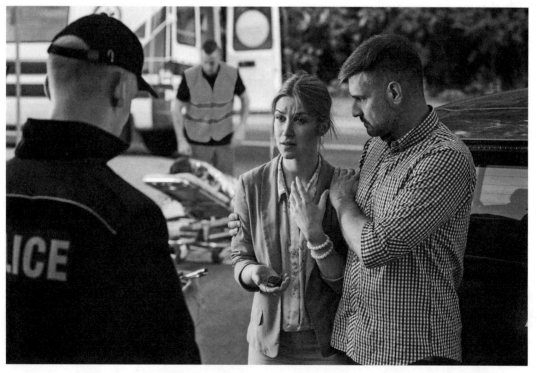

If you are in a major car accident, you must file a police report, even if there were no injuries. Follow police instructions to the letter.

File a police report just to be safe and avoid someone coming back months later claiming they were severely injured or that their car was further damaged.

In a Major Accident

Do all of the above, but focus on checking to make sure everyone is fine. If anyone needs medical attention, call 911 and begin giving any first aid you are capable of.

You must file a police report in a major accident, especially if there were injuries.

Cooperate with the police, and tell the truth. Often they are trained to tell who hit whom from damage location and marks on the vehicles. Do not admit fault, even if you think it was your fault, as the other driver may also have been at fault. The insurance companies involved declare fault.

Do *not* sign anything unless it is a police report or insurance company paperwork.

Stay calm and do not get involved in blame games and fighting, as this can escalate into a violent altercation. Document the damage, and follow police instructions on what to do next.

Brake Failure

One of the scariest things that can happen to a driver is to lose your breaks. Keeping up on maintenance is important, but if it does happen:

Stay calm and put on hazard lights to let other drivers know there is a problem.

If the brakes are not working, check to make sure there is nothing like a plastic water bottle lodged under the brake pedal.

Downshift the car to low gear, and reduce speed, but do it in stages.

If your car has an ABS, or anti-lock breaking system, press hard on the brake pedal. After a few seconds the brakes should begin to work. If you have an older car with no ABS, pump the brake pedal.

Move the car to the side of the road as you slow speed.

Put on your parking brake to help you reduce speed.

Look for a place where there is a lot of gravel, sand, or even grass to help slow the car down.

A small hill or incline can also help slow down the car and get speed low enough to bring it to a stop. You can even steer towards bushes or hedges to drive into, but beware of driving into a large tree, which can be fatal.

Do *not* put the car in reverse to slow down.

Do *not* put the car in park to slow down.

Once you are safely stopped, call for help and take the car to have the brakes fixed immediately. Don't assume it was a "one-time" thing.

STEERING FAILURE

Although power steering failure is rare with today's vehicles, it can happen. Follow the same rules as above, but realize that you will have greater and greater difficulty steering the wheel and getting it to turn as the power steering system fails. Use what strength you can to turn the wheel enough to get yourself off the road and stop the car.

DRIVING IN RAIN, SNOW, AND ICE

So you are driving on an icy road and your car begins to skid. What do you do? Don't panic! Skidding can occur when you over-steer and the front wheels begin to turn, but the back wheels spin out, causing the back end of the car to fishtail. A skid can also occur when you under-steer and the car makes a wide turn, usually on wet pavement. The car can also slide side to side in a skid. If you have your foot on the brake, let up slowly.

If your foot is on the gas pedal, take your foot off the gas, and steer in the direction you wish the wheels to go, not the direction of the skid.

If you have standard brakes, pump the brakes gently as you steer the car.

If you have ABS brakes, do not pump. Apply steady pressure to the brakes.

If your car hydroplanes after driving through a puddle of water, you will lose both tire traction and your ability to steer the vehicle. Once you feel your tires have regained traction on the pavement, there will be a small jolt forward in the direction you are steering, but don't be alarmed. Follow the above rules and hope that others are aware of your car's situation and can assist in getting out of your way.

STUCK!

If your car gets stuck in mud or snow, do not spin the wheels, as this will dig you in deeper.

Try turning the wheels from side to side a few times to dislodge mud and snow.

Step lightly on the gas pedal, and try to ease the car out of the rut.

If you have to, use a shovel or your hands to clear mud and snow away from the tires, and use sand, cat litter, or even salt in the path of the wheels to assist them with traction.

You can try to rock the vehicle loose by shifting from forward to reverse gear and tapping on the gas as you do, but this can cause damage to your transmission, so use that as a last-ditch effort.

WHAT TO DO IF YOUR CAR IS SINKING

If your car becomes submerged in water, you must take steps to help yourself because help may not find you, especially if there is no one around to call 911. Within thirty to sixty seconds, water can reach the top of your windows, and you could drown in the time it would take you to place a call. You must act fast!

Stay calm and focused. Every second counts.

Undo your seat belt first.

If there are other passengers such as children, undo their seat belts if they haven't done so.

Open the window *as soon as you hit the water.* Do not try to open the door and waste time fighting the pressure of the water. Focus on the windows. The car's electrical system should be working for two to three minutes after being in water, so try opening them with the button on the side of the door first, then try manually.

It takes about one to two minutes for a car to fill with water. Move fast, but stay calm. Breathe normally until the water hits chin level, then hold your breath while making your escape.

Break a window if you have to, and escape through the open window. You can try ripping off the seat headrest to break the window, or keep something in the car such as a tire iron or crowbar.

Swim to the surface and get to land, then call for help. If it is night, look for the light in the water, and swim towards it, or follow the direction of any bubbles in the water, as that will be the surface.

If you or someone else cannot swim, use what objects you can to push yourself up to the surface, including getting on top of the car.

If you have an infant, you will have to carry the infant as you escape.

Try to quickly remove any heavy clothing you may be wearing, so you don't sink.

Please note that you can escape through the car doors under certain circumstances, such as before the entire car is immersed, if you can open the door without wasting too much time to do so. But if the car is fully immersed, the pressure against the doors will be incredible, and you need every second to get out.

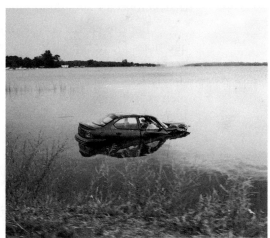

If you're in an car accident and find yourself in the water, the priority is to take off your seatbelt, open the door before you are too deep (or break the window), and get everyone to shore.

If your car is being swept away in rushing water, you may be tempted to stay inside if the water hasn't engulfed the inside of the car, but you still need to escape as quickly as you can. The fast-moving waters may slam the car into a wall or pipe or take you into deep waters.

The steps are: *remove seat belts, open the windows, get out!*

PULL OVER!

Do you know exactly what to do if you are pulled over by the police? The first thing that will happen is you will see the police car behind you with its siren and lights on. Pull over to the right of the roadway, and come to a complete stop. Be sure to use your signal when pulling over, and if you feel comfortable driving to a more lighted area, do so. Sometimes, as on busy freeways, the police are interested in a car in front of you and will drive right by, but you must pull over anyway if you see the lights and hear the siren behind you.

Stay in the car until the officer approaches, but turn off your engine. *Relax.* You can roll down your window part of the way (don't roll it down any further, even if they ask you to) or wait until the officer instructs you to. Being courteous and following instructions will go a long way. If it is dark out, turn on an interior light so you can see and the officer can see into the car. You may be scared, but realize that the officer may be anxious too.

Keep your hands on the wheel when the officer approaches, and keep them visible at all times afterwards.

A police officer may just be giving you a warning about a broken tail light, so don't get belligerent ahead of time, or you may create more trouble than you needed.

Let the officer do the talking, and respond simply and directly to any questions. Do not speak first or offer information they did not ask for. If the officer tries to "trap" you with the question "Do you know why I pulled you over?" simply respond by saying, "No, I don't." If the officer begins to ask questions such as "Where you are going?" or "What you are doing tonight?" do not answer. If you choose to answer, do not lie. You are not obliged to give answers to these types of probing questions.

Wait to be asked for license and registration. Let the officer know you are going to open the glove box and reach in to retrieve your paperwork. Move slowly. You will not be subject to a car search unless the officer has reason to do so. This can include open bottles or cans of alcohol, the smell of pot, or a visible gun or weapon.

Depending on your state's laws, a police officer can ask you and your passengers to get out of the car; otherwise stay inside. Getting out without being asked is looked at as an attempt to flee the scene. Officers make a visual sweep of your car the second they look inside, so if they suspect you or another passenger may be carrying a weapon or be a threat, they will make you get out of the car.

Officers can do a pat-down search if they suspect you are carrying drugs or a weapon. Check your state laws on whether this is legal or illegal. The pat-down will be over your outer layer of clothing, but if they do feel a gun or object, they can reach inside clothing to retrieve it. They can also search the car at this time. All moving vehicles in the United States are subject to search if there is reasonable suspicion associated with the traffic stop. Officers are also permitted to have a K-9 dog sniff the outside of your car for explosives and drugs.

In general, police officers cannot search your cell phone without a warrant or without your consent.

If you are given a ticket, do not argue. Accept it, and leave when the officer tells you it is safe to go.

If you are arrested, make sure you do not say anything that might incriminate you. Understand your rights in your state. You can be arrested if you were driving erratically, breaking road laws, or driving a stolen car. Once the officer sees you, he can often tell by your pupils and by smelling your breath that you may need to be tested for drugs or alcohol with a field sobriety breath test. There must be probable cause for the arrest, but you can ask if you are indeed being arrested, or if you are free to go after a search. This is the most important question *you* can ask. Hopefully it won't get that far, but for an officer to *legally* detain you, there must be probable cause that you committed, or are about to commit, a crime.

If you are interrogated without having been read your rights, they cannot legally use your answers in a court of law as evidence against you. Do not speak without a lawyer present.

Most of the time, when the police pull you over, they have a reason. With all the news stories of police brutality, and brutality against police, both sides of the equation may be fearful and on edge. The best thing you can do is follow instructions and accept responsibility if you were doing something wrong. Arguing, hitting, or threatening a police officer over a ticket is just not worth the jail time.

If you feel threatened by the officer, tell them you want to call 911 and have backup assistance. Police often wear bodycams and try to avoid scaring you, but it does happen, and it has to be considered, especially for women driving at night alone. If you feel your life is in danger, demand the officer follow you to a lighted, populated area to continue the ticketing.

Be smart. Often police hang out near bars and restaurants, knowing that people will be leaving them intoxicated. Have a designated driver. Do not swear at police or use obscene gestures, and don't try to lose them by outdriving them. Not only can you get ticketed for speeding, but you can also be charged with resisting arrest!

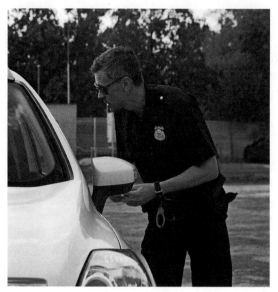

If you are pulled over in your car by a police officer, do not argue with the officer. If you feel a ticket was improper, you can argue your case in traffic court.

It comes down to common sense and remaining calm and courteous. Are there bad cops? Yes. Are there bad citizens? Yes. But most of the time, you did something that warranted being pulled over, and the best thing you can do to avoid trouble is accept the warning or ticket and move on. There are police officers who use routine traffic stops as an opportunity to search the car, and you, more closely. There are police officers who enjoy arresting people even on shaky grounds, but the vast majority are doing their job and doing it correctly, aware of the growing negative public sentiment towards the bad cops that make the nightly news. The public has been trained to fear authority, but even if you are afraid, do know your rights, stand up for them courteously, and know what rights the police officer has so you can follow the rules respectfully—on both sides.

If you feel you have been violated by a police traffic stop or wrongfully arrested, contact a traffic ticket attorney in your area.

Road Safety Tips

Some additional tips to keep you and your family safe while driving are:

Never pick up hitchhikers, even if they look "friendly." You can assist them in calling for help if they've had a breakdown.

Drive with doors locked at all times.

Always have more than a quarter of a tank of gas, preferably more.

If someone bumps your vehicle, don't get out of the car. Stay inside, and call the police if the other driver tries to engage you. This can be a very dangerous criminal scam.

When you come to a stop at a traffic light, leave enough space between your car and the car in front of you in case you need to pull away quickly.

Never allow children to go into fast-food or rest-area bathrooms alone.

Only stop at night at a well-lit and populous rest stop or fast-food joint, and keep an eye on your car.

If you have to stop your car and need emergency help, raise the hood and tie a white cloth to the antenna or door handle, and get back in the car.

If you are driving and another driver motions that your tire is flat or a light is out, wave thanks and do not get out of the car until they are gone or you can drive into a service station.

Safety Before and During a Trip

Does your house give away the fact that you are gone on vacation? Mail piled up at the door? No lights on? No car in the driveway? Criminals know exactly what to look for when someone is away.

Have your mail stopped temporarily while you are gone. Ask a friendly neighbor to take in any packages left at your door.

Keep a light on outside and inside on timers so it looks like someone is home. Do not think crooks are fooled by a porch light left on all day. Try to mimic what you would do if you were at home.

Invest in a good home alarm system.

If you leave the car for a few moments, lock the doors.

Back the car into parking spaces at night so that you can pull away fast if needed.

Stay alert in a parking garage or lot at night, and do not get into your car unless you can see there is no one nearby. Check the back seat.

If you are being followed by someone as you walk back to your car, run past the car and get help. Scream if you have to!

Carry valuables on your front, not behind you in your pocket or backpack. Keep your purse or laptop case close to your body.

Leave expensive jewelry, furs, and other items at home if they may attract the unwanted attention of criminals. This includes expensive camera equipment.

Be wary of who you talk to! Not every fellow traveler is a friend!

Always look back when leaving a restaurant or café to make sure you have not left anything valuable behind.

Avoid using a credit card at an Internet café.

Think about getting traveler's insurance before you go. Don't assume your health insurance covers everything on an international trip.

Know what travel warnings and advisories there are for your destination, and be aware of your surroundings at all times.

Avoid getting into an elevator alone with anyone you feel unsure of. Trust your instincts. Do not use a dark stairwell alone. Use common sense and good judgment.

HOTEL SAFETY

It is always a good idea to stay at a hotel with a good rating (and good reviews!) and to book reservations in advance rather than assume there will be vacancies. If you use something like Auto Club or a travel agent, they can steer you to the best and safest places to stay.

If traveling with children, look for hotels that have amenities such as playgrounds, play areas, pools, and media rooms. Try to avoid getting an upper-story room with a balcony, but if you do, keep the sliding doors locked that lead out onto the balcony. Larger chain hotels are more kid-friendly than expensive luxury hotels.

When you get to your hotel, carry your own luggage in, and watch for people lurking too close by when you check in.

Hotel room numbers should not be spoken aloud at the check-in desk or written on the key directly. The envelope or key sleeve will have the room number.

When you go to and from your room, be sure that no one is following you. This is especially important for women traveling alone. If someone is too close for comfort, pick up speed and move to a common area where there are other people. Do not try to get into your room quickly or you may get shoved inside with no protection.

If someone is bothering you by following you to your room, ask for a different room or for a security escort.

If you leave your room, make sure you lock the door behind you.

If you leave the room, do not hang the sign out for the maid to clean up. That is basically announcing that the room is empty. You can hang the Do Not Disturb sign to indicate the room is occupied.

If a bag or something is stolen from the room, it will most likely be a hotel staff member who stole it. Ask that the object be searched for within the hotel.

If you like to go for a morning or night run, let the front desk or hotel security know, and try to go with a buddy if you can.

Do *not* assume valuables are safe if left in your locked hotel room. Ask the hotel staff to put them in the hotel safe.

If someone knocks on your door, ask that they identify themselves, and look through the peephole to ensure it is room service or a friend.

Never leave ID or a passport in the room. Keep those and other important documents on you at all times or locked in the hotel safe.

Do not carry all your cash and personal items in your purse or in your back pocket or wallet. If they are stolen, you will be left with nothing. Keep some cash and important ID you don't need in the hotel safe, and take with you only what you need at the time.

Even in the most luxurious hotels, we can forget that valuables are still valuable to someone who wants them. You can feel at home, but think of being at home with potential thieves, and don't let down your guard just because the hotel got five stars on the best review sites. There may have been a few reviews in there by people who got ripped off. In fact, review sites are often paid money by hotels, restaurants, and other businesses to scrap bad reviews or elevate good reviews to the top, where they will be read the most. People often don't take the time to scroll through a hundred good reviews to find the ten that say the place sucked. Businesses also pay people to write fake reviews. The best thing you can do is ask friends and colleagues where they have stayed before in a particular city and how safe it was.

TRAVEL AND VACCINES

Going abroad? Be sure to think about what vaccinations you may need at least three months before you plan to leave. Some countries may even require proof in the form of an International Certificate of Vaccination or Prophylaxis. Find out in advance what the region you are visiting requires, and ask your general practitioner if they can administer the proper vaccines or direct you to a source that will. Some of the vaccines must be given well before your travel date, so don't wait.

The Centers for Disease Control and Prevention has a great online source that will tell you what you will need, depending on where you are going are:

Traveler's Health: http://wwwnc.cdc.gov/travel/destinations/list

There are certain conditions where vaccinations may not be advisable, such as pregnancy, HIV/AIDS, or an autoimmune disease, even chemotherapy, so check with your doctor first. Too many people think they can wait until a week before their trip to get the shots they need, only to find out they won't be able to leave if they haven't been inoculated for the required period of time per vaccine type.

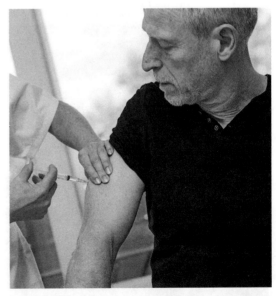

AIRPLANE SAFETY

Traveling by plane safely begins at the airport. You want to make sure that your luggage is locked and tagged, but think about using an office address instead of a home address. Once your baggage is checked, it is out of your hands, so secure it as best you can, and follow all airport rules, or risk having your luggage opened and left behind.

Going through security, listen to instructions and follow them. Keep calm, and do what you are told to avoid problems. Make sure you packed your liquid items

Make sure you are up on your vaccinations when you travel abroad. You can visit the CDC's website for information on which vaccines are required depending on your destination.

properly ahead of time according to the current rules enforced by the Transportation Security Administration (TSA), which can be found on its website: www.tsa.gov. Keep an eye on the items you place in the security bins as you go through the detectors. If you are subjected to a physical search, don't complain or resist, as it will possibly end up in your being detained and missing your flight.

Report any unattended baggage you see at the airport to security. Also report anyone carrying a firearm. If someone asks you to take an item on board the plane for them, report them immediately, and do not take the bag.

Be careful entering airport bathrooms. You may want to take your carry-on into the stall with you, if it will fit, to avoid having it stolen.

Once you are on the plane, stow your carry-on close overhead, and keep with you only what is allowed by the airline. Keep purses close to your body or directly under your seat, with your foot over the strap to keep it from sliding away or being grabbed. Be sure nothing you stash under your seat might trip you if you need to make a fast exit in an emergency. Also be aware that items under your seat can turn into deadly projectiles in a crash, so make sure they are firmly secured.

Don't be one of those pesky travelers who insist on using electronics when told not to. Yes, they can interfere with plan signaling devices in the cockpit. Wait until you are told it is okay to use them. Respect other passengers and use headphones when listening to music or a movie, especially at night when others may be sleeping.

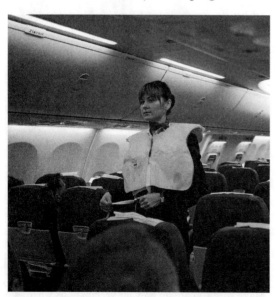

Most travelers don't listen to the flight attendants giving safety instructions, but even if you have heard them before you should pay attention!

Do you listen when the flight attendants go through their safety routine? Most flyers tune them out, but it is critical you pay attention and know where the emergency exits are, how to use the oxygen masks, and other pertinent information that could save your life! That same information will be on a card in the seat pocket in front of you. Take two minutes to review it. Don't trade your life for a few moments of laziness.

Look around for the emergency exits, and look beneath your seat for the flotation device. Just knowing these two things can make a huge difference in an emergency.

Did you know that you can select your seats in advance? Passengers who sit in the tail end of the plane actually have a 40 percent higher survival rate than those who sit up front in the first several rows. Passengers who sit over the wings report less nausea. Do you need to use the bathroom often? Pick a seat near the restrooms, preferably the back of the plane. Choose your seat wisely!

Pay the extra money and get your baby or small child their own seat so they can be properly restrained. In the event of a crash, having a baby or toddler on your lap could lead to death.

Try to wear flat shoes and comfortable clothes while on the plane. If there is a crash, you may need a jacket to keep warm. Imagine trying to run from a plane in high heels, which, by the way, are not permitted on evacuation slides. Keep your fancy shoes in your carry-on, and opt for sneakers instead.

Always keep your seat belt on when told to. Keep it properly tightened too, so that in the event of a crash, it can keep you from flying forward. Keep your belt on while you are napping or sleeping.

IN THE EVENT OF A CRASH

Try to stay as calm as you possibly can and assess the situation. Is the plane over water or land? If an impact is imminent, clear your area of things that can fly in your face and injure you. Stow all loose items safely away. Listen as the flight attendants tell you what crash position to assume. You will want your feet flat on the floor and a bit in back of your knees to best brace your legs. Keeping your legs under your seat may help avoid broken bones or injuries so you can get out of the plane quickly.

You will be told to brace your upper body and protect your head. If you don't hear the instructions, put one hand on the back of the seat in front of you, then the other hand on top of it, interlacing fingers. Rest your forehead on top of your hands, face down. If the seat in front of you is too far, or there is no seat, bend forward and put your chest against your thighs with your head between your knees. Grab your ankles tightly.

Once the plane impacts, if in water, put on your life jacket, but do not inflate it until you are instructed to do so. Hold your breath if water is at face level, swim out, then inflate the jacket. If you inflate it in the plane, it could act against you by pushing you up into the top of the plane.

If the plane impacts the ground, or during a hard descent, oxygen masks will drop. Put yours on first before assisting anyone else, including children. Do it fast, because once the plane's cabin has broken apart, you have about fifteen seconds to put the mask on and breathe in oxygen or risk losing consciousness.

If the plane catches fire, you need to get out. Don't worry about luggage and purses and laptops. *Get out.* The only thing you should try to grab is a blanket or jacket, which you may need. According to the National Transportation Safety Board (NTSB), over 60 percent of fatalities in plane crashes are from the fire and smoke and not the actual impact. Cover your mouth and nose with a cloth, and stay low to the ground as you make your way to the emergency exit. Follow instructions and exit the plane, running at least 500 feet (150 meters) to safety in case of an explosion.

Keep your eyes open at all times, because the emergency exit nearest to you may be blocked or on fire. Go to the next exit quickly. Never try to push your way over or through other passengers, as that slows down the line and can get everyone killed.

Once you are safe, treat any wounds you can on yourself and others, and wait for further instructions.

The vast majority of flights each day occur without event, or possibly with some turbulence. But too often flyers ignore the very instructions that can, in the rare event of a disaster, mean the difference between panicking and surviving.

What if your plane crashes in a cold, snowy environment? What would you do to survive the crash and the elements? Because of your location, it may take rescuers a while to find where the plane went down and get help to you. Once you are free from the crash, get away from the plane in case the fuel ignites, causing an explosion. Hopefully, any fire or explosion will be seen by rescuers in planes or on foot. Once the crash site seems safe, stay near it, because that is where rescuers will go first, and you want to be there when they show up.

Use food and water from inside the plane to survive on. You can also melt snow for water. Take shelter under a large piece of fuselage, and look around for blankets and other coverings you can use for warmth.

If you are there for a while and realize you may need to go get help, assess your surroundings, and head downhill if on a mountainside, or look for signs of civilization such as fireplace smoke. Listen for sounds of far-off traffic and head towards it. Beware of the possibility of avalanches, extreme cold and hypothermia, and falling on ice. Never leave the crash site at night, and use flares from the plane's emergency kits or any means you have of making a fire to signal rescuers.

Huddle together for warmth with other passengers. This is a time for everyone to work together to survive the elements until help arrives. Share food and water and body heat, and pay special attention to the needs of the elderly, children, and pets in the cargo hold. Don't forget that the luggage can provide ample clothing and jackets for warmth. People may at first be angry at having their clothing appropriated, but in a do-or-die situation they will understand why it is necessary.

Many of the same rules apply to a plane crashing in a desert or forested area, although in a forest you may have more access to food and water sources and the shelter of overhead trees. The desert will be unforgiving during the day, so this is one instance where it will be better to move away from the crash site in the early morning or twilight hours. Pay attention to the ground: snakes and scorpions will be under foot. If there are any roads nearby, watch for passing cars and make signs if you can, letting them know to call police. Indicate with an arrow where the plane crash site is located. Don't expect people to stop and take you to the next town, but you can at least ask them to call 911.

In a plane crash, the decision to stay with the wreckage is usually best, because rescuers will know where the plane went down, and help will be forthcoming. But if you must leave the area, be smart about it, go in groups, and take what food and water and protection against the elements you can carry between you.

BOATING/CRUISE SHIP SAFETY

Taking a cruise anytime soon? Like planes, cruise ships offer safety instructions that are often overlooked in the excitement of getting out on the water. On any given day, there are hundreds of cruise ships traveling the oceans and seas, and very few of them experience an emergency situation. But it does happen.

The biggest issue on a cruise is sickness, whether motion sickness or norovirus. While motion sickness can be addressed with some type of medication, an outbreak of norovirus can have hundreds of passengers sick within a day or two. The Centers for Disease Control and Prevention says your chances are slim of getting this debilitating stomach virus that can cause severe diarrhea, but it does happen, and we hear about it in the news media quite regularly, even if the outbreak involves just a handful of passengers.

Norovirus and food poisoning may be hard to avoid completely, but washing hands regularly with soap and water, being careful not to touch the eyes, nose, or mouth, and staying out of contact with sick passengers can help you stay well.

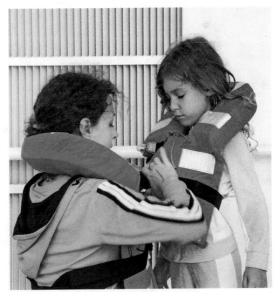

Now and then we hear about some type of engine or mechanical failure on a cruise ship, but be assured that if this happens, there will be help on the way. The best thing to do is listen to the instructions of the crew in any situation.

Know the emergency rules and drill. Listen when the crew gives the safety address, and know what the evacuation plan is should something happen.

Make sure your passport and documents are with you, and use the same common sense as you would in a hotel, not leaving valuables in your room. The ship will have a safe for valuables.

The International Convention for the Safety of Life at Sea requires that all cruise ships instruct passengers on ship safety within twenty-four hours of departure from port.

Scan and email your important documents to yourself so you have a backup copy.

Have travel insurance before you board, and book when the weather is likely to be at its best.

Keep any prescription meds on your person in case you need them and are locked out of your room or blocked from reaching it.

Know where the ship's medical quarters are.

Know where your life jackets are located.

Be wary when going off the ship at a port or on a tour, and stay with a group if you can. Stay away from prohibited areas, and try not to attract unwanted attention, especially being careful to not carry expensive cameras and flashy jewelry.

Always ask your cruise director any questions you have, and don't guess, including what parts of a particular city to avoid.

In the event that your ship needs to be evacuated, stay calm. Follow the crew's instructions on how to put on your life jacket and disembark quickly. Don't rush back to your room to grab valuables; it isn't worth risking your life if the ship is sinking or on fire.

Cruises can be a tremendously relaxing way to see the world and enjoy good food, views, and company. You may want to ask friends and check review sites to see which cruise lines have the best reputation for safety and customer satisfaction.

IF YOU ARE THE BOATER

Follow boating safety just as you would if you were in a car. Take a basic boating course to understand the rules of the waterways and how to control your boat on calm and stormy waters.

Check to see that your boat is in good mechanical working condition before you take it out and that you have adequate fuel.

Be sure to have extra food, water, and medical supplies on board, even on a short trip.

Make sure you have the correct, valid boating license/permits needed in your area.

Try to arrange boating trips during good weather, and watch the forecasts.

Have a backup person who can handle the boat if you should fall ill or become incapacitated.

Have life jackets for all passengers, and make sure they know how to use them.

If you have an accident or emergency, report it and radio for help immediately.

RAIL SAFETY

Whether you take a subway or a train, like millions of other passengers, you probably don't think too much about something going wrong. But there are basics to rail safety just as there are with a plane or a boat. Obviously, you want to stay off the tracks and far enough away, and thankfully the platforms are marked to assist you. Trains travel at amazing speeds, even when slowing into a station, so be sure to keep children away from the tracks at all times. An approaching 200-ton train is always coming faster than you visually guess it is, so don't take chances with safety. Trains cannot slam on their brakes and stop as easily as a car, and they have the right of way 100 percent of the time!

Never lean over a platform to see if the train is coming, and if you drop something, leave it or ask a police officer or station personnel to fetch it for you.

Walk on platforms. Running increases the risk of tripping and possibly going down onto the tracks.

One of the biggest issues at subway and train stations and on platforms is crime, so be alert, keep your valuables close to your body, and hold onto luggage until it is time to load it in the cargo areas. After hours, wait for the train in the designated wait areas and not off hiding in the shadows.

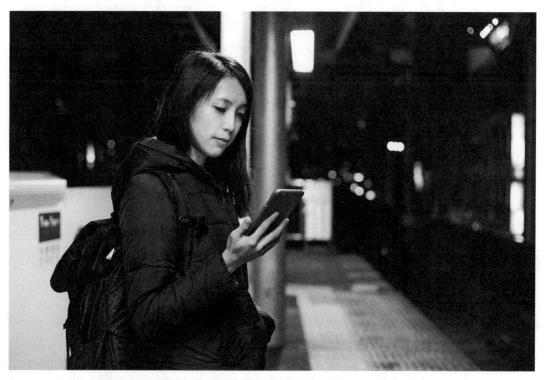

Be extra vigilant when traveling the subways, especially at night. Be aware of your surroundings, get off the cell phone, and keep your possessions close to you.

Try not to use the subway late at night, and if you are alone and feel uncomfortable, find a police officer or station personnel to stay with you until the train arrives. Also be aware of getting into a train car alone or with someone you feel anxious about. *Trust your instincts.* Better to wait for a more crowded car than be sorry.

Avoid napping on the train, but if you must sleep, keep your purse and valuables close to your body and strapped or tied tightly on to avoid pickpockets and thieves.

As the train leaves the station, stay away from closing doors to avoid getting something trapped in them.

If you are traveling with children, understand that they may take longer to walk to the train, get on and off the train, and settle in for the ride, and be aware and patient. Try not to sit next to doors where a child may run out or get caught. Go over emergency and bathroom signs with your kids so they know what to do if you are incapacitated. Locate emergency exits together, and make a game out of finding the first aid kits, fire extinguishers, and other emergency supplies.

Go over your route ahead of time with your group of travelers in the event you get separated. Write down the route for children so they can show a station attendant which trains they need to take if you are not able to be in communication via cell phones. Have a plan in case a child accidentally gets stuck on the train and must go to the next station. Have them get off the train and sit on the first platform bench they see or alert station personnel until you can get to them.

Never walk or run around or in front of crossing areas unless the train is at a full stop and passengers are disembarking. Listen for whistles and bells to alert you that the train is getting ready to move. Even if the track is empty at the time, you could decide to cross, get stuck, and be sorry when the oncoming train cannot brake in time. Cross only on designated crossing paths or tracks, and do so *after* the train has left the station if possible.

Use the station's "customer assistance intercom" if you need help for any reason or feel unsafe.

Only use the emergency cord in an actual emergency, such as seeing someone being dragged in a closed train door. Do *not* use the cord if you or someone else becomes ill or you accidentally miss your stop while texting a friend. Wait until the train is at the next station, and get off then.

WHERE SHOULD I SIT?

On any form of public transportation, there are safer seats than others. Whether a bus, plane, or train, the seats next to emergency exits are always a better choice than a main exit. If something happens, you will be able to get out quickly before a stampede of panicked passengers. Tables on a train or bus may seem like a great place to set up your laptop and work, but keep in mind that these tables can be deadly if the vehicle gets into a collision and the table is pushed into your torso as a result. You may choose aisle seats near the emergency exits instead, or even a main exit where you think you can be one of the first out the door. In long trains, you want to sit nearer the rear of the line of cars, but avoid the last two cars. Sticking to a middle car is safest, as the front and rear cars will sustain the most damage from any kind of collision.

Sitting in the back of a bus near the large rear window can also provide you with an exit if you need it, but be ready to break the window, and be careful of passing traffic when you get out.

In a plane, seats over the wing may be the strongest and most stable in a crash, but they have the disadvantage of being closer to the fuel tanks. The front of a plane often is the most comfortable, but will sustain the most damage during impact, so it's better to sit in the back and put up with a little extra turbulence and noise. Seek safety over comfort in any transport system.

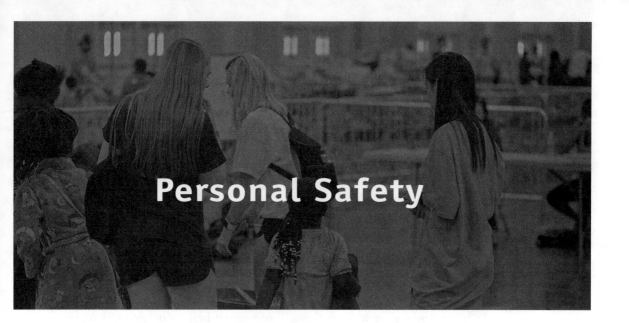

Personal Safety

Nobody wants to be a crime statistic, yet being the victim of some type of crime is a much higher risk than suffering through most major disasters. While not all situations are preventable—a bank robbery, for example—there are things you can do to stay safer and increase the odds of surviving.

ASSAULT

Whether you are jumped by thugs on the street or the victim of a sexual attack, an assault comes out of nowhere with little to no warning. We don't have time even to process what is happening, let alone react to it in the most desirable way. The best way to diminish the odds of being hurt or raped in an assault is to take a self-defense course and know what to do in a variety of situations, because no amount of reading and watching instructional videos can compare to hands-on practice. Many self-defense courses are cheap and local, and some are geared towards women or children or entire families.

But if you are the victim of an assault, you must act fast and on instinct. Most assaults occur as a part of a robbery attempt. If someone jumps you for your purse or wallet, give it to them. It's not worth losing your life over. If you can scream to attract attention, do so.

A good self-defense class will teach you some basic skills that can stop an attacker and incapacitate them long enough for you to get away. Invest in a class.

If you are walking alone and live in an area that allows open carry, keep your weapon in your hand or visible to anyone who might attempt to attack you. But make sure you are abiding by local laws or *you* could be the one who ends up in jail.

Never walk or run alone at night. Go with a buddy. A large dog can act as a deterrent. Keep valuables in a pouch or sack close to the body.

Try to get a good look at your attacker without them being aware of it. When they run off, call police or get help quickly so you can better describe the person to police.

Immediately call and cancel bank cards and credit cards, and contact the Department of Motor Vehicles and Social Security office if you were carrying ID and your wallet or purse was stolen.

SEXUAL ASSAULT

No one wants to think about it, but sexual assault is rampant. Usually the attacker is male and the victim is female, but not always. The elderly and children can also end up victims of sexual assault.

It is critical that women think about never being out alone at night, whether driving or walking or running. It isn't fair, but the world we live in dictates that women think about carrying some type of weapon, which we will discuss later in this chapter. Do not walk or run alone at night or early in the morning. Do not walk into underground parking garages alone at any time if you can get someone to walk with you. If you must be alone in a dangerous situation, exercise situational awareness, and hold your head up high. Criminals are much more likely to attack someone who looks weak, scared, and distracted than someone who appears to be on the lookout and ready to react.

If you are the victim of sexual assault, the choice is yours as to whether you feel you can fight off your attacker or should do as they say. No one, including the author of this book, can tell you which choice might be better in what circumstances. Unfortunately, it may come down to instinct. You must do what you believe is necessary to survive the attack.

If you have been assaulted, call 911 or get to the hospital immediately. Do not bathe or clean off any part of your body. Do not change your clothes. Keep the scene of the assault intact. If you choose to file a police report, do so immediately. Police will need every clue they can get to help find your attacker and bring them to justice.

At the hospital, ask for a SANE, a Sexual Assault Nurse Examiner, to assist you and administer a rape kit if the assault involved intercourse or any form of rape (oral, anal). Often hospitals have rape crisis counselors on hand to help you.

Get counseling or therapy immediately, even if you feel good about surviving the assault, because post-traumatic stress disorder will occur. Rape is a violent crime, and even if the victim is accepting the situation on the surface, the damage runs deep and must be addressed.

Know that it is *never* your fault. If anyone shames you or disrespects you, remove them from your life. If you have a doctor or counselor who shames or guilts you in any way, fire them. *Rape is never the fault of the victim. Ever.*

If it is someone you know, do not be afraid to turn them in. Get a restraining order if you feel it might help. Tell close friends so they can watch out for you.

Talk about the assault/rape to close loved ones and trusted friends, but do not continue to dwell on it and go deeper into depression. Take steps, however small, to begin to take back control of your life and your thoughts and move forward. If you are not able to stop ruminating, get professional help. You deserve to heal, and there is no shame in asking for help to do so.

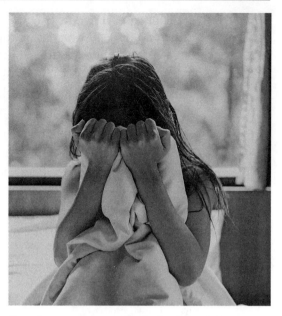

Rape is *never ever ever* the fault of the victim.

Consider carrying a weapon in the future to give you confidence, but be sure to learn how to use the weapon and what the laws are in your state.

Often rape and assault victims find some healing in helping other victims get through what they have dealt with. If you feel this might be something that would help you, offer to volunteer at a rape crisis center.

The most important thing to remember in any crime, and especially in rape, is that you are not at fault. Do not try to "go it alone," and get the help you need to begin the healing process.

RIDER SAFETY

Today people can call a taxi if they need a ride somewhere, but they also have new options such as Uber and Lyft, companies that provide fast and often cheap transportation where you need it, when you need it. But with these new options come new potentials for crime. There are definitely some things you can do to protect yourself when using one of these services.

Do not stand alone outside waiting for your ride. Wait indoors or with others until your car has arrived.

Make sure it is the exact same car you ordered on the app or service, and do not get into a car that looks different, even if the driver claims they are with the company. When you use the apps to order a car, you will be given the driver's first name, a photo, a copy of their driver's license, and a picture of the vehicle with license plate number. You can also see the driver's rating. Make sure it all matches perfectly, or refuse the ride. Many college students have reported "imposter drivers" when using these services, so be careful, because a fake driver will have only one thing on their mind: committing a crime against you.

If you are riding alone with the driver, sit in the back seat. This way you can get out of the vehicle on either side if you need to. If you can get a friend to accompany you on the ride, do so, and both sit in the back seat.

Keep your cell phone in your hand, and have 911 on speed dial.

Let others know where you are going and how you are getting there. These apps allow you to share your status while you are en route so that others know exactly where the car is and what it looks like too.

Do not give your phone number or other personal information to the driver. They don't need it! The apps will actually make your phone number anonymous when you order the car to protect your privacy.

Use your judgment and gut instinct. If you don't feel right, don't get in the car. If you are being aggressively flirted with or bothered by the driver, call 911.

STALKING

If you suspect someone is stalking you, keep a record of every email, text, phone call, message, photograph, or conversation. Document *everything*, including times and dates.

If a stalker is nearby, either walking by your home or workplace, sitting in a car watching you, or following you at a distance, get video evidence.

Do not ignore emails and letters, as they may contain actual threats you can go to the police with.

File a restraining order, and let law enforcement know you are being stalked. They may not be able to act unless there is a viable threat, but they will have your report on file.

Consider carrying a weapon, and beef up the security in your home or apartment.

Alter daily routines to keep stalkers off guard. If you are going away on business or a vacation, let others know your plans, and ask them to check on you regularly.

Tell people. Even neighbors you are friends with can be extra pairs of eyes and ears.

Do *not* confront or engage the stalker in any circumstance.

CARJACKING

Cars can be hijacked just as a plane or semitruck can. Often carjackings are perpetrated by an organized ring of criminals or gangs that steal cars and resell parts for a profit. While you can look up the criminal "value" of your car online or in your *Consumer Reports* magazine, it can happen to anyone at any time. Carjackers don't usually work alone and often drive up to a victim at a stoplight, and one gets out and holds a gun to the victim's head. The victim may be dragged out of the car and left on the pavement or shot in the head to prevent them from identifying the attackers. It is a terrifying crime that happens fast, and the best advice is to let them have your car without a fight.

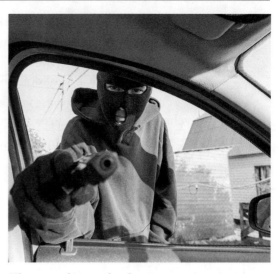

They may also take your purse or wallet. Let them. You can always call and cancel cards and notify the Department of Motor Vehicles and Social Security. The key is to survive.

The smart thing to do when someone is trying to carjack you is to get out of the car and let the thief take it. A car is not worth your life.

The best way to avoid a carjacking is to be aware of your surroundings. Lock your doors, and if a car pulls up beside you and you feel anxious, *move*. Even through a stoplight if it is safe. Get to a populous, lighted area, or lean on your horn as you drive.

Always wear a seat belt. It may sound crazy, but carjackers are all about getting your car fast and getting out of Dodge. A seat belt complicates matters.

At any stoplight, keep enough room between the front of your car and the rear of the car in front of you to be able to speed away quickly if something looks wrong.

Never open your door or even roll down your window to talk to anyone. The person you think just needs directions could be a carjacker. Don't take chances!

If you are told to get out of the car, you can choose to throw your keys as far as you can and run. Some believe the carjackers will go for the keys, as the car is their main goal.

Have proper car insurance that covers theft, and think about investing in a car tracking device that police can use to find the car if it is stolen, such as the LoJack system.

Above all else, give up your car and your belongings instead of your life. One can be replaced, the other cannot.

If you have a loud car alarm installed, trigger it manually if you can. Noise can deter a crime, especially when there may be witnesses around.

If a vehicle bumps you in the rear of your car, *do not get out*. Call 911 immediately. Drive away fast if you can.

Keep car keys separate from house keys so that, if they grab your wallet and car keys, they at least don't have easy access to your home too.

You can try throwing keys and cash or jewelry out of the car, then exit the vehicle and run away.

If you have children in the car, reach back and get your child, and exit the car together. Never assume that if you get out, the carjacker will be nice and let your child out the back door while you stand there.

If you have your cell phone near you, try to dial 911 (which should be on speed dial) without the carjacker noticing as you try to get out of the car, throw your keys, or speed away. This will enable the 911 process to begin as the crime happens.

KIDNAPPING

Whether a stranger grabs you in a local shopping center parking lot or you are held hostage by a group of terrorists, kidnapping happens all over the world and in many different situations. Sometimes gender makes a difference, as in men kidnapping women for sexual assault and rape. Other times, it is adults kidnapping children for sexual purposes. Often it might be for money, especially if you are known to come from a wealthy or important family. Whatever the reason, being kidnapped is an absolutely terrifying situation that would cause the bravest among us to freeze.

Kidnappings occur abroad and can then be especially dangerous because often the victim doesn't have the ability even to communicate with the attackers. But assume that most kidnappings occur close to home, and start there to protect yourself. If you work late and come home at night, or jog in the evening, you must be aware of your surroundings at all times. If you come into your garage, do you close the door before you get out of the locked car? Anyone can slip into the garage while you are unloading bags or your work items.

When shopping, do you park away from the entrance? Try to park close to the main entrance and in a well-lit area, and go to your car with others. If you are alone, ask the store manager if they can have security accompany you to your car. Look inside your back seat before you get in!

When driving, day or night, know where you are going. Kidnappers and criminals can tell when someone is lost and will prey on them. Use your phone's GPS, and if you miss a stop, try to know an alternative route ahead of time to avoid having to stop and ask someone, which could lead to trouble. If you do need to ask for directions, go to a well-lit gas station, and ask the attendant.

In a hostile environment, you want to become somewhat invisible and have your phone in your hand ready to dial 911. If you suspect someone is following you, have your hand on your mace, pepper spray, or alarm whistle if you have one, and be ready to use it. If you live in an open carry state, show that you are armed and it may deter the attacker.

Preventing a kidnapping is your number one choice. Yell, scream, kick, run, use your weapon if you have one. Just get away and get to safety. But if it does happen, and you are kidnapped, you can survive. You have to quell the panic first and foremost. The rush of adrenaline and panic won't help you. Try to be as observant as possible, and look for any chance there might be to escape. You want to observe:

- How many people there are
- If they are armed, and with what types of weapons
- Where you are being held and if there are exits visible
- Are they young, old, foreign?
- Do they speak your language?
- What is their emotional state?
- Do they show any kind of respect or compassion, or are they cruel?
- If they have not covered your eyes, try to remember visuals along the way to where you are being taken. If you can later get to a phone, this will help rescuers.
- What type of security is there around the facility you are being held in?
- Is it a home, building, warehouse, garage?
- Are you injured?

Ideally, if you can find out their motivation for kidnapping you, it will give you an advantage in keeping tensions lower. You want to be strong and positive, but also keep the attackers at ease and not lead them to believe you are a threat to them at any time.

You can choose to try to establish some kind of rapport with your kidnappers. This is a matter of instinct and discernment. But at the very least, do not insult or threaten them. They have the advantage now, not you.

Listen to their conversations, and identify what their plans are for you.

Keep track of time and behavior patterns and who leaves which exit when.

If there are other people being held captive, try to engage them in conversation, and look out for each other. When trust is established, you can devise a possible plan of escape. Try to blend in with other captives, though, as you don't want to stand out and be thought of as "difficult."

If you have children or loved ones, you can try to appeal to the attackers' own feelings of love for their families.

Keep your mind sharp and alert, and gradually begin to try to communicate by asking for water or a bathroom to use.

If you are restrained, don't visibly struggle to free yourself. Test the restraint and try to loosen it when you are not being observed.

If they bind your wrists with duct tape, you can escape by raising your arms over your head and bringing them down with extreme force while pulling your wrists apart. The tape will split if you use enough force.

Don't make it too obvious that you are watching and listening to their plans.

If you see a potential weapon, try to take it and hide it from their view.

If and when an opportunity for escape presents itself, take it and run for it. You may be better off waiting through negotiations and rescue, but you must use your discernment, especially if you sense you will not be kept alive even after any ransom is paid. If you do escape, make sure you can get away for good, because if they capture you again, they probably won't keep you alive for long.

If rescue is imminent, stay out of the way of gunfire, and follow the rescuers' instructions to avoid being mistaken for another kidnapper and fired upon.

Once you are free, don't think the ordeal is over. You will experience symptoms of post-traumatic stress disorder and need someone to talk to. Don't be afraid or ashamed to get help.

If they hold you in the trunk of a car, you can escape! Try to pull the trunk release if there is one. Pull it up or down accordingly. It might even have a glow-in-the-dark handle to find it by. Not all cars will have this, so you may have to try to pull the trunk release cable instead. Pull up the floor carpet beneath you and feel for a cable. It may be beneath a piece of heavy cardboard. It also may be along the side of the trunk. Find it and pull it to open the trunk.

If you can escape via the backseat area, wait until the driver is out of the car. Push or kick the seat down, and crawl out into the back seat, then make a dash out the door.

Maybe you can reach the tire iron or car jack inside the trunk and use that to pry open the door or push out the brake lights so they drop down outside the car. This way you can attempt to signal to motorists that you need help. If you hear noises indicating you are in a populated area, kick and scream and bang on the door with all your might to try to draw attention to anyone who might hear you and call 911 on your behalf.

The minute you are free and clear, if you can call 911, do it right away while you still have descriptions and observations fresh in your mind. The trauma and fear of the situation could make your memory fuzzy if you hold off too long. If you don't have your cell phone, find a business or store that is open,

If Your Purse or Wallet Is Stolen

Having your personal items stolen can be more frustrating and debilitating than having your car stolen. When someone takes your wallet, they now have your money and identity in their hands. Once you know your wallet or purse has been stolen or gone missing, there are steps you can take to reduce the damage:

- Contact your bank immediately to have your ATM card disabled and replaced with a new account number. The same applies to your checking account if your checkbook was taken.

- Contact the Department of Motor Vehicles to let them know your driver's license was taken and to take steps towards getting it replaced.

- Contact your credit card companies to let them know your cards were stolen and have them frozen or have account numbers changed. Have them also put a fraud alert on the cards and watch for suspicious activity.

- Contact the credit reporting agencies to let them know your identity and financial accounts have been compromised and to put a fraud alert on your accounts and freeze new activity.

File a police report if you notice money has been stolen from any of your accounts. The author of this book did just that when her checkbook was stolen, and it resulted in the arrest of a career identity-theft criminal. Do not trivialize your wallet or purse theft as unimportant. The police want to know, as the person who stole it may be someone wanted for other crimes, and reporting helps build a case.

If your keys were also stolen, have home locks replaced immediately. Car keys are a bit trickier, but you can go to your mechanic or your local car dealer and ask for their help in getting the lock mechanisms changed.

Contact the Social Security Department in your area to let them know if your card was stolen.

Contact your cell phone provider if your phone was taken, and have them assist you in rectifying the situation.

Never carry PINs or account numbers and passwords in your wallet or purse. If you do, and you are a victim of theft, change them immediately!

Document everything in your wallet, and make a physical copy of any important papers you carry with you.

If you are traveling abroad and your passport is stolen, and you don't have a clean color copy of the main page, contact the nearest U.S. Embassy for assistance.

Obviously, the best way not to lose a wallet or purse is to keep your eyes on it at all times, but theft happens, and thieves can be tricky. All it takes is looking away for five seconds for them to nab and grab. If they do, just don't let them get anything out of it other than the contents.

and go inside. Tell them what happened, and ask to use their phone. Remain inside until the police arrive.

If you are gagged and chained, your options for escape might be zero. Then it comes down to doing whatever you can to stay alive and survive and possibly escape from the location you are being taken to. Kidnapping is a horrific situation with few options, but they are there if you can keep calm enough to be observant of them.

If your child is kidnapped, call 911 immediately, and do what you can to observe the kidnappers, what gender they are, how they are dressed, how tall they are and their build, any identifying tattoos, the make and color of the car, and the license plate number. The sooner an AMBER Alert or other type of child abduction alert can be put out to the public, the better. Also observe what direction the car was heading and any other identifiable marks. If you can follow the car on your own, you must consider that they may be armed and shoot not just at you, but at the child if they feel the situation puts them in danger of being caught. Most parents would instinctively want to chase down their child's abductors. If you do so, be well aware of the risks.

Avoiding kidnapping comes down to situational awareness and trusting your gut not to take chances with your safety and override a concern just because it "probably is nothing." Act as if it is something.

ROBBERY

A robbery can occur in your home, while you are at the bank, or at your workplace. Anywhere there are money and valuables to be had, a robbery is a possibility. You can be jogging in the park and become a victim of robbery. Situational awareness is a huge factor here. If you go into your local bank and see two big, burly guys in overcoats looking nervous, stay away and alert a security guard. If you are home, lock windows and doors, and consider a home alarm system. If you are working where robberies may occur, such as a retail shop, be aware of customers and watch them carefully.

If a robbery happens, rule number one is *do as they say*. If they tell you to get on the floor, get on the floor. If they tell you to face the wall, face the wall. Do not say anything or make any sudden moves. Do not try to talk the robbers out of it or try to disarm them. Often the robbers want to get what they can in the way of valuables and not add murder to their list of crimes. Stay quiet, don't panic, and don't be stupid.

Never stare at a robber. They will think you are trying to memorize their appearance to tell police later.

If you can hide, hide. Call 911 and stay quiet.

Once robbers have what they came for, they will usually leave fast without incident. Call 911 and set off the store alarm *after* they are gone.

Keep all witnesses there until police arrive. Do not touch anything the robbers touched, and leave the crime scene intact.

Do not speak to the media after a crime. You could botch the case.

Robbers may take hostages. If you have a medical condition that is life-threatening, you can try to reason with them, but don't expect compassion. If

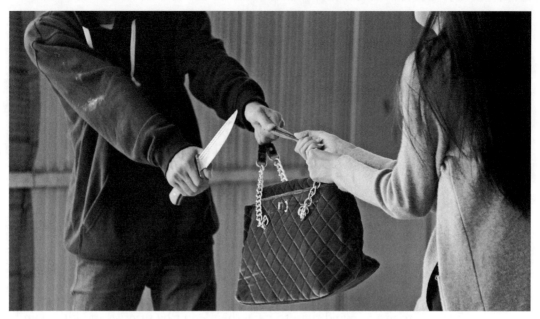

During a robbery, it is not wise to try to keep your possessions when the thief has a gun or knife. Let them take your purse or wallet and get away with your life.

they decide to spare you, it will be because they don't want a murder on their rap sheet. You can try things such as letting go of bodily functions or using extreme emotion to show the robbers you would make a terrible hostage, but be aware that these techniques may also backfire on you and anger them. Hostage situations tend to be rarer because they put more pressure on the criminals to keep people under control. It is far easier for them to grab and dash.

If anyone is injured during the robbery, help them after the robbers leave and 911 has been called. Treat the most severe injuries first, using the ABCs.

After a robbery, go home and rest. You will need to be on the lookout for possible symptoms of post-traumatic stress disorder. Many robbery victims report horrible nightmares and a constant state of hypervigilance. *Get help if you need it.* Find a counselor or therapist skilled in PTSD who can help keep you from ruminating and playing the "what if they had done this or that" tapes over and over again in your mind.

There is a lot of discussion nowadays about being the "good guy with the gun" in the event of a crime. This book and this author do not attempt to make a judgment call on whether or not pulling a weapon on a robber or robbers will work, or result in your death. Every situation is different, and there is no blanket answer to the question of whether being armed or not would stop a crime or add to it. Use your judgment, but be very aware of the gun laws in your state and how you might be held liable for pulling a weapon.

If robbers enter your home, let them have what they want. Do what they say. If you see them enter the home before they see you, hide and call 911.

Do not try to call 911 if the robbers can see or hear you. They will choose to protect their own lives by taking yours.

Listen to their orders and follow their commands. Let them have anything they want, and if they ask you where valuables are kept, tell them. If they ask for something you don't understand or have, state simply that you don't understand or do not have the items in the house they want. Tell them they can take whatever they want in the house.

Do not stare at them to get a good visible description. When they are looking for valuables, you can mentally create visuals to tell the police. Do try to take notice of anything the robbers touch, especially if they are not wearing gloves, to tell police later.

Keep your hands visible at all times. Fast movements may cause a robber to react with gunfire.

If there are others in the house, tell the robbers. It is better they know which rooms to avoid than to have them enter by surprise and kill a family member.

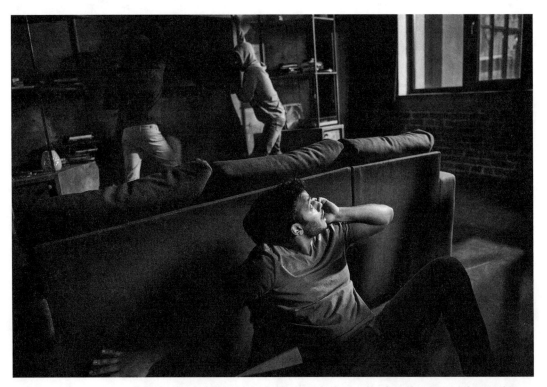

Do not call 911 or anyone else if the robbers might hear you when they are inside your home.

Do not put up an argument or try to resist. Remember, robbers want *things*, not dead bodies.

If you feel your life is in danger and you can get to a weapon, it's your call. Again, be aware of gun and self-defense laws in your state. Often, firing a warning shot is enough to send them on their way fast. If there is one robber and you can disable them without risk to your own life, do so.

Call police after the robbers have left and you have locked all doors and windows.

If you are selling something online or via a phone app, make sure you meet the buyer in a common area with other people around, and be careful when going back to your car if you did not make the sale. If you have valuables, have a friend go with you to the meeting place.

Do not give a buyer any personal information, and do not allow them to make a direct deposit into your bank account. Get cash or a cashier's or bank check for payment, or if your phone allows a credit card, use that instead. Cash is always best for the cleanest transaction.

Never invite a stranger into your home if selling something online, even if they appear nice and harmless. They could be working with others in a crime ring. This is a warning especially for seniors, who tend to be more trusting of people coming to their door. Do not open the door for a child, teenager, or adult unless it is someone you are expecting and know!

If you are having a garage or yard sale, try to have others with you, and do not leave a door open leading into your home. Keep the cash in a cashbox away from the main action of the sale, and have one person designated to retrieve change while others watch the customers.

If someone pulls a gun, give them your money and whatever they want to take. Usually garage sale crime involves people stealing items or trying to get to the cashbox when you are not looking, so stay aware of the situation at all times.

The truth is, it always comes down to survival. Do what you must to survive and keep your loved ones alive. Sometimes that means doing nothing. Sometimes it means fighting back. No one can tell you what will work in any and all situations.

SELF-DEFENSE BASICS

Yes, take a self-defense course, and sign up your loved ones while you are at it! The more you can do to help yourself during a crime, the better. There are some basic techniques you can learn by reading or by watching a video, but nothing beats good old-fashioned hands-on training. There are a variety of courses in different techniques, but some take a long time to master. Taking a karate or martial arts class may be fun, but a class designed specifically for defending yourself in a crime will be the most helpful.

Self-defense doesn't have to be rocket science. It is about doing something to hurt, distract, or disable another person quickly so that you can get away. During a crime, you will be experiencing panic and fear, but knowing some techniques that you can use to get away or buy yourself some extra time will give you an edge on the panic. Your mind and memory may be muddied with the immediate need to survive. But if your body is relaxed and ready, you can deter an attacker long enough to run and call for help.

Some of the basics are:

Chop/Smash—Flatten one hand with the palm facing downward. Strike the person's throat or nose with the edge of your hand in a quick thrust.

Jab—Use the heel of your hand to jap upward at the attacker's chin. Do this at as close range as possible. Use as much strength as you can muster to hurt their jaw area.

Stab—Use your hand, stiffened with fingers together, as a "knife," and strike at the side of the neck where the carotid artery and jugular vein are located.

Poke/Thrust—Use your fingers to thrust into the attacker's eyes or nostrils. The harder the better.

Box—Take the edge of the palms of both hands, and box the attacker in the ears as hard as you can.

Groin Impact—Kick in the groin, hard and fast. If they grab you from behind, raise one knee, then back the leg foot-first into the groin area. If you are facing the attacker, try to kick or raise your knee up hard and fast into their groin.

Side Kick—If you can, raise one leg to knee height, then snap it outward fast and hard into the attacker. Go for the kneecap, groin, or stomach.

Whack—If you have the space between you and the attacker, you can try whacking them in the face with a purse or other object you may have (umbrella, laptop in case, etc.), including your own elbow.

Stomp—Yes, stomp as hard as you can on the attacker's foot.

Go for the feet, knees, stomach, groin, face, eyes, ears, and nose. These are areas sensitive to pain. Leverage your weight by throwing your body forward. If you are tall enough and strong enough, you can also employ things like chokeholds, bear hugs, and grabbing the attacker's wrists to bring them behind their body in a hold, while kicking their legs out from underneath them.

If the attacker has you pinned on the ground, you can try to knee him in the groin to wiggle out from under, or pivot to the side or on top of him.

Ultimately, though, getting good training is best, because it will show you exactly how these moves feel to perform them and will perfect your technique. Look for classes at local colleges, women's and men's clubs, private companies, even many gyms. In the meantime, there are many great videos online that can show you tips such as how to get out of zip ties and ropes, how to free your hands from duct tape, and even how to memorize pressure points on the body to disable another person.

WEAPONS

Sometimes you feel like you need to have a weapon to secure your safety inside and outside of the home. Women especially are learning how to use guns properly to protect them from assaults. A weapon can be anything from a whistle to a shotgun. You alone must decide what your needs are. The most important thing to remember is this: if you choose to buy a gun, learn how to use it, keep it locked and away from children, and know what the gun carry and operating laws are in your state.

Anyone can carry a whistle, noise alarm, or even a small air horn in a purse or pocket to deter an attacker. Noise tends to attract attention and will also alert a police officer in the area of a problem. But if you need something more, consider getting a canister of Mace, pepper spray, or a Taser gun if legal in your state. Some states do not allow possession of self-defense sprays. Don't

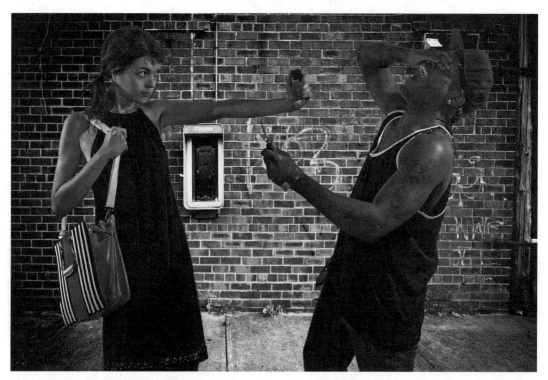

Mace or pepper spray may be effective in fending off a robber in some circumstances; of the two sprays, pepper is often preferred as more effective.

just assume yours does and buy one online, only to find yourself behind bars for using it.

Often Mace or pepper spray will also be permissible as reasonable force for self-defense. It cannot be used to punish someone or to deter a flirtation at a local bar! Mace is a chemical that is a classified irritant, similar to tear gas used by police. Pepper spray is an inflammatory agent that can incapacitate someone when sprayed in the eyes. Mace may not stop someone who is under the influence of certain drugs or alcohol, but pepper spray will affect anyone it comes in contact with. Only pepper spray will cause someone to be temporarily blinded with intense burning. It can also cause extreme nausea. Because of this, pepper spray may be the more effective choice.

"Mace" is actually a trademarked name of a tear gas and is not to be confused for the cooking spice of the same name!

Contact your local law enforcement to see what is legal and recommended in your state and area, as local laws may also be different. Stun guns and Tasers may be completely illegal, or particular types may be allowed. People under eighteen are not permitted to carry a stun gun. Some states may require a background check to carry either one. Other states outlaw both for use by private citizens. Don't buy one online without first making sure that it is legal, as some online sellers may tell you it is just to make the sale.

Also beware when buying from a third party or an individual. They may not have purchased the item legally, and as the new owner, you will be responsible if caught using it.

KNIVES AND GUNS

A knife is an option, but is it something that can be easily used? Obviously you cannot carry around a huge knife, but does a smaller pocket knife provide any protection? In some cases it might, but keep in mind state laws as to what you can and cannot carry. Using a knife to deter an attacker may depend on how much time you actually have to retrieve the knife and extend the blade. Remember, a knife is more of an "up close and personal" tool for fighting and protecting yourself. Unless you know how to throw one like a ninja master, it won't help unless you are close enough to use it.

If you are at home, even a heavy frying pan can be used as a weapon. Don't forget to look around at what you already have on hand, such as crowbars, heavy fire extinguishers, and pots and pans. A butcher knife or pair of sharp scissors is better than having no weapon at all, but use with discernment and only if doing so doesn't put your own life in danger.

For many people, a gun will be a better option. Firing a single bullet at an oncoming attacker, if you have good aim, will do the trick in keeping the attacker away. But if the gun gets knocked out of your hands and into the hands of the attacker, what then? This book in no way attempts to decide whether you should purchase and carry any kind of gun. This is a hugely personal choice and one that must comply with state laws. People are choosing to keep guns in the home for security purposes, and many states now have open carry laws that make it easy to show a potential attacker you are armed.

The best way to be comfortable with owning and using a gun is to buy one from a professional store, sign up for lessons on how to use it, and keep it locked and away from children to avoid unnecessary harm and suffering. If you go to a gun store, you can ask the store employees or owner what type of gun might be best for you, based again on the carry laws in your state. Some people opt for a small handgun. Women may like the idea of keeping a handgun or pistol in their purse at all times, as long as it is locked so that it does not fire at the wrong times. There are plenty of gun ranges around that can allow you to get your hands on a particular size and style of gun to see what works best and what you can use with ease and accuracy.

For out and about, some states do allow larger guns such as shotguns, rifles, and even assault weapons to be carried. The reality is, you do not need to carry anything extreme. The goal is self-protection. If you choose to buy a shotgun or rifle, get good advice, and get trained in how to properly use, clean, and store the

weapon. A conceal-carry gun usually means a length of 4.5–6 inches and is generally light and small, also known as a "compact" or "snub-nosed" pistol. Larger pistols are often called "duty" or "combat" pistols.

Keep in mind your physical size and strength too. This comes into play when choosing a particular gauge of, say, a shotgun. The gauge is the bore diameter of a shotgun (called the "caliber" for handguns and rifles: the larger the number, the smaller the bore diameter). When choosing which gauge shotgun, you must consider the powerful recoil and how easy it will be to handle if you are of a smaller build. Know the difference between a rifle, shotgun, and semi-automatic shotgun and the types of ammunition and how to load it before you commit to buying anything, and make sure what you choose makes sense for you. When you walk into a gun retailer, they will often have guns displayed by type, and in the case of handguns, by caliber. Ask—don't just read a few reviews

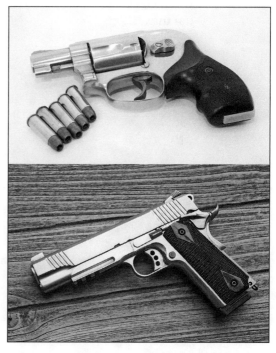

There are two basic types of handguns: double-action revolvers like the .38 special shown at top and semi-automatic pistols such as the .45 at bottom.

online and think you know which gun is best for your specific needs. Even the area where the trigger finger goes can vary in length and work for or against your finger size! You also want to make sure a gun fits your grip so you can have the most control while using it, and know what capacity the ammunition has in case you need to use more than a few bullets to take down a threat.

Guns and knives can be taken from you and used against you. They can also save your life. Get educated before you buy, and learn the proper way to use the gun you are investing in. No matter the type or size or style, those basics never change.

Being prepared for any crime is a plus. Deciding whether or not to take a class or buy a weapon is a personal choice that requires a bit of research, but it can be a great decision that may save your life or the lives of your loved ones. Ideally, we want to do whatever we can to avoid attracting a crime in the first place, but that's in a perfect world. Many families are choosing to take survival classes together. It is not only fun but incredibly empowering and can ensure that everyone knows exactly how to handle themselves and any weapons in the home if needed.

A final suggestion is to join a neighborhood watch program, even if you live in a condo complex or apartment building. It's a great way to get to know your neighbors and have everyone on the same page when it comes to potential threats.

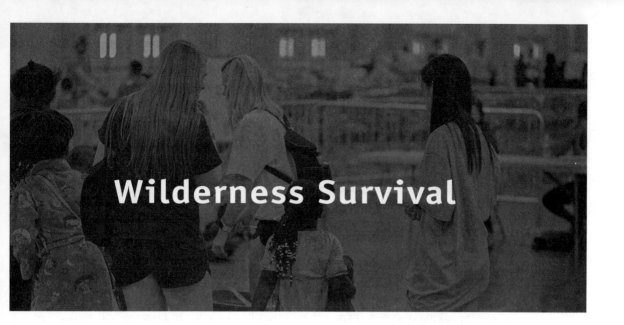

Wilderness Survival

Whether you are out on a day hike, a weeklong family camping trip, or bugging out of the city after a major disaster, surviving and thriving in a wilderness setting involves finding adequate shelter, having plenty of food and drinkable water, and knowing what to do in an emergency. Without the comforts of home, it is critical that you know your surroundings, especially if you've never camped or hiked in that area before. Don't just count on trail markers and fellow hikers to direct you back to base camp or to the safest source of water.

CAMPING AND HIKING

Before you even leave the house, check with the National Weather Service to see what the chance of rain or snow will be in the area you plan to camp or hike in. Rain could even lead to flash flooding if you will be on a hillside or near a creek or river. The last thing you want is to be trapped in a slot canyon during a sudden flash flood. Even if the weather is great when you leave, continue to listen for updates and possible changes that might affect your choice of where to set up camp.

Unless you have serious wilderness survival training, stick to designated campsites and hiking trails, and be sure to check in at base camps or with park rangers to let them know where you will be and how many are in your party.

Map out your route both on your cell phone and on paper, because out in the woods you may not have any cell phone coverage to rely upon. Beware of venturing off into unknown territory. If you get lost, no one will know where to look, and you won't have a method of contacting anyone. Consider having a flare gun on you when hiking in case you do venture off the maintained and marked trails.

If it is legal in your area, invest in a few canisters of bear spray, which is a form of pepper spray that you can use in a chance bear encounter.

Whether camping or hiking, have extra food, water, and a good first aid kid stocked with the basics. Include warm clothing and a blanket and a waterproof raincoat or plastic poncho. If you are going on a long hike or rappelling, go in a group. Be careful on trails with steep cliffs, and observe all posted warnings. If you are hiking with children, consider taking a longer, less steep route. Keep the weather in mind at all times to avoid having to deal with hyperthermia or heat exhaustion.

Snakes and poison plants are rampant in the wilderness. Consider wearing long pants, or socks that pull up to your knees, and sturdy closed-toed shoes. Some hikers like to bring along a ski pole or stick, which can be used to assist walking as well as clearing brush immediately ahead and possibly uncover a snake in the waiting.

Speaking of shoes, if you are an avid hiker or want to become one, make sure to invest in a good pair of comfortable hiking boots. Visit a specialty sporting goods store to get the best advice. The last thing you want or need is to be stuck in the middle of nowhere with feet too sore to stand on.

Similarly, do some research and choose the best hiking and camping gear you can afford. Buy a tent that is both easy to assemble and strong enough to withstand some rain. Don't forget about a sanitation system. Yes, you can "relieve yourself" in the woods, but if there is a danger of running into wild animals or snakes, bring a large bucket and some hefty trash bags and ties and some toilet paper.

In case your phone GPS isn't working, consider buying a compass to help you keep your directions straight. You may also want to mark your trail as you go so you can easily get back to camp. This can help when you are hiking with children, and you might become incapacitated and need to send them back for help. Invest in a light pair of binoculars as well for searching from hilltops and high points.

Honor the code of the trail when hiking. Don't leave behind litter. Do not damage trail markers and map stations. Serious hikers live by this code because they know and respect nature and understand how easy it can be to get lost and become disoriented. There is a trail saying: Take nothing but pictures, leave nothing but footprints.

According to the U.S. Forest Service and the Centers for Disease Control and Prevention, recreation activities should be planned just as for a trip abroad. Some of the tips they suggest are:

Think about any vaccinations you might need before you head out, such as tetanus, pertussis, meningitis, or hepatitis A. Ask your doctor if you are concerned.

Travel with someone, and leave your itinerary with a responsible third party.

Before you take on a long hike, make sure you are in good physical shape! If it is a group hike, plan it around the *weakest* member of the group and what they are capable of. If you are traveling with a disabled person, take into account what they are able to do, and perhaps let faster hikers form a separate group.

Watch the weather and plan accordingly.

Avoid cliffs! This especially applies if you and others have been drinking, it is dark out or wet from rain. You are not a sure-footed mountain goat!

Know the basics of first aid, and have someone carry a first aid kit. Know your ABCs too.

Make camp before dark, or you run the risk of falls, accidents, and getting lost in the woods.

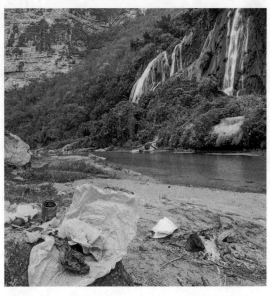

Here, the beauty of the La Conchuda waterfall in Chiapas, Mexico, stands out. Unfortunately, not all hikers honor the trail and nature's beauty.

Don't assume a clear brook offers clean, drinkable water. Boil it, or use your water purification tablets to avoid water-borne parasites. If you have diarrhea, stay out of any water areas others may be swimming in. Do not swallow any water that you are fishing, bathing, or swimming in.

Pack a lot of energy bars, which are a great and compact source of carbs, proteins, and fats, and carry plenty of water.

If you are bringing your dogs, keep them leashed, and be sure to have food, snacks, heat protection, and water for them too. Clean up after them if they poop in the middle of the trail!

Protect yourself against the sun with a hat, sunglasses, and sunscreen. Use a broad-spectrum sunscreen that will protect from UVA and UVB rays, and don't forget a sunscreen lip balm or stick!

Assign tasks, if in a group, so everyone can be in charge of something specific and one person is not expected to remember everything.

Take breaks if needed, but give yourself a two-hour window to set up camp during daylight.

Never leave a fire unattended. Drown it with plenty of water, and look for any burning embers.

Never use fuel-burning equipment such as stoves, heat devices, lanterns, or grills inside a closed tent or shelter because of the risk of carbon monoxide poisoning. Keep them outside.

Out in the Storm

If you are out in the middle of the woods or hiking up a mountain, and a storm approaches, obviously the ideal situation would be to get back to camp. If you are on a lake fishing or boating, or out playing golf on a Sunday afternoon, a storm can mean flash flooding and lightning.

While you want to avoid being near waterways or areas where flash flooding can send water downhill towards you, you also want to descend from exposed, high places to avoid getting struck by lightning. This applies to locating your camp too. Don't pitch tents right next to the tallest trees around or isolated trees in a clearing. They act as lightning rods!

If you are on a mountain bike or horse or in a golf cart, get off immediately and drop anything metal you may be carrying, such as an umbrella, ski pole, or golf club. If you are out in the open, find a low spot and crouch with your head low or covered. Don't sit or lie down, because the more of your body that is in contact with the ground, the more chance you have of being injured if a lightning bolt hits nearby. If you are with a group of people, spread out 15 feet (4.6 meters) apart to avoid all of you getting struck. If you are in the woods, stay put until the storm is over.

If someone is hit by lightning, tend to them immediately for the ABCs. Unlike in the movies, a person hit by lightning will not carry and transfer a charge to you. Help them!

Once the storm appears to have passed, wait a bit before going out into any clearings to avoid lightning that may still be lingering. Make sure that the area you are in is not in the path of a potential flash flood!

Beware of wildlife, and keep foodstuffs put away in containers to avoid visits from bears. This includes garbage, cooking grease, coolers, and even utensils that haven't been washed yet.

If you need to relieve yourself outside at night, go with a buddy and bring a flashlight. Animals feed at night, and the noise and light may drive them away.

Know the difference ahead of time between regular and poisonous plants!

Wear long-sleeved clothing, long pants, and sturdy shoes.

Stay away from alcohol, as it can dehydrate you and add to clumsiness on steep trails.

Apply some type of bug repellant to skin that will be exposed.

Wear light-colored clothing if you are concerned about ticks, as they will be easier to spot.

Do not eat wild berries, mushrooms, or any other plant!

Do not approach or pet wild animals such as raccoons, possums, mountain cats, and coyotes. They may be small and look harmless, but they are not, especially if they feel threatened.

THE DISASTER SURVIVAL GUIDE

One of the biggest problems is campers and hikers who go out into the woods thinking they will remember the trail they took and then find themselves lost as darkness falls. Always have a map and a compass at the very least. A cell phone with GPS and trail markers is great, but there may not be any service in the middle of the woods or up on a mountain. Don't take that risk. Mark the trail as you go, and do *not* use bits of popcorn or food, because they won't be there when you go back. Use strips of cloth or trash bag ties on branches, or something in bright colors that you can easily see. Avoid using green and brown, as they will blend in too much with your surroundings. If you are injured, you may be better off finding a somewhat sheltered area with brush and trees and waiting until morning, or sending the person you are with for help. As a very last resort, if there is a nearby stream, creek, river, or even a drainage waterway, follow it downhill. Again, make camp before dark, getting back at least two hours before it starts to get dark. Better safe than sorry.

If you want to take a night hike, there are guided hikes in groups that you can sign up for.

Survival in the wild can come down to protecting your body temperature and staying warm when it's cold, and cool when it's burning hot. Any shelter you find must block the elements and insulate you for warmth and away from the cold.

ANIMAL AND PLANT HAZARDS

A walk in nature can turn into a nightmare if you are not prepared for a potential problem. Let's start with bears. Do you know what to do if you encounter a bear, mountain lion, or other large predatory animal out in the wild? Many national parks and camping areas do not allow you to carry bear spray, which is a type of pepper spray. You have to remember that, when you enter the woods and mountains, you are on their territory and need to act with respect.

If you spot a bear or other large animal at a distance, avoid it. The same applies if you come upon babies or cubs. Stay away. The parent animals can be nearby and look at human interaction with their babies as an act of aggression. Leave the area and try to report the location to a park ranger. The closer you get, the more you are actually allowing bears and wild animals to become less fearful of people. In designated sites, park rangers will be on the lookout and have their own methods for dealing with animal intruders.

At a campsite or on the hiking trail, the key is to present yourself as being "big" and making a lot of noise. If a bear is nearby or coming toward you, do not run from it. Stand tall, arms linked with others, and scream, yell, bang on things. Never surround the bear, as this will make it feel threatened and launch an attack. Scare it away. Clap, stomp, wave your arms high to intimidate the bear with your size, and make all the ruckus you can until the bear backs off. If any of you are holding food, drop it or toss it out of the way of the campsite. Do not

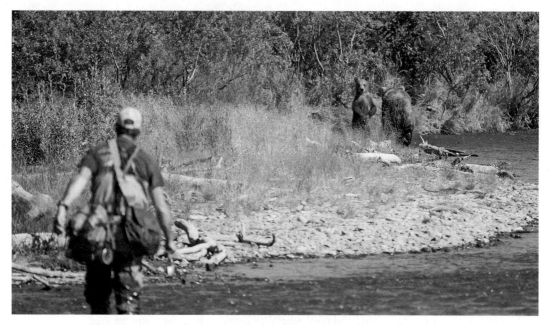

If you encounter a bear or bears while hiking, camping, or fishing, do not approach them; move away from them as quickly as possible. If you are hiking in an area where bears are known to roam, make noise by clapping, singing, or talking loudly and the bears will avoid you.

stop to take cell phone pictures, because the bear may change its mind and attack.

Beware of areas where there are a lot of dead animal and bird carcasses around, as you may be entering a bear's or other wild animal's feeding ground and will be seen as a competing predator. Also, look for aggressive behavior from the start. Bears will snort, paw the ground, and pop their jaws as signs they feel threatened or ready to lunge at you. These behaviors may be to get you to back off and leave the area. Do not turn your back and run screaming. Just quietly back up and away until you feel you are at a safe distance.

However, if you do get attacked, the best thing you can do is fight with all your might, protecting your face and neck. Punch, kick, slam your hands into the bear's ears, jab at the eyes. Do whatever you can to break the bear's hold on you. If there are several bears, try to climb a tree. Use legal bear spray if you have it, pointing the nozzle just above the bear's head level so that the spray actually falls in its face, which will sting the eyes, nose, and ears and send the bear off in the opposite direction. If not, do your best to fight it off while screaming for help.

Bears attack for two reasons: defensively, to protect themselves and their cubs; and offensively, to get your food or to get you as food. Black bears tend to

Bear Spray

Bear spray or bear Mace is *not* the same as regular pepper spray. Bear spray is much stronger and is highly effective. You might not be able to fight off a bear with regular pepper spray. Nor will you deter a bear by spraying it on your cooler, tent, or backpack. It works well because bears have a sense of smell about 2,000 times stronger than that of humans. Just getting the spray in their noses works wonders, but it also causes extreme distress if you get it in the bear's eyes or mouth.

It is not lethal, but it will work long enough for you to get away. You take the can out of the holster and remove the safety clip, then point and spray. You may want to aim the spray just above the bear's head, as it will arc down to the face. Spray in short bursts for about two seconds each. If it is freezing or raining, the spray may not work as well reaching its target, as the pressure in the canister will decrease, so try to keep the canister in a warm place when you are outside.

Bear spray or Mace is easy to get, but you may want to go to a camping or survival store and ask for a recommended brand, or check online reviews. There is no rating system for quality control, so see what others have said about using it.

be more predatory and will attack humans more than brown bears. Grizzlies are more predatory than black bears. Female bears will be more concerned with protecting their cubs. Know what kinds of animals are common in the area where you are hiking or camping. Both black bears and grizzlies can outrun a human, so don't run away. Often bears do what is called "bluff charging," which is to charge without actual contact to allow the enemy a chance to back down and leave. Slowly back away if a bear bluff-charges you.

You can also try playing dead to deflect a defensive bear or animal attack. If you must do this as a last resort, get into a fetal position with your body tightly curled, and cover your head with your backpack if you have it with you, or bury your head between your legs and stay still and quiet. If a bear sees you as a threat only, this may cause them to take off, feeling safe. This is a *last-minute* choice, though. Until you feel you cannot out-dodge the bear any longer, stay standing and moving.

Even wolves and coyotes, which may not seem big enough to worry about, can attack you if provoked. Often they travel in packs, and you may not see the pack right away. Back away from the animal slowly, and if you must fight, go for the head area. You can try to block the animal's mouth with your non-dominant arm, then use your other hand to smash the heel against the animal's nose, ears, or head and stun it enough to get away. Don't treat your bite wounds until you know you are safe and the animal can't find you.

Avoid issues with bears or any other wild animals that may be predatory, aggressive, or even rabid as much as you can by staying away from areas they are sighted in, avoiding coming into contact with cubs, and not leaving food and garbage out in the open or uncovered in tents. You can also avoid a potential attack by respecting a bear or other animal's space and not trying to get close to get a photo for social networking. Leave them alone and you have a better chance of being left alone in return.

PLANTS

Know what poison plants are indigenous to your area, whether at home or out camping in the woods. The best way to deal with poisonous plants is to avoid exposure by wearing long pants and sleeves while out in the woods.

The big three are poison oak, poison ivy, and poison sumac. Poison oak is found primarily in the western United States, but there is an Atlantic poison oak found in the southern states. Poison ivy is found throughout the country, with western poison ivy in the West and eastern poison ivy in the eastern United States. Poison sumac is found in swampy regions of the eastern United States, but also in Texas and the southern states.

Poison ivy and oak share the "leaves of three, let them be" status of having leaf clusters in threes. Leaves may be notched or smooth, and the plant itself will have a reddish tinge in spring, green in summer, and more of an orange/yellow tone in fall. They may also have greenish-white berries and green/yellow flowers. Poison sumac grows as both a vine and a shrub, with seven to thirteen leaflets per stem. Leaves are smooth with pointed tips.

They all produce urushiol, a very potent oily resin that is highly irritating to exposed skin. Symptoms of contact to all three include redness, rash, itching, blistering, and systemic infections if left untreated. Initial reactions may be mild, with symptoms worsening over time, so treat the problem once you realize there has been exposure. If you can identify the type of plant, that helps. Even if you were wearing long sleeves and pants, the oil will be on your clothes, so if your skin is fine, be careful when removing clothing! Touching someone else that has been exposed, even a pet, can get the oil on you too.

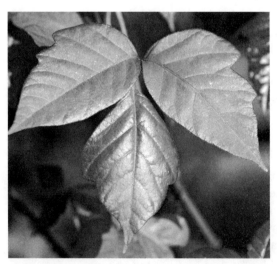

Both poison ivy and poison oak have a distinctive, three-leaf configuration that makes them easy to spot and avoid if you are vigilant.

Immediately wash the exposed area with cold water and soap. There are commercial products you can use, but rarely do we have them on hand. Call your doctor or ask your pharmacist if you want more protection than water and soap. Launder your clothing right away, including sleeping bags if you were out camping. Scrub under fingernails to remove any oil deposited there.

Cold packs can help relieve pain. Benadryl or an antihistamine will help with some of the itching, as will cold compresses, calamine lotion, or hydrocortisone cream. Do not apply anything on open or blistered skin.

Severe symptoms may require a steroid shot, so seek your doctor's help.

HOW TO START A FIRE

Ideally, you should have dry matches or a lighter and fuel source in your gear. But if you are without these items or they don't work (matches wet from unexpected rain), you need to know how to start a fire to keep warm and to cook food and boil water. Fires require oxygen, fuel, and a spark. Look for dry twigs, branches, and dry leaves, and put them in a pile. Now you have your fuel. Oxygen is in the air. So how do you make the spark light it all up?

Can you find a flintstone and something with steel? Strike the flint against the steel until a spark or two ignites the fuel source. You can even buy a flint/steel kit to bring with you if matches and lighters aren't your thing. You can also try rubbing two dry sticks together or striking a rock against another rock to make a spark, but that may take a lot longer.

If you have a small magnifying glass, you can use the sun's rays to start a fire, but if you don't, try putting some water in a clear plastic bag. Tie the bag off, and make it as round as possible, like a round balloon. Hold it up to the sun. See how the rays spread on the ground? Focus the light about one or two inches over the kindling to light the fire.

Use pine needles to make a fire if they are around, as they contain a highly flammable material called "pitch" and will even keep a fire going in light rain. Split larger pieces of wood into smaller pieces, which burn better. If the only wood around looks wet, try peeling off the bark to get to the dry wood underneath.

To start and feed a fire, you need the right amount of food. Start with tinder and kindling. Tinder is anything that gets the fire started, which burns the kindling, which in turn lights the fuel or the wood.

Tinder can be anything that is highly combustible and only needs a spark to get it going. Think things like dry leaves that are crushed, bark and bark shavings, fallen pine needles, paper, strips of newspaper, strips of rubber, cotton wool, charred fabric, dried grasses, and wood shavings. Once the spark gets the tinder going, then it will ignite the kindling.

Kindling can be dry, crisp leaves, pine cones, dry bark chunks, twigs and branches and is usually some type of wood. Softer woods flare up faster, and if the wood has resin it will burn even faster. The kindling must be more substantial than the tinder, so that it creates high flames, but not as big as your main wood logs. Kindling must be dry when collected or it won't take the flame. If all you see around you is damp kindling, then shave off the outer layer to get to the dry interior.

Wood is the largest part of the fire and is usually large branches, logs, and chunks of wood. Softwoods will burn out more quickly, so they may not be good for cooking over a fire. Hardwoods burn hot for a long time, so they are great for cooking and roasting. All wood used must be dead, dry, and not from something man-made like a telephone pole or fence post, because those will contain paint and other chemicals that will be released upon burning. It helps to know the trees in the area you will be camping or hiking in, so you can identify hard and soft woods. If you plan to camp and hike often, consider investing in a good field guide to trees and plants for your region.

Have any hand sanitizer in your first aid kit? They usually contain alcohol, which is flammable. You can rub some on leaves or a cloth and place on the tinder to assist the kindling in catching fire off a spark.

If you wear thick coke-bottle eyeglasses, you are in luck. You can use the thick lenses like a magnifying glass to make a fire. Spit on the lens, and then angle the lens at the pile of kindling you have. Hold steady awhile and blow on the fire to get it going. You can also do this with a glass water bottle. The idea is to focus the rays through the water to create a single point of intense heat on the dry kindling.

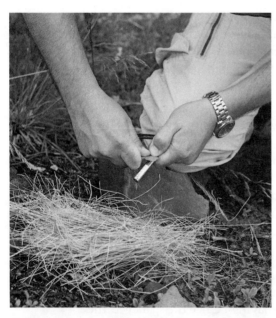

A man starts a fire using a fire striker (carbon steel to start a spark) over dried grass. If you don't have this tool, or a match, or a cigarette lighter, you might try a piece of glass or even a polished aluminum soda can bottom.

You may want to use a larger log of wood for your base, and then, when the tinder on top of it is lit, stack your kindling against the larger log, almost like a lean-to, which will allow oxygen to pass through and feed the larger log's flames. Keep adding larger kindling until the fire grows really hot, then add larger logs of wood.

You can also use your fire, once it's roaring, to make smoke signals for other campers or hikers to see if you need help and don't have a flare gun. Burn something that creates thick smoke, then use a blanket or board to wave over it to create puffs of smoke. Pine and spruce leaves make thick smoke. Obviously, this works best if you make the fire on a high spot that isn't hidden by tall trees.

Alert! SOS!

You can use fire and smoke to alert other campers and hikers, or even a helicopter flying by, that you are in distress. Do this out in the open so it can be seen, preferably at the top of a hill or in a clearing where high winds won't disperse the smoke before it can be spotted. Make a platform with twigs and branches that will raise the actual fire up higher. This can look like a teepee made of wood planks and branches. Using your most easily combustible materials, get the fire going at the base, and pile on greener branches to keep the smoke thick and visible.

If you think you will need to make a fire again the next day, here is a wonderful way to make it a lot easier. You can make a "char cloth." This is done by taking a small piece of cloth and putting it inside some kind of metal box or container. Then you seal the container and put it in the fire for a few minutes. Carefully remove the container from the fire, let it cool, and keep closed until the next time you need a fire. When you open the case, you will have a piece of black cloth that is not burned but can be used to create a much easier spark from. Also, if you have petroleum jelly and cotton balls, you can soak the cotton balls in the jelly and use them for fast and long-burning fuel.

But if you don't have the ability to make a fire, find something that can reflect sunlight into the sky, such as a mirror, eyeglasses, a magnifying glass, or a glass or plastic bottle. You can even use your cell phone screen. Hold it up to the sun, and move it back and forth to reflect light in "flashes." If there is a boat or plane you are trying to target, try making a peace sign with one hand. Line up the boat or plane between your two raised fingers, and aim the flashes back and forth between those fingers.

SHELTER, FOOD, AND WATER

The weather can be enemy number one in the wilderness. Finding shelter might be as easy as popping a tent, but if you are stuck without cover, you can succumb to heat, cold, and even predators. You can, with the right materials, build your own shelter. Rules of thumb, though: do not ever build on wet ground; do not build on top of hills or high areas, where strong and cold winds can become a hazard and blow your shelter away; do not build in low and narrow valleys, where wind also blows hard. A shelter can be a quick pile or mound of leaves and twigs you can crawl under or put your sleeping bag under, or something more elaborate built with sticks and brush that mimics a tent. To do this, you would need long sticks that can be put into an A-frame and covered with leaves and twigs. No matter how fancy your shelter is on the outside, make sure to have a dry bed of leaves to sleep on to avoid the cold ground.

In the woods or mountains, the idea is to keep warm and dry. If you are stuck out in the middle of the desert, the goal will be to keep cool and avoid the punishing sun's rays. Heat stroke is the second most common cause of death in the desert. Dehydration is first. If you are stuck with no shelter, not even a broken-down car to get out of the sun in, you may have to walk to find something to hide in or under. A tip, if water is scarce, is to use your own urine to soak a cloth, bandana, or anything you might have on you that you can then wrap around your head.

Finding water in the woods is easy, as long as you follow steps to boil or disinfect it. In the desert, where the average annual rainfall may be less than ten inches, you may have to get creative. You can keep an eye on any wildlife or birds to see what direction they are moving in, which will often be towards a water source. Fly and mosquito swarms are an especially good indicator of nearby water. Even bees fly towards and away from water. There may be some water deposited from previous rains under rocks or near dry riverbeds and streams. Green plants in the desert imply rain has fallen. The key is to not use up all your own water supply walking long distances to find water.

When it cools down a bit, you can dig for water under areas where greenery is growing or in low valleys and rock crevices. Water might be found about twelve inches from the surface. It may take a while for the water to collect into the hole, but once it does, be sure to disinfect before drinking if you can. Also look for water in the form of dew on plants and in the hollow trunks of dead trees. You can also eat cactus fruit to get water, and you can eat the pads of prickly pear cactus by cooking them over a fire.

In North American deserts, we also have barrel cactus, which has water inside, but this is only a last resort if no other water source can be found. The liquid inside can cause severe reactions such as vomiting, nausea, and even paralysis. The only really safe barrel cactus is the fishhook barrel cactus, found in the southwestern part of the United States and into Mexico. It may have little red or yellow flowers on top and can be cut at the top to reveal the white interior "meat." Mash the meat up until you can squeeze a liquid from it to drink, and only drink a very small amount.

Out in the woods, if you cannot find a creek or other water source and have run out of water, you can get water from the trees around you by collecting it from leaves. You need to work with leaves that are directly exposed to sunlight. Early in the morning, rap a plastic bag around a chunk of these leaves and the sun will force water inside the leaves to evaporate, trapping the residue inside the bag. All you need to do is poke a hole in the bag and use the water. Make sure the plastic bags are clear and also clean when you use them.

You might also camp near a snowy mountain that will have run-off, but be careful not to be right up against the base in case of flash flooding. Most designated campsites and hiking trails have access to water sources, but when you choose to go out on your own, it might be helpful to check a map of the area beforehand to spot any creeks, lakes, ponds, rivers, or brooks.

Although we can get some of that much-needed water from food sources, drinking it or liquids containing it, such as juice and milk, is much better.

How Long Can You Go without Food and Water?

Yes, you can survive without food far longer than you can without water, possibly even a few months! According to "Who, What, Why: How Long Can Someone Survive without Food?" a February 20, 2012, article for BBC.com, there have been instances of people subsisting on next to nothing but snow or water for two months. Water is far more critical to our survival. Many of us tend to have enough body fat on us for our brains and metabolic system to use as fuel.

Surviving two months on next to nothing is of course the extreme, but according to Dr. Mike Stroud of the Department of Medicine and Nutrition at Southampton University, the body's metabolism can slow down to conserve energy. He feels that body fat is not that great an indicator of how long you can survive, but it would be about sixty days before organs would begin to shut down in an extreme case. Two months is a lot of time, and no doubt we could find food during that period, even if it came in the form of bugs and plants.

The body will use glucose, which is stored in the muscles and the liver, as glycogen, the primary fuel source. But once that is used up, the body will convert fat into ketone bodies, which can fuel the brain as well as the muscles and organs. But once the body fat is gone, then you have the wasting of important tissue reserves, and worse.

So while the body does slow down to accommodate the lack of food, you can still only go so long without finding some source of nourishment.

When it comes to water, things don't look as good. We can last up to a week without water, but even that limit is more oriented to studies of people who are on their deathbeds, when food and water needs slow to a crawl. Three to four days is much more reasonable. Because over 60 percent of the body is made up of water, and every cell we have needs water to function properly, as do our organs, joints, muscles, and skin, we need to find it more quickly than food. If we lose too much water, our blood volume may drop dangerously low and cause blood pressure levels that are fatal. If the weather is hot, we need to find it even quicker because of the amount of water we lose in the form of sweat.

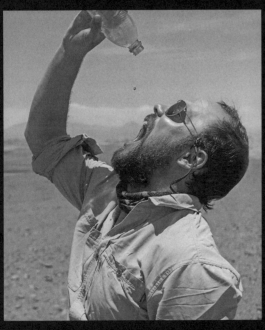

The human body can go without food for a few weeks, depending on body fat, but surviving without water for more than four days is unlikely.

What about food? If you have enough with you to last the duration of your stay, good for you. But if you end up being caught out of doors for longer than you hoped for, do you know how to fish? Hunt? Trap animals? Do you know how to clean them, skin them, and cook them?

If you are lucky enough to be near a body of water with fish in it, and you don't have a fishing rod and gear, find a long stick and poke at the fish you can see to try to catch one. When you get a fish back to your campsite, you will need to clean it and take out the bones, using a sharp knife, and dispose of anything not to be eaten in a sealed trash bag. You can make a makeshift grill to put the fish on over the fire, using interwoven greener twigs that are flexible, or you can poke a stick through the fish and cook it over the open flame.

You can also make a type of "dam trap" to put in the water and catch fish in. This can be a metal box with a fishhook and bait inside, or a stretch of fabric that can act as a net. If you don't have bait hooks, make one with a sharp piece of wood or metal, and stick a worm on the end. Safety pins make great hooks, as do paper clips. Rough them into a hook, find anything you can use as bait, and if you have string or rope, you can use that as a makeshift fishing pole. If you don't plan to hold the rope or line, attach it to a stick, and place it in the ground with a small bell or noisemaker to alert you when a fish bites.

If you have a hunting rifle or a crossbow or some other type of hunting gear, you won't have to worry about catching food by hand. But you do have to clean the carcass and remove all inner organs and body parts that won't be eaten, dispose of them in a sealed trash bag, and cook over the fire long enough not to get sick from undercooked meat. The truth is, if you are out of food and starving, you will do what it takes to trap and catch food, even if it is something you wouldn't have otherwise considered eating, such as squirrel or raccoon, even insects, which can provide protein and keep you alive in a pinch.

You can make a spear out of a tree branch or stick and use it to kill small animals. Traps work too, but you have to place them in high animal traffic areas. They can consist of a box rigged with a rope that will pull the cover down when something gets inside, or a net attached to twine or rope on either side that can be lifted up when an animal steps into it. Get creative. A pit trap is an option too, if you have the ability to dig a hole and then cover it with twigs and brush, but you have to get the animal to walk over it for it to work. In any trap, put some kind of bait inside, like water, to attract the animal inside in the first place.

Never eat an animal carcass you find on the ground, no matter how fresh the kill may look. It may already be infested with maggots and fly eggs. Or it may be the meal of a nearby predator that won't take too kindly to having its dinner stolen.

One way to find potential animals to hunt is to follow heavily used trails and look for tracks and droppings. Water sources are great because birds and other animals will use them as watering holes. Also look for visible signs of dens, nests, and holes where animals could be hiding.

You can sun-dry meat you catch by cutting it into long, thin strips, like bacon. Stick two large sticks or branches into the ground about a foot apart, and then tie a cord, rope, or twine at each end to form a line between the tops of the sticks. Hang the meat over the string or twine and keep each strip from touching other strips of meat or from folding over on itself. Do this in a place with plenty of sunlight, and protect the meat from bugs and predators as best you can. This works great if you are in the desert camping or hiking, as there is ample sunshine.

When it comes to foraging for food, if you are not familiar with the types of plants, grasses, mushrooms, and berries that grow in the area, you run the risk of eating something not meant for human consumption. But foraging doesn't require the effort of hunting and fishing, so if you find edible goods like nuts, berries, and greenery that you can survive on, more power to you.

According to the U.S. Air Force guidelines, listed in the *Special Forces Survival Guide* by Chris McNab, which were created by downed pilots who needed to identify what they could and couldn't eat, the following rules apply:

- Avoid plants with umbrella-shaped flowers (but vegetables like carrots, celery, and parsley are fine).
- Avoid bulbs.
- Avoid white and yellow berries.
- Avoid plants with milky white sap.
- Avoid legumes, as they may lead to stomach issues.
- Avoid plants that irritate the skin.
- Avoid plants that smell like almonds on their leaves or woody areas, as this can indicate the presence of cyanide.

But …

- Eat plants growing in water or moist soil.
- Eat aggregated fruits and berries.
- Eat single fruits on stems.

Also look for acorns from oak trees. The nut is edible, and they are small and easy to carry back to camp. Pine trees have nuts too, and their inner bark can also be eaten. Other edible nuts include walnuts, almonds, chestnuts, and beechnuts. Tall grasses and ferns can be eaten. Go for the base, where the starchy carbohydrates are focused. You can also eat cattail, the stalk of which is similar to celery, clover, and daisies. You can eat fungi, but not all are edible, so it helps to know which is which. In general, you can eat tree fungi and many varieties of puffy mushrooms found growing in the ground. However, if a mushroom stains yellow when cut open, it is poisonous.

Try testing the plant first. You can do this by separating the parts of the plant into a pile. Leaves, stem, flowers, etc. This way you can test one part at a time. First, smell the plant parts for an acidic odor that may mean they are not safe to eat. Try not to eat anything else for eight hours before you test the plants. Touch each part of the plant to see if there is a skin reaction. If not, you can try a part of the plant along with a mouthful of purified water. If you feel any burning sensation at all when you touch the plant part to your lip, don't eat it. Hold a bit of the plant on your tongue for up to fifteen minutes. If there is no reaction, you can try eating that plant.

Spruce and pine needles can make a great tea. They contain a lot of vitamins C and A. Bruise the needles first with a rock, then put them into a pot of boiling water. Remove from the fire, and let steep for ten minutes before drinking.

Look for dandelions, which grow wild, and eat the leaves.

Look for the youngest plants when you are picking them. They will be easier to digest.

When it comes to berries found in the wild, here is a general rule: "White and yellow, kill a fellow. Purple and blue, good for you. Red, could be good, could be dead!" With blackberries and cranberries, not only can you eat the berries, but the leaves are also edible.

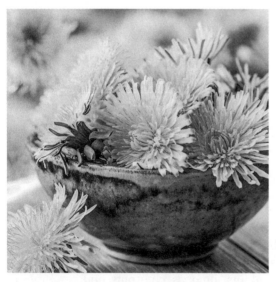

Quite a few plants that are common to see are edible, including cattails, clover, chickweed, and dandelions. Dandelions are best when boiled; you can eat every part of this "weed," and you can even make dandelion wine!

Even wild plants that are edible may have parts that shouldn't be eaten, such as stalks and leaves. You can try the poison taste test if uncertain. You obviously want to avoid plants that are afflicted with pests or mold/fungi, and plants in contaminated or filthy water, unless you plan to boil the plant.

You can eat a variety of insects, but avoid eating bugs like spiders, bees, and millipedes. Ants and crickets are fine to eat. Crickets can be roasted over the fire if the thought of eating them live doesn't appeal to you. You may want to cook ants too, to remove any toxins from the ground they were found in (especially if the soil was damp).

Other edible insects and bugs include worms, grasshoppers, termites, slugs, and snails. You can skewer them with a stick and cook them over a fire. If it has a stinger or is brightly colored, leave it alone.

When it comes to finding insects, they are often most abundant beneath rocks and on the ground in shaded brush areas. Older trees can be havens for termites too. Look for a termite nest, and use a stick to poke the nest and retrieve insects. Scrape them into a jar or container, and cook them over the fire back at camp.

Some pointers when foraging for bugs:

Be careful when searching for insects that you don't accidentally get bitten by something hiding beneath the rocks or brush, such as a snake! Wear work gloves if you can. Never jostle or disturb a wasp's or hornet's nest or you will be sorry.

Brightly colored insects tend to be poisonous, even if they are easy to spot. Go for the dull in color and appearance.

Grubs found on the underside of leaves are not good to eat, as they can excrete a venomous fluid.

Cricket and locust wings, heads, and legs should be removed before eating, even if you plan to cook them.

When it comes to finding food, look down and around, but also look up. Most birds can be eaten, if you can catch them. You can also eat the eggs in

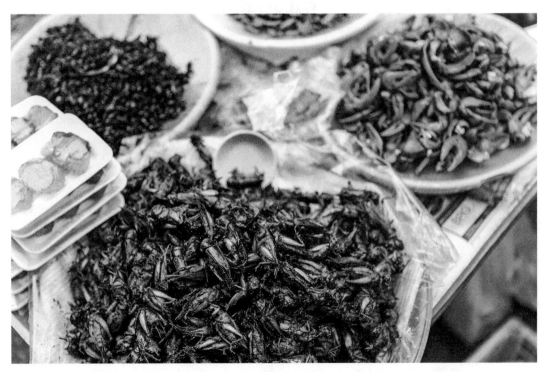

A Thai vendor offers a spread of various insects to eat. Insects are a great source of protein that you can take advantage of yourself if necessary.

their nests. Be careful not to eat dead birds, as they may be infested with maggots or carrying diseases.

Nonvenomous snakes are also something you can fall back on—again, if you can catch them. You can make simple ground traps or, if you have seen them around, hunt them down with a sharp stick or butterfly net. Skin them and throw them over a fire roasted. Frogs can be cooked and eaten, but not toads, which may carry toxins in their skin.

When creating your shelter, keep in mind that a big problem is setting up shelter in a danger zone and finding out too late. Watch out for potential overhead "widowmakers," old tree branches that can fall on you in high winds. Also try to stay away from dried out and dead trees that, if they catch fire, will go up fast and furiously around you. If you are in the mountains, avoid being right at the base or in foothill areas because of possible flash flooding from snow runoff.

Oh, and take some time to survey the area you may camp in for at least twenty yards in every direction before you begin to set up tents and start a fire. Look for bee and wasp hives, ant colonies, claw marks on trees that indicate large predators may be around, and signs of animal nesting places that can cause you trouble later if mama or papa returns.

WILDERNESS HACKS

Toothpaste can be used on bug bites to help relieve itching and stop minor pain and swelling.

Tampons can be used to absorb blood from wounds.

Even a dead lighter can be taken apart for the cotton inside, which is dry and can assist in catching a spark to make a fire.

Have a roll of aluminum foil? You can make bowls out of it and also lay a sheet down on damp ground to start a fire on.

Keep a line of big rocks around the campfire to trap in some heat long after the fire has died out. Smaller rocks hot from the fire can be put inside aluminum cans filled with water to purify it.

Large aluminum sheets can be draped outside your tent to reflect sunlight away and keep you cooler inside.

Those crazy glow sticks kids get at Halloween make great makeshift lights if the flashlight runs out of batteries.

There are many unusual and creative ways to make being stuck out in the wild more survivable and comfortable.

Animal organs such as bladders and snake skins make great makeshift water carriers. Be sure to rinse them out first.

You can make a torch out of a stick with a rag tied around the top end. Soak the rag in a fuel source, and light it on fire. It may not last long, but it can help when you need extra light.

Lost in the Woods?

If you are without a compass or phone with GPS, you can still find your way back if you pay attention to nature's signals. The easiest is to watch for sunrise and sunset to tell east from west and then north and south. Some other tips include:

- Look at tree trunks for moss growth. Moss usually grows away from sunlight and is often found on the northern side of trees. The same goes for moss-covered rocks.

- The thickest part of the moss will be on the north side.

- Make your own sundial by sticking a twig in the ground and watching the direction of the shadow on the ground to indicate east-west movement.

- In the northern hemisphere, your shadow will point northward at noon. In the southern hemisphere, it will point southward.

- Spiders will build their webs on the southern side of trees.

- In the desert, look for barrel cactus. They lean south.

- On mountain slopes that face the sun, look for trees. There will be more snowmelt on the side of the trunk facing south.

- Ideally, you will have a general guess as to what direction you were moving in when you left your campsite, so you can then redirect yourself back.

- Don't forget your watch if you wear one! Often watches, especially men's sportier watches, have compasses in them.

If you hunt and cook your own food, be sure to prepare the dead animal away from the campsite and put all uneaten parts in a sealed bag or container. Remember: bears.

If you plan to stay outdoors awhile and fish and hunt your own food, know how to make some basic snares and traps if you are not using a gun or bow and arrow. For smaller animals, you can use funnel traps that direct them into the hidden trap. This works well for rabbit, squirrel, and smaller mammals.

Buying a new sleeping bag? Look for a U.S. military Gore-Tex modular sleeping bag system. It comes with a sleeping bag liner inside that will keep you warm. If you are going camping in colder weather, look for a sleeping bag with goose down that is in a layer of Gore-Tex liner to protect against moisture. Synthetic bags also keep you warm, but tend to be a few pounds heavier than goose down.

Invest in a sturdy tent that won't tear or leave you with a broken zipper in the cold and rain. Look for a tent that is rated for use in places such as Mount Everest if you want to be extra sure of protection.

Invest in a good compass, and learn how to use it. Don't opt for cheap plastic compasses that may have polarity issues and be less than accurate.

A headlamp makes a great flashlight that allows you to stay hands free for cooking or cleaning.

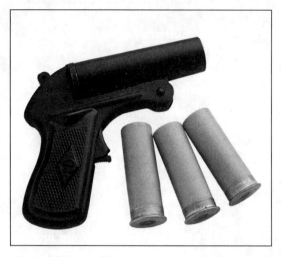

A signal flare gun like this is an optimal tool to signal for help when you are lost in the wilderness or even at sea.

Ladies' lipstick can be used to mark trees on the hiking trail in case you get lost.

Get both a signal flare gun with extra flares and roadside safety flares. You can use the signal flares if you are lost or trying to signal to others in your group. The safety flares can be used if you need something to start a fire in a pinch. Handheld flares will burn for a good half hour and can be stuck into the ground to light campsites.

Consider bringing an air horn. Not only can it work wonders warding off bears, but it can also act as a noise signal to others if you are lost in the woods.

If you are stuck outdoors for a long time, you need to pay attention to your hygiene. Dental plaque can build up fast and become painful, leading to infections. If you didn't bring toothpaste or floss, you can even wipe your teeth with a clean cloth or pick at the plaque with a piece of twig. Remember that if you go without bathing for a while, you run the risk of bacteria and fungal growth in the more dark, moist places on the body, including armpits, under breasts, groin areas, in between fingers and toes, and in the folds of skin. Bathe when you can, and air-dry, and wash clothing in a creek or river, even if the water isn't sparkling clean.

Potty tip! When there is no toilet paper around, you can use leaves, or you can squat instead of sitting low. By spreading your, um, "cheeks," you have less of an area that needs cleaning.

Being out in the wilderness requires some creativity when you don't have the items you are used to at home. You may find yourself wishing you had packed with more common sense, but don't fret. There are hacks and tips you can use to make the outdoors less intimidating.

Whether you are outdoors for a day, for several days, or bugging out for good after a disaster sends you running from your home, knowing the basics of where to set up shelter, where to find water and food, first aid, and survival hacks is a must. Not only will you be contending with other people and wild animals as well as bugs and plants and the weather, you will be away from the comforts and conveniences of home that we all have become so used to. Everything from cooking to sleeping to going to the bathroom will suddenly become something that requires thought and planning. It's always best to do that sooner rather than later.

Using Tools

One of the best investments you can make for your home emergency kit *and* your bug-out or camping kit is a multipurpose tool. This one item alone will allow you to do so many things and is compact enough not to take up much space. A multipurpose tool doesn't weigh a lot either, so it can be kept in a backpack for a hiking expedition. There are a variety of these tools on the market, and you can choose which one fits your needs best.

The basic tools include a corkscrew, tweezers, pliers, Allen key, wire cutters, a tiny saw, a bottle opener, and a straight blade. More complex tools may include a small magnifying glass, a whistle, a flashlight, and even a tiny noise alarm. Aim for practicality, but consider buying one tool for your home kit and a different one for outdoor use, as needs may be different.

There are larger tools with a compass, dry container, and even a starting flint inside the container to help with fires. These would be ideal for camping and outdoor kits.

If you are stuck without a can or bottle opener, you can improvise with a small knife. For a can, take the knife and poke holes all around the top lid until you can slip the knife point under and pry up the lid.

For a bottle, use the knife tip carefully to get under the cap and apply pressure, lifting the cap upward while pushing the knife downward.

If you don't have a knife, you can use a rock to poke holes in the lid of a can or do enough damage to the can by repeatedly smashing the rock against it that you can get to what's inside. Don't try this on a glass bottle, though, for obvious reasons.

If you have a metal spoon, you can position the edge of the spoon under the bottle cap and push the cap up while pushing down on the spoon handle. A spoon can also open a can if you place the tip of the spoon against the inner edge of the top lid where there is a small, raised lip from the crimping process that seals the can shut. Hold the spoon with the inside bowl facing the can's lid, and continue to rub the tip of the spoon back and forth over the lip area. The friction should eventually thin the area enough for the spoon to break the lid. Then pry it open with the spoon.

PART 4
BEFORE, DURING, AND AFTER FROM A TO Z

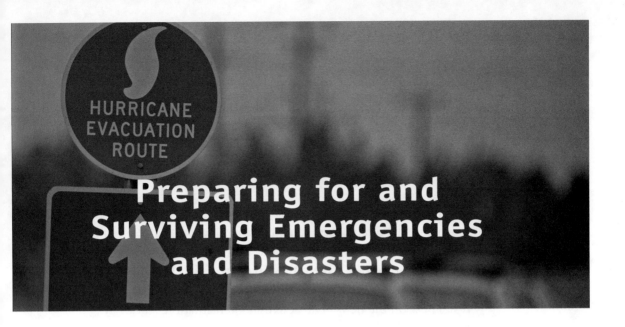

Preparing for and Surviving Emergencies and Disasters

Every hurricane season, there are stories of people who refused to evacuate and later needed to be rescued by emergency personnel, putting all of their lives in danger. There are stories of those who rush to the store to stock up on food and water days before a predicted blizzard, only to complain that the shelves have been emptied. There are stories of those who decide to chase tornadoes, only to have the tornadoes take a direction that was unpredictable and threaten lives. There are stories of people who decided they had to play golf during a thunderstorm and got struck by lightning, and those who never got around to shoring up their heavy furniture before that 6.5 temblor struck.

It doesn't take much to get prepared. It takes time, which we all complain we don't have enough of. But it also takes the common sense to know that if we do the few things on each of these *before* lists, many of which apply regardless of the disaster or emergency, it will not only save time later when we get to the *during* and *after* lists but save lives as well.

This section offers some great tips, in alphabetical order, on what we can do before, during, and after a variety of situations. Again, notice that most of the *before* preparations are the same: mainly getting our emergency kits ready, having a plan of action, and knowing where to go if we need to get out and how to communicate with our families. Each disaster/emergency also requires specific things that we can and must do to get ready.

It is scary to think about the *during* part, when panic takes over and we feel helpless, even hopeless. But knowing ahead of time what to do once "it" happens can empower us not only to help ourselves, but to take action to help those around us. Then we can do what needs to be done *after* and learn from what we did right and what we did wrong. Both can offer valuable lessons for the next emergency—and there will be many more.

They say "hindsight is 20/20," and that may be true, but foresight is where we want the clarity and focus. It's worth the time.

ACTIVE SHOOTER

BEFORE

Sign up for active shooter training, or watch YouTube active shooter response videos from law enforcement and the Department of Homeland Security.

See something, say something. Be aware of your surroundings and know your environment. If you see something suspicious, call 911 or report it to a security guard or the nearest person in authority.

If you hear on the news of an active shooter situation, stay away!

Have a family plan that ensures every member knows what to do in an active shooter situation.

Wherever you go, be aware of the two nearest exits, make a mental escape path, and look for potential hiding places. Be sure to keep disabled individuals in mind when looking for places to hide or escape, as stairs may not work for them.

DURING

You have three choices. Run, Hide, Fight.

If You Can Run

- Get away from the shooters as soon as possible.
- Don't worry about purses, laptops, or belongings. Just *run*.
- Help others escape, but if they are not cooperating, leave them and go.
- Warn anyone about to enter the area to stay away.
- When safely away, call 911.

If You Must Hide

- Find a hiding place out of the way of the shooting, and be quiet.
- Lock doors and windows, close blinds, turn off lights, block entrances.
- Spread out, as trying to hide in groups will be less successful.
- Hide along the walls, under windows, and out of the shooter's direct path of fire.
- Call 911 or text an alert. If you need to, call the police, but stay quiet and try to whisper the details, but don't do this if there is a chance the shooter can hear you or your phone.

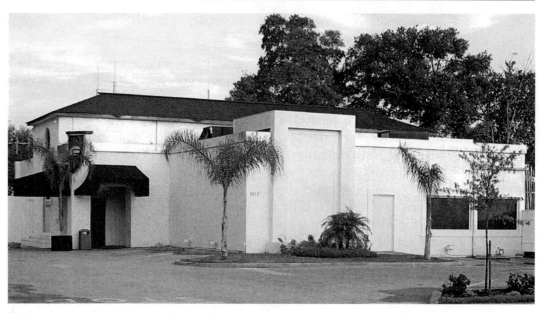

The Pulse nightclub in Orlando, Florida, was the site of a horrific shooting when security guard Omar Shateen—a man who hated all kinds of minorities—killed or wounded over a hundred people. In this day and age, it pays to be prepared for the unpredictable.

- Do not leave your hiding place until law enforcement arrives and tells you it's clear.

If You Must Fight

- Be aggressive and act fast.
- Try to knock the shooter off their feet with your body weight or another object.
- Try to work with others to ambush and disable the shooter. Yell to distract the shooter, and then rush them. Get the gun away from them by kicking it while you keep them held down until police arrive.
- Throw items at the shooter to knock them off balance.
- Use lethal force if you have to.

AFTER

Wait for law enforcement to come to you. They may not know you are a victim and not the shooter or an accomplice.

Keep hands visible, empty, and raised so law enforcement knows you are not the shooter!

Follow all law enforcement instructions, and hit the ground if told to. Do not run or you may get shot!

If first responders are not on site yet, try to help the injured.

Apply first aid where needed.

Seek professional therapy or counseling after the event, even if you don't think you need it. Watch for nightmares, panic attacks, and other signs of trauma.

One of the greatest dangers in a mass shooting may not be the shooter, but the mob of people trying to get away from the gunfire. People can turn into stampeding, panicked animals as they try to find the exits or get out of the facility. You could die under foot in a mob scene. If you can get out quickly, do so, but if you are caught in the mob, try to keep on your feet and let the bodies carry you to the exit. Hold on fast and tight to children, carrying them if you can. People will not care about you or your kids and knock you to the ground just to get themselves to safety. Go with the flow. As soon as you see a break, if you can duck for cover, get away from the mob, and stay covered until you reach an alternative exit.

Once you are outside or away from the shooting area, do not assume you are completely safe. Shooters will track people down in parking lots and outside venues they've just shot up. Get as far from the area as you can, call 911, and if you can get to your car safely, get out of Dodge. If you see the shooter coming, you can choose to hide, run, or fight, but be aware that if you are outdoors in the open, you may have fewer options.

BIOLOGICAL ATTACK

BEFORE

Stay tuned to news if there is a possibility of an attack.

Have your emergency supplies up to date, and be sure to have plenty of duct tape, plastic sheeting, and face masks should you need to shelter in place.

Know your evacuation routes.

Have a plan for family members who are not at home at the time of an event.

Report any suspicious activity to your local authorities, especially during high terror alerts.

If you are traveling, *do not* accept any packages or bags from strangers, even children! Keep track of your own luggage, and lock it before you turn it over to the airlines.

Talk to your family about the possibility of a biological terror attack. Though the risk is low compared to many other disasters and emergencies, it can happen. The more you know and learn, the more power you have when it is time to respond.

DURING

Listen for news and instructions on local news and emergency channels.

If told to evacuate, do so immediately, and wear face masks and medical gloves if told to.

If the attack occurs, leave the area immediately.

If you think you have been exposed to a biological agent or may be at risk, cover your mouth and nose, shield your eyes with goggles, and cover any exposed cuts or wounds to avoid contact with a contaminant. If you don't have a mask, use a cotton cloth, folded T-shirt, or thin towel. Wash any potentially exposed areas as soon as possible, and change clothing.

Put contaminated clothing or items in a bag or container. The container should be approved for bio-hazards, but if you do not own one, use any container or thick plastic Ziploc bag. You may have to improvise.

Know that a gas mask may not protect you from the biological agent, but it can help give some protection.

Keep an alcohol-based disinfectant in your emergency kit.

In the case of a contagious bacterial agent, stay home and stay away from potentially infected people.

Seek help immediately if you were directly exposed or if you are experiencing any strange symptoms.

If you feel you have been exposed, take a cold shower with plenty of soap. Wash your eyes with warm water or a saline solution.

Depending on the suspected agent used in the attack, authorities may have different instructions on how to respond. Do not assume all biological agents are the same!

Consider installing a HEPA (High Efficiency Particulate Air) filter in your furnace return duct.

AFTER

Have clothing and contaminated items destroyed or professionally cleaned. Do not wash them in your washing machine.

Watch for post-attack symptoms in yourself and others who were present.

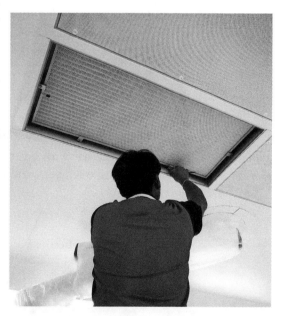

A maintenance man installs a HEPA filter in an operating room. High Efficiency Particulate Air filters remove fine particulates, including allergens, from the air and can be installed in the home, too.

BLIZZARD/SNOWSTORM

Before

Have a family plan of action, especially in case someone gets caught out on the road during a storm.

Prepare your home with insulation and weather stripping around doors and window sills.

Test your carbon monoxide detectors and fire extinguishers.

Have firewood stocked, and make sure it is kept dry.

Have space heaters with automatic shut-off switches and non-glowing elements, and keep them at least three feet away (one meter) from flammables, furniture, and drapery.

Make sure everyone knows how to turn off the main water valves in case a pipe bursts.

Have the chimney cleaned and inspected.

Keep cell phones charged, and have a charger on hand that is not dependent on electrical power (solar, battery, hand crank).

Have extra blankets, heavy coats and sweaters, gloves, scarves, and other warm clothing.

Try to stay home! If the weather is too extreme, it's not worth going to school, work, or anywhere else and risking getting caught out in the cold!

Plan on keeping pets indoors, and make sure they have warm bedding.

If you use medical devices, have a backup plan in case you lose power.

Keep your car prepared by having fluid levels checked as well as lights, brakes, heater, defroster, tires, and windshield wipers.

Keep at least half a tank of gas.

Stock the car with emergency essentials such as jumper cables, water, food, blankets, ice scrapers, and sandbags that can be opened and used for traction on ice.

During

Stay inside, whether you are at home or work, until you are told by officials it is safe to travel.

Travel only if absolutely necessary, and try not to travel alone in case you get stuck.

Be careful walking outside on driveways, walkways, and steps.

Only shovel snow if you must. Do not exert yourself in extreme cold.

Wear dry, thick clothing, and protect hands and feet. Mittens are much warmer than gloves, but gloves work better for moving objects or working.

Cover your head to reduce heat loss. The head is a vital area that must be kept warm. Also try to keep extremities warm and dry to preserve body heat.

If exposed to cold, watch for symptoms of frostbite: skin that is white or grey-yellow, numb, and has a waxy and firm feel. Seek emergency care if you can.

Watch for hypothermia symptoms: shivering, extreme fatigue, slurring of speech, dizziness, confusion, and loss of memory. Take the person's temperature, and if below 95 degrees Fahrenheit (35 degrees Celsius), seek emergency help immediately. You can also wrap the person in a sheet or blanket and soak it with cold water to draw heat out of the victim's body. Keep pouring cold water on the sheet or blanket.

Do not use generators, grills, stoves, or other items that use gas, propane, natural gas, or charcoal in a closed space. If you do, use them outside, and keep them away from windows, doors, and vents that might allow the spread of carbon monoxide.

If you must leave, make sure the visibility level is safe. Otherwise, stay put until the storm abates. It won't do you any good to get lost even deeper in the wilderness and make your situation worse.

AFTER

If you don't have power, and the roads are paved, go to the nearest shelter.

Protect yourself against the elements if you go outside to clear the driveway and other exit paths.

Knock snow out of rain gutters to keep them clear should more rain come.

Look for any structural damage from heavy snowfall to the roof, awnings, carports, and other exposed parts of the home.

If anyone is feeling ill, continue to watch for symptoms of hypothermia. Call for help immediately if they develop.

CHEMICAL DISASTER

Like a biological attack or pandemic, you may not know what is happening until you experience symptoms such as burning eyes and throat, loss of coordination, nausea, and difficulty breathing or see dead birds, insects, and animals all over the street outdoors. Chemicals in the form of poisonous gases, vapors, liquids, solids, and aerosols can spread their potentially lethal toxins before the local authorities have a chance to get the right information to the public, especially in the case of a terrorist or other intentional attack.

BEFORE

Have your emergency kit ready, with plenty of face masks, medical-grade gloves, plastic sheeting, scissors or knife, and duct tape for possibly sheltering in place.

Carbon Monoxide: The Silent Killer

Every year, approximately 430 people die in the United States from carbon monoxide poisoning, with thousands more going to the emergency room from exposure. Carbon monoxide is the silent killer. It strikes more often during the coldest months of the year but can kill at any time. Most of these deaths are preventable.

Because carbon monoxide is colorless, odorless, and tasteless, most people don't know they've been exposed to high levels until it is too late. It is the result of burning fuels in your home, car, and elsewhere—from auto engines, stoves, grills, gas ranges, fireplaces, furnaces, and gas lanterns—that build up indoors and affect people and animals. Symptoms include:

- Headache
- Dizziness
- Vomiting
- Weakness
- Upset stomach
- Confusion
- Flu-like symptoms

Breathing in too much carbon monoxide can make someone faint or kill them, which is why many deaths occur during the night when people are sleeping.

Installing battery-operated carbon monoxide detectors throughout your home will alert you to increasingly dangerous levels. Some detectors have digital readouts that tell if the levels are too high.

Be sure to keep all appliances, stove, furnace, fireplaces, chimneys, and other fuel-burning sources checked for optimum efficiency, and make sure none of them are near flammable objects when in use. Never use these items for heating in a closed space, and *never* run your car engine in a closed garage. Ventilation is key when using anything that could emit carbon monoxide, but having working detectors is your first line of defense. If you are on a lower income, check with your local gas and power company to see if they offer discounted or even free carbon monoxide detectors (and smoke detectors too).

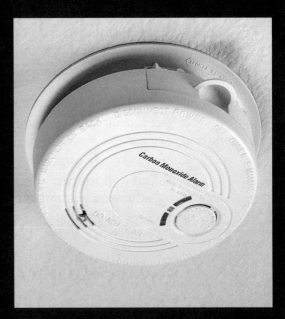

In addition to smoke alarms, you should have a carbon monoxide alarm in your home.

Know your emergency plan, and learn how to properly shelter in place.

Tune in to local news if there is word of a disaster, and do as you are instructed.

DURING

If you know the impacted area, get out and away from it immediately.

If the event occurs inside a building, get out, and avoid passing through the contaminated areas.

If you are at home, get out if you can. If you are told to stay, shelter in place.

Close doors and windows, and turn off any forms of ventilation, including furnace, air conditioner, air vents, and fans. Block the fireplace or close the chimney flue.

Seal off the room with sheeting and duct tape, but make sure to first get your emergency supplies like food, water, and first aid.

Listen for instructions on radio, television, or cell phones.

If you are outside in the contamination zone, try to immediately get to an area upwind with clean unaffected air.

If you or anyone else is directly exposed, call 911 or get to a hospital.

Try to avoid anyone who has been exposed to the chemicals.

Remove clothing and items exposed to the chemicals. *Do not pull your shirt/top over your head.* You do not want to contaminate your mouth, nose, or eyes. Cut the shirt/top off with a knife or scissors if you must.

Put all contaminated clothes and items in a sealed bag or container.

Flush your eyes with water, and wash your hands with soap and water. You can also wash your face with soap and water. *Rinse thoroughly.*

Eyeglasses must be put into bleach for decontamination. Rinse and dry before wearing.

Contact lenses should be thrown away, as they will be contaminated.

AFTER

Watch for symptoms of exposure, and get help immediately in the days after an event if any pop up.

Clean all surfaces of the house with a bleach product, and wash clothing, even if you were not directly exposed.

You can call the National Poison Control Center at 800-222-1222 if you believe you or someone in your home has been exposed and get information about what to do.

Household Chemicals

Even as we fear a nearby chemical disaster at a local manufacturing plant or a terrorist attack using chemical weapons, we are more likely to experience a chemical emergency involving household products we use every day. Products considered hazardous include:

- Spray paint
- Aerosol cans of hair spray
- Flammable fluids, kerosene, and propane tanks
- Pesticides
- Cleaning products
- Batteries
- Mercury thermometers
- Fluorescent light bulbs
- Lawn and garden herbicides
- Paint and paint thinners

Hazardous products should be kept in a cool, dry place and away from living areas. Keep them in their original containers so you know what they are. Never store them in unmarked containers, especially with children around. Do not mix cleaners and products, as this can be deadly. Dispose of hazardous products properly. Instructions are on the packaging.

Never use aerosols such as hair spray, cleaners, and paint products near an open flame. Check the product to see if it is flammable.

If you spill a chemical product, clean immediately with dry rags. Put the rags outside to allow the fumes to evaporate, then wrap the rags in newspaper or put them in a sealed plastic bag, and put them in your trash can. *Never reuse rags used to clean up a chemical product spill!*

If any of the product gets on your clothing, throw it away, as the chemicals may not wash out. Wash exposed hands or body parts with water and plenty of soap, and rinse thoroughly. Call the poison control center if concerned, or go to the hospital, especially if your skin burns, itches, or breaks out in a rash or hives.

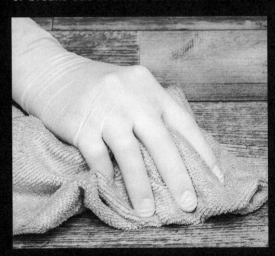

You should never reuse a rag for other purposes after it has mopped up chemical spills.

CYBER ATTACK

BEFORE

Only connect to the Internet using secure, password-protected networks.

Never click pop-ups, open attachments, respond to spam emails, or download files from strangers.

Type in the URL of the site you want to visit rather than copy a link someone sent you.

Constantly review and update all privacy settings, and change passwords regularly.

Never give out personal information by email.

Password-protect phones, pads, and any device that uses your accounts.

Choose difficult passwords that mean something to you, but are not common, and never use the same one twice.

Watch for any suspicious activity on bank statements and credit reports.

Make sure all software is up to date.

Run a scan to make sure your computer or phone is virus-free.

DURING

Report the incident to the police and the FBI.

If in a public place such as a library, let the librarian or person in charge know immediately.

Disconnect your devices, and power down. Then perform a full system restore to clean out the virus.

If at work, contact the IT department immediately.

AFTER

Change all passwords.

Close any accounts that may have been compromised. Let your banks know.

Contact credit card companies and credit reporting centers to let them know of the incident.

File a report with the police.

Report identity theft to your social security office and to the Department of Motor Vehicles. Also contact the Federal Trade Commission to report identity theft.

EARTHQUAKE

BEFORE

Know your risk. Where are the closest fault lines? Are you in a highly active zone? Are you in an area that experiences major quakes of 5.0 and above? All fifty states now have experienced earthquakes, so you are not immune!

Have all your necessary supplies. Have supplies for the home or office but also for the car if you need to evacuate.

Learn first aid, because there is a risk of injury during a quake.

Make a plan for getting to a safe part of the home, preferably in an interior doorway, up against the door frame, or beside a bed or table (do *not* get underneath or you can be crushed!).

Know the plan for your workplace or school. If there is none, figure out the evacuation routes, know where fire extinguishers are, and if the elevator is down, be aware of other escape routes.

Retrofit your home by bolting heavy furniture to the walls and using putty to keep breakable vases and decorative objects from flying through the air. Fit cabinets with magnetic door latches or other latches that prevent them from flying open during a quake. Consult with a structural engineer if you suspect your home needs to be evaluated for weaknesses.

If your city has an earthquake drill day, participate! California has a yearly Great ShakeOut day when all participants statewide practice their "drop, cover, and hold" drill for one minute, no matter where they are at the time.

Move objects that have the potential to block exits once shaking begins.

During

Stop, drop, cover, and hold. If near a bed or table, duck beside it a few inches below the surface so falling debris hits the surface and not you.

Stay calm. Do not rush for the doors!

Get away from windows and glass cabinets or cabinets with glass inside.

Stand against a wall or sit in a corner, and cover your head.

If in bed, cover your head with pillows, and stay until the shaking stops.

If outdoors, get away from power lines and trees with branches that might fall. Get away from buildings, as the brick and glass may fall. Stay away from overpasses and bridges. If possible, get to an open, clear area, and ride it out.

If you are in your car, stop driving, and stay inside until the shaking stops.

Stay out of elevators!

Once the initial shaking stops, be ready for aftershocks!

Do *not* use candles or matches. Open flames and gas leaks can lead to explosions and fire.

Stay away from chimneys and brick structures.

If on the beach, get inland as quickly as possible should there be a potential tsunami.

After

Be ready for aftershocks.

Try to get safely outdoors, and watch for broken glass and sharp items.

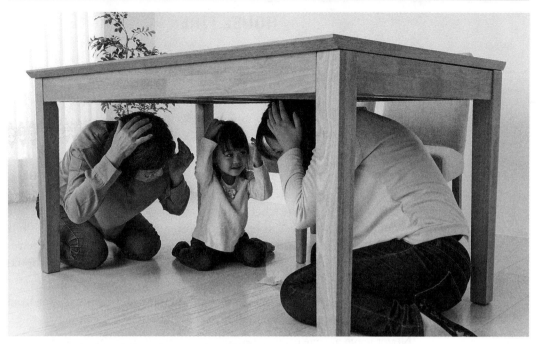

During an earthquake, hide under a sturdy table or doorway if you can.

Stay out of working elevators, as aftershocks might strike.

Check for gas, water, and electrical damage, and shut off gas if you can.

If injured, treat yourself. Check to see if others are injured, and apply first aid.

Do not re-enter a building to get property. Aftershocks may hit, and you could be trapped.

Manually open garage doors and get cars out if there is no power.

Turn on a battery-operated radio for information, or a ham radio if you have one, and do not clog phone lines trying to call people.

If you are trapped and cannot move, shout and bang on objects to get someone's attention. Do not try to get yourself loose, as you may make your situation worse.

If someone is trapped, and you know how to use leverage/cribbing to remove heavy objects, get help to do so. Otherwise get help.

During cleanup, wear protective gloves, long pants, sturdy shoes (no open toes), and face masks to avoid dust. Do not try to move heavy objects or debris without help.

HOUSE FIRE

BEFORE

Have a fire escape plan with your family, and practice. Update as needed. Make sure every family member can identify two exits from the rooms they may be in when the fire breaks out.

Make sure windows are not jammed or stuck in any way.

If you own security window bars, make sure everyone knows how to open them and get out.

Make sure all home smoke alarms are in working order. Test batteries every month. Replace batteries that are not working, and in general replace any batteries once a year. It is best to have both an ionizing smoke alarm, which is more responsive to flaming fires, and a photoelectric alarm, which is more responsive to smoldering fires. Equip your home with both. Smoke alarms should be replaced every ten years.

Keep home heating equipment, including small space heaters, away from flammable materials such as drapes and tablecloths.

Never leave a stove on unattended, and keep cloth potholders away from the flame or burners.

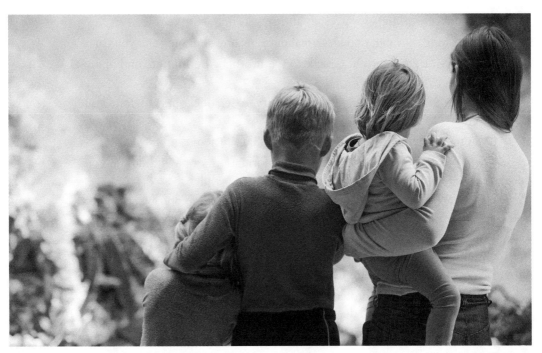

If smoke alarms go off in your home, don't wait until you see flames; get everyone out as quickly as possible and call 911.

Keep bedroom doors closed at night.

If barbecuing outside, keep the grill at least ten feet (three meters) away from the home and out from under awnings, eaves, and tree branches.

Stay in the kitchen while cooking. If you have to leave, turn off the stove. You can always turn it back on later.

Do not smoke in the home, especially at night, as a cigarette butt that is not completely put out can cause a fire.

Do not *ever* smoke in bed or burn candles overnight.

Check light switches, and replace any that are hot to the touch or faulty.

Inspect fireplaces and chimneys once a year, and make sure your fireplace screen is strong enough to prevent a log from rolling onto the floor. It should also be able to catch sparks.

Keep matches, lighter fluids, and hand lighters stored safely away from children.

Make sure all combustible and flammable materials are kept away from any heat sources, including those kept in the garage.

Have a few fire extinguishers around the house, and know how to pull the ring and use them!

Have digital backup copies of computer data, personal documents, and professional documents if you work at home, and keep them in a fireproof safe.

DURING

If you smell smoke, and the alarm has not sounded, check out the source of smoke quickly. If you are behind a closed door, put your hand on the door to see if it feels too hot to open. Make sure not to burn your hands on the hot metal doorknobs.

If the alarm sounds, get out even before you see flames.

Crawl low to the ground to try to avoid heavy smoke, and use a cloth to breathe through if you can find one.

Get out of the home, and call 911.

If you are unable to help someone trapped in the fire, you must get out and call for help. Assist firefighters by letting them know who is in the house and where, including pets.

Be careful about trying to be a hero and rushing back in to save someone or a pet, because you may lose your life as a result.

If your clothes catch fire as you try to exit the house, drop to the ground and roll, covering your face with your hands. Roll back and forth until the fire is out. If this is not possible, or if someone else is on fire, you can smother the flames with a blanket or towel and treat any burns by washing gently with cool water for up to five minutes.

Fire FAQ

According to the National Fire Protection Association, an average of seven people die each day from fires in the home. Approximately one of every 338 households report a fire each year, and half of the deaths caused by those fires occurred between the hours of 11:00 p.m. and 7:00 a.m. The leading causes of house fires, from most to least frequent, are: cooking equipment, heating equipment, and smoking. Smoking fires are the leading cause of home fire deaths. In the year 2015 alone, fire departments in the United States responded to over 365,500 home fires, which caused over 2,500 deaths and $7 billion in damage.

Chances are, before any other emergency strikes, you or someone you love will experience a fire in the home. Many people still don't have a plan of action to take in a fire and/or don't have working fire alarms. Between the years 2010 and 2014, three out of five fire deaths occurred in homes without smoke alarms. Having a working alarm can cut the risk of death in half. The more time you have to be warned and get out, the better.

It only takes about two minutes for a fire in the home to become life-threatening, and only five minutes before the entire structure can go up in flames. Remember, fire is *fast, hot, dark,* and *deadly.* It goes from a small fire to a raging inferno much more quickly than you think; it can be 100 degrees Fahrenheit (37.8 degrees Celsius) at floor level and over 600 degrees Fahrenheit (315.6 degrees Celsius) at eye level; fire produces thick, black smoke that makes it impossible to see; it is more likely you will die from smoke and toxic gases than the actual flames.

Do not take elevators in a burning building. If stairwells are clear, use the stairs, or use an outdoor fire escape if the stairwells are filled with smoke.

Do not impede firefighters from getting to the building.

Use a clean, dry cloth to cover burns, and never use butter, oil, or an ointment.

Get burn victims to a hospital or call 911.

After

Do not go back inside your home after a fire unless cleared by the fire department.

If your home is unlivable, call the Red Cross for temporary housing, food, and care.

If your home is destroyed, contact your insurance company right away to get instructions for inventorying the contents and getting in touch with fire restoration companies. If not insured, there may be charitable aid organizations you can contact by asking your local fire department.

Contact your mortgage company, and let them know about the home fire damage.

If your house is livable, let the fire department test and restore lost water, gas, and power. Do not try this yourself, as there may be burned wires and mechanisms that could cause another fire or electrocution.

Get professional assistance cleaning up after a fire, as some clothing and other items may not be salvageable even after being washed off. This is especially true for electrical and other fires that release toxic chemicals that do not wash off with water or come out with traditional cleaning methods.

If anyone displays any strange symptoms after a fire, including rash, coughing, sore throat, sores, burning eyes, weakness, and vomiting, get help immediately. This is especially important if the fire was electrical in nature (appliance fires can cause toxins in smoke).

SENIORS AND FIRE

If you have senior citizens living with or near you, pay attention to their needs during a fire. They may react more slowly and not be able to move as quickly, so you must exercise patience, especially if their mobility is limited. Most likely, they will have some type of medical aid, device, or even prescriptions drugs that they must have to ensure their health, so have those in a place they can easily be retrieved from.

Also take into consideration that the physiological makeup of the skin does deteriorate with age, and therefore elderly people are more prone to be injured from burns, as well as smoke inhalation due to limited lung capacity. Sadly, according to the U.S. Fire Administration, 75 percent of seniors who die in home fires did not have smoke alarms or had alarms that weren't in working condition. If you have a senior relative who lives alone, make sure they have working smoke and carbon dioxide monitors in all rooms. Also be sure they can cook and use a stove and oven without incident, as many seniors may become forgetful and leave the stovetop burner or oven on after they've gone to bed.

Many state and local agencies offer free smoke alarms for senior citizens. Ask your local fire department or emergency services office if they can direct you to such a program.

Consider that even in senior living facilities the alarms may not be in working condition, and check the batteries. Talk to facility personnel about what precautions they take for fires and other emergencies and whether the seniors living there have knowledge of the evacuation procedures and locations of emergency supplies. Just because there is someone caring for your senior loved one doesn't mean they will be available to do so in a disaster.

SCALDING

Although it doesn't involve actual fire, do you know what to do if a child or someone in your home is the victim of scalding? Scalding liquids are the num-

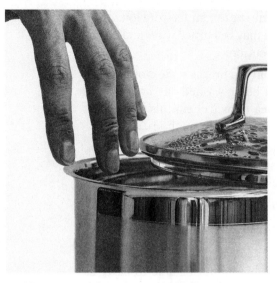

Scaldings commonly occur around boiling water in the kitchen. To treat the burn, run the wound under lukewarm water for twenty minutes, make sure no clothes or jewelry are touching it, and wrap in cling film to protect it. Do not use ice water or creams on the wound.

ber one cause of injuries to children in the United States. Often it is just the result of having the hot water temperature too high at the water heater. Look at the temperature setting, and turn it down to a lower or warm setting between 120 and 130 degrees Fahrenheit (48.9 and 54.4 degrees Celsius), or follow the lower, energy-efficient settings on the water heater manual.

Scaldings can occur in the kitchen, with boiling water, or in any sink in the home. Children should be kept away from stovetops when food is cooking and water is boiling. Always check the temperature of an infant's or child's bathwater before you let them enter the tub. Use a thermometer or your hand, and make sure their skin is not exposed to high temperatures. Because the skin of children is thinner, they can burn faster than adults. Never leave children unattended in the tub either, as they can turn the faucets on themselves.

How fast can scalding hot water seriously burn the skin?

120°F / 49°C	5 minutes
130°F / 54°C	30 seconds
140°F / 60°C	5 seconds
155°F / 68°C and higher	1 second

Pediatric scaldings, or any scaldings for that matter, are totally preventable. Check your water heater, and keep an eye on any situation involving hot liquids, baths, and sink usage.

FLOOD

BEFORE

Have sandbags to place around your home. You can buy them at a big box home store, or ask your local fire department where to get them. Often they will give them away for free in a potential flood zone.

Check around your home for items that should be brought indoors, such as patio furniture and decorative items.

Listen to your TV or radio for flood alerts and flash flood warnings. Evacuate, if you are told, to higher ground, but often it's best not to wait until mandatory evacuations. Have an exit plan!

Fire Extinguisher Use

There are several types of fire extinguishers for a variety of potential fire types. Before you buy a few for your home and emergency kits, be sure to know the difference.

Fire Type A: ordinary solid materials. Use a fire extinguisher marked A that uses both water and foam. Water removes heat, and the foam removes oxygen and heat. Use on cloth, wood, rubber, paper, some plastics, and regular combustible fires.

Fire Type B: flammable liquids. Use a fire extinguisher marked B that uses foam and CO_2 to remove the oxygen source, and dry chemical Halon to break the chain reaction of fire. Use for gasoline, grease, and oil fires.

Fire Type C: electrical equipment. Use a fire extinguisher marked C that uses CO_2 to remove oxygen, and dry chemical Halon to break the chain reaction. Use only on electrical equipment.

Fire Type D: combustible metals. Use a fire extinguisher marked D that uses special agents to remove the oxygen source.

Fire Type K: A special extinguisher for fighting kitchen oil, fat, or grease fires, using a wet or dry chemical.

There are fire extinguishers you can buy that are Type ABC or a combination thereof. It pays to have several extinguishers around the house and in your emergency kit.

How to use a fire extinguisher:

- Call 911 or have someone call 911 as you fetch the extinguisher.
- Stand with your back to the nearest exit and approximately 6 to 8 feet (1.8–2.4 meters) away from the flames. Fire extinguishers have a range of between 8 and 12 feet (2.4–3.6 meters).
- PASS! Pull, Aim, Squeeze, Sweep.
- Pull the pin that is inserted into the handle of the extinguisher. Grab the ring and pull the pin out.
- Aim the nozzle away from you and at the base of the fire. Holding the carrying handle with one hand, use the other hand to grab the hose or nozzle. Go for the base of the fire and not the flames themselves.
- Squeeze the levers together to release the extinguishing agent. Apply even pressure as you sweep the agent across the base of the fire from side to side until the flames are out. You can move closer to the fire as the flames die down.

If the flames rise up again, repeat the aim, squeeze, and sweep until they are out for good.

If the flames are too high and you feel in danger, leave the scene and wait for emergency help to arrive.

Only use fire extinguishers for smaller, contained-area fires such as in kitchens.

Disconnect electrical appliances, and turn off gas and power at the main switch/valve before you leave.

Know whether or not you are in a floodplain or flood-prone area, and always be ready to either shelter in place in the case of a flash flood, or evacuate.

DURING

If you are driving, *turn around, don't drown*. Never try to drive on a flooded road, especially through moving flood waters. Even still water can be a lot deeper than it looks.

Get away from rivers, and do not drive over bridges that are over flooding water. You can get caught on the bridge when fast-moving flood waters begin to erode its infrastructure, taking you down with it.

If in your car and the water is rising, *only* get out and move to higher ground if the car is not rising with the waters. *Never enter moving water*. It is safer to stay in your car until help arrives.

If you are camping near a waterway, stream, river, or lake, get to higher, drier ground as soon as possible, as water levels can rise quickly with heavy rainfall.

If indoors, move to the highest floor and stay put. Even six inches of moving water can knock you down, so if you must go outside, do so with extreme caution.

Never walk through standing water, as you can get electrocuted from downed power lines or exposed underground lines. Try to find a way around it.

AFTER

Do not go back to a flooded neighborhood to check on your home until you are told it is safe to do so.

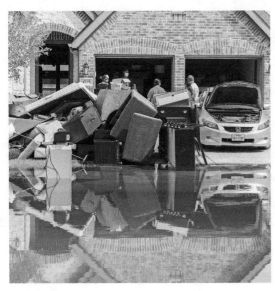

After authorities give the all-clear to return to the flooded area, make sure you wear protective clothing and watch for underwater debris to prevent injury.

Floodwaters can harbor contaminants, so use protective clothing and a mask when going through your home.

Watch for underwater debris, and wear long pants and sturdy shoes to walk through the water.

Call your insurance company immediately, and begin inventorying items damaged and destroyed. Even items not immersed in water can become infested later with mold. Catalog everything on your cell phone with pictures if you can.

Call an expert to service cesspools, septic tanks, wells, and potentially damaged sewage systems and water pipes on your property.

Report downed power lines to the power company and the local police/sheriff.

DAM FAILURE/FLOODING

All of the above applies, but if you live near a dam, you must have an evacuation plan ready, because fast-moving waters could prove deadly. You can find out in advance whether you live near a high-hazard dam by contacting your city emergency services or even your local fire department, as they are also responsible for helping to rescue people during flood events.

Watch local news carefully for information about how close the dam is to capacity, and make plans to leave beforehand.

Have an evacuation plan in order to get you away from the dam and to higher ground. Never head downstream from the flow of water from a burst dam!

If the dam does fail, you will most likely need to evacuate immediately and take with you what you can grab. Have a kit ready near the door or in the car, and follow all directions from law enforcement and emergency services as to where to go and where to avoid rising waters and flowing debris.

HAZMAT

Hazardous materials incidents are similar to both biological and chemical emergencies, with some exceptions. They usually are the result of an accident at a chemical plant, a transportation-related accident, or a leak at a nearby facility and thus are more likely to be reported to the media and law enforcement quickly. Knowing where the incident happened and what it involved right off the bat helps emergency services better tell the public what to do.

BEFORE

Know how to shelter in place, and have an interior room picked out with as few doors and windows as possible.

Show everyone in the family how to operate the home's ventilation system and close off vents.

DURING

Tune in to the radio, television, or cell phone news service for instructions.

If told to evacuate, do so *immediately*.

Immediately close windows, doors to the outside, vents, attic fans, bathroom exhaust fans, fireplace dampers, and other openings to the outside.

Shelter in place.

If outside, get uphill, upstream, or upwind from the location of the event. A half mile away minimum is best; go further if you can.

Stay away from and do not come in contact with spilled fluids, liquids, mists, solids, strange gases, fogs, fumes, and smoke. Cover your mouth with a face mask or cloth when passing by a hazmat area.

Seek shelter in a building nearby if you cannot walk at least a half mile away.

If you are stuck in your car, close windows and air vents, and shut off heat or A/C.

Avoid eating and drinking near the contaminated area, as hazardous materials can be airborne and invisible.

If exposed to the hazardous material, use a cloth or face mask, and take shallow breaths. *Get help immediately.*

AFTER

Follow decontamination instructions by local law enforcement or emergency services personnel.

Seek help if you feel sick or have skin or eye issues such as rashes, itching, and burning.

Put exposed clothing, shoes, and other items in sealed bags or containers.

Once authorities allow you to go home, if you have evacuated, open all doors and windows to ventilate the home. Turn on fans to assist ventilation.

If you need to clean up a contaminant in your home or on your land, make sure to ask local authorities about the proper cleanup methods.

If you smell any strange odors or vapors in the following days, call 911 immediately.

HEAT WAVE

BEFORE

If a heat wave is predicted, be ready. Stock up on extra water, and make sure your emergency kit is up to date.

Be ready for power outages due to high use of air conditioners.

Be aware of seniors, children, pets, and sick people in your family or neighborhood who might need extra help during extreme heat.

Make sure air conditioning ducts are clear and working properly.

Check on your home's insulation to make sure you have weather stripping that will keep hot air out and cool air in. Check doors and windows.

If you don't have central air conditioning, install a window air-conditioning unit, and insulate snugly.

Know ahead of time the symptoms of heat exhaustion and stroke, and be aware and ready with first aid training.

Cover windows that receive a lot of sunlight to keep the indoor area cooler, and consider having outdoor awnings and louvers on windows to prevent heat from entering the home.

Pay attention to weather alerts for heat advisories and warnings. The National Weather Service will issue alerts as follows:

Heat Wave—prolonged, excessive heat, sometimes combined with high humidity levels

Excessive Heat Watch—Indicates that conditions for an extreme heat event are high within the next 24- to 72-hour period.

Excessive Heat Warning—At least two days of an extremely high heat index, heat along with humidity, that exceeds daytime highs of 105–110 degrees Fahrenheit (40.6–43.3 degrees Celsius).

Know where the "cool zones" are in your neighborhood in case you need to get to them.

In extreme heat events, consider keeping children home from school, as many schools have inadequate air conditioning. Many schools do close early in heat waves.

DURING

Stay indoors if you have fans or air conditioning. Avoid all activity outdoors, especially in direct sunlight.

Drink water and stay hydrated! Avoid caffeine and sugary drinks! *No alcohol.* This has a dehydrating effect.

Dress in loose-fitting, light clothing.

Never leave a child or pet unattended in a hot car even for a few minutes!

Avoid exercise during peak hours of sun and heat, or exercise indoors.

Avoid using the oven for cooking.

Be sure to replace salt and minerals with energy drinks or electrolyte drinks, because sweating causes the depletion of electrolytes.

Stay on lower floors of homes or offices, as heat rises.

Check on any family, friends, or neighbors who may need extra care during an extreme heat event, especially the elderly and sick. Look for symptoms of heat-related issues:

Heat Exhaustion Symptoms

- Dizziness
- Headache

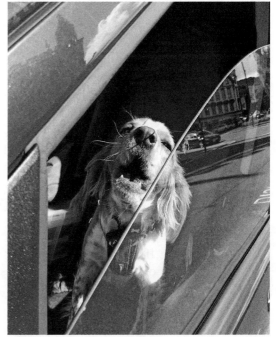

Never, ever leave a pet or child locked in a car, even with a window cracked open.

- Sweaty skin
- Weakness
- Cramps
- Nausea, vomiting
- Fast heartbeat

Heat Stroke Symptoms

- Red, hot, dry skin
- High temperature
- Confusion
- Convulsion
- Fainting

If you or anyone else exhibits these symptoms, call 911 or get to a hospital. Heat exhaustion must be treated as soon as possible, or the condition will worsen. Heat stroke can be deadly, so you must act fast because of the potential for brain damage if the body is not cooled quickly. Move the person to a cool, shaded area, and fan them or spray with cool water. You may want to get them into a tub or shower of cool water. Monitor their temperature until help arrives or until you can get them to a local hospital, but *do not give them fluids to drink*. This may sound counterintuitive, but it can cause even more stress to the body, and that can be dangerous. If instructed by a 911 operator to give fluids or try any other cooling method, follow their guidelines for what to do.

After

Restock water in your emergency kits as well as other supplies used during the heat event. Be ready for the next wave, especially during the summer and early fall months. Monitor local news for future weather alerts.

Continue to monitor others for belated signs of heat exposure, and get help. Ask children how they feel, because they may appear drowsy but in fact be reacting to extreme heat.

HURRICANES

Before

If you live in a hurricane region, you should have at least two weeks' worth of food, water, and supplies. A month's worth is even better.

Have a bug-out bag filled with supplies in case you are asked or ordered to evacuate. Be sure to include medical information and prescriptions in case you need to be at a shelter for more than a few days.

Know your evacuation routes, and have alerts on cell phones. Once the local news begins reporting a potential hurricane, be ready to leave, and *leave* when told. Don't put yourself in danger trying to "defend" your home, and please don't put first responders in danger by making them rescue you when you realize later you should have left. *Evacuate*.

If you are not in an evacuation zone, board up or cover windows, and get into a center room or a strong room with no windows to avoid broken glass from high winds.

Charge all cell phones, and keep chargers and batteries with your bug-out bag/kit.

If the power goes off, you may still be able to text and use your cell phone and social media to communicate with others, but be prepared to be out of communication during the peak of the storm.

Remove tree branches that can fall onto your home ahead of time. Clean out gutters, and use sandbags near your home if heavy rains are expected.

Bring patio furniture, planters, garbage cans, decorative items, and other outside objects that could become dangerous projectiles in high winds into the garage.

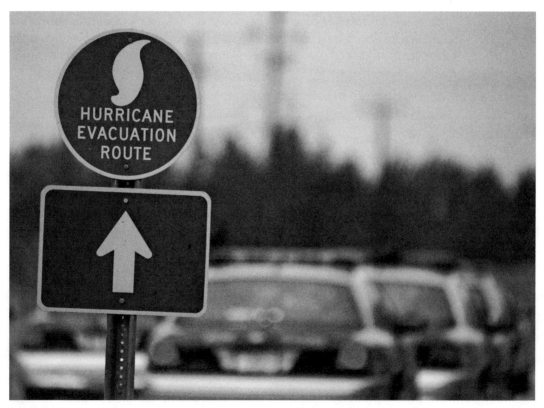

States where hurricanes are fairly common will have predetermined evacuation routes marked by signs such as this one along roads and highways.

Retrofit roof tiles (and look for potential leaks), windows, and doors, including garage doors, to withstand heavy rains and high winds. The roof is most critical, as a strong roof serves as your first line of protection against the high winds and flying debris.

Consider a generator for power, and follow all safety instructions.

DURING

If told to evacuate, even if it is not mandatory, do so. Better safe than sorry, and if there is a worst-case scenario, better alive and away from home than at home and without aid. *Do not put first responders in danger by making them come for you when you were told to leave.* Please consider the safety of others as well as your own.

Stay tuned to weather reports on television, radio, cell phone, or ham radio.

If you are stuck inside a building, close windows and doors to the outside, then get away from windows, watch for flooding on bottom floors, and hunker down in an interior room with no windows if possible.

Close all interior doors of the house or building you are in. This helps compartmentalize the tremendous pressure inside the home into smaller areas during high winds and can keep strong upward pressure from blowing the roof off.

Stay away from coastal areas, as storm surge can be deadly.

Do not go outside during severe thunderstorms and high winds.

Watch for tornado alerts, which often accompany hurricanes.

AFTER

Let family and friends know you are alive and well. You can do this via text, social media, or any other method.

Do not go home unless cleared by authorities. Flooded neighborhoods may be too dangerous to enter.

Avoid walking or driving through floodwaters, as downed power lines could make them electrically charged. Never drive through moving floodwaters.

Take pictures or video of damage to your home for your insurance company.

Restock any emergency supplies used during the hurricane immediately.

Be ready for additional rainfall and flooding if the hurricane downgrades to a tropical storm and is slow-moving enough to deposit heavy rains.

Clean up any debris and water damage, and wear protective gloves, clothing, and a dust mask.

Natural Gas

Though it may not qualify as a disaster, natural gas incidents can cause devastating explosions and destroy homes and lives. Natural gas is a fuel, and it is safe during normal transportation and use. But when natural gas leaks from pipes or appliances, it becomes deadly, so you must know what to look for. Add to that the carbon monoxide produced by natural gas, and because these gases are often colorless, odorless, and undetected, you may not know there is a problem until it is too late.

Tips: Check pilot lights and burners, and make sure the flame light is approximately 90 percent blue. If it is yellow, that means the appliance is not working correctly. Call a service tech immediately, as it could be giving off fumes. However, not all gas appliances will have a visible pilot light. Ash and soot around pilot light openings and air ducts, any strange odors or noises from the appliance, and a long warming time are signs of a problem. Nowadays, a chemical called mercaptan is added into natural gas so that there is an odor you can identify when there is a leak, but in its natural state, natural gas has no smell.

Keep kitchen ranges clean, and never use a gas stove to heat a room, as it can produce carbon monoxide.

Have larger gas appliances serviced regularly.

Keep children away from gas appliances.

Do not wear loose clothing that can be ignited by flames while you are cooking.

If you smell a strong odor, leave the home and call 911 immediately.

If your pilot light has gone out, you can relight it by turning the appliance off, then following manufacturer instructions. If it won't relight, or you are uncertain what to do, call your local gas company for assistance. Don't try to tamper with it yourself.

PANDEMIC

BEFORE

Get a flu shot if your doctor so advises. Flu shots are not advisable for everyone and don't fight the most current mutation of the flu, but they can be effective at stopping the most common flu bugs and decreasing the severity of the current strain.

Stay healthy and keep your immune system strong. Consider taking vitamins and minerals. Obviously, eat healthy foods, get enough sleep, and exercise your body to maintain a powerful immune system. Sometimes common sense is the best advice.

Keep a supply of over-the-counter drugs that fight colds, fevers, and pain, stomach remedies, and cough and cold medicines. Also keep some fluids with electrolytes, such as Gatorade, Powerade, and electrolyte waters, as these can be helpful if vomiting and diarrhea become a problem.

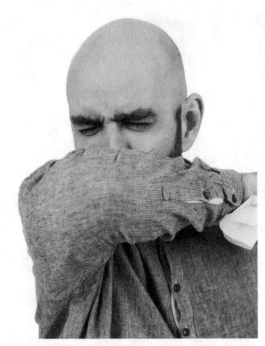

When you sneeze, sneeze into the crook of your arm. If you sneeze into your hands you might forget there are germs there when you shake hands with someone or touch objects that others may use.

Have copies of your updated medical records, and keep them on a flash drive.

Buy some N95 face masks to keep on hand in case a pandemic breaks out.

DURING

Stay away from areas where large groups of people gather. Wear your N95 if you must come in contact with others.

If you know someone who is sick, keep your distance, and wash your hands if you must handle anything that belongs to them.

Wash your hands often during a pandemic, and try not to touch your eyes, nose, or mouth.

Cover your mouth and nose when you cough or sneeze.

Call for help if you suspect that you or a loved one has been infected.

Drink plenty of fluids, especially water and electrolyte drinks if you are vomiting and sweating.

Once the virus or agent is identified, follow the instructions of local authorities, including where and how to get a vaccine if one is available.

If symptoms are severe, call 911 or go to the hospital, but wear your mask to avoid spreading germs to others.

AFTER

Keep your immune system strong by eating right, drinking fluids, and getting adequate sleep, because you may be taking care of others who are still sick.

POWER OUTAGE

BEFORE

Have enough emergency supplies for a short- or long-duration event, including food and water.

Remember to plan for pets.

Check home circuit breakers and fuses if the power is only out in your home.

Stock up on batteries for flashlights, cell phone batteries and chargers, solar powered chargers, and candles and matches.

Buy a small generator, but learn about different fuel choices, some of which are dependent on electricity.

Know how to open your garage door manually if you need to leave.

Freeze water in bags or make extra ice ahead of time to help keep perishables cold. Buy dry or block ice to store in the freezer.

Keep your car's gas tank as full as possible. Do not run the car engine in the garage or near the home in a partially enclosed area if you are using it to charge devices and appliances.

If you need power for medical devices and don't have a generator, know where the nearest hospital is.

Make sure your exterior home address numbers are visible from the street for emergency vehicles should you need them.

DURING

Use flashlights first. Candles are for backup only, as they can cause accidental fires if left unattended.

If you have a ham radio or battery-operated radio, or if cell phone service is on, listen for instructions and information about the outage and how long it might take to restore power.

Keep refrigerator and freezer doors closed. If you must take out food, do so quickly. An unopened refrigerator can store food safely for up to four hours, and each time you open it, you cut that four hours down.

If the outage occurs during a heat wave, go outdoors or to a cool zone, a theater, or a restaurant where there is power to stay cool.

Drink water and stay hydrated, even if you are not thirsty. Avoid liquids with caffeine and sugar. Do not drink alcohol.

Dress according to the weather, especially at night, when you will not have power to heat or cool your home.

Do *not* use a gas or charcoal grill inside a home or building.

Disconnect appliances, computers, and equipment to avoid the power surge when power is restored. That surge can be damaging to components.

If using a generator, keep it outside the home. Do not use it in a garage.

If driving, remember that traffic lights will be down, and use rules of the road and common sense.

Check on elderly or sick neighbors to see if they are doing okay, especially if they use medical devices that rely on electricity.

AFTER

Throw away food that has been exposed to temperatures above 40 degrees Fahrenheit (4.4 degrees Celsius) for more than two hours. If it looks, feels, or smells bad, toss it. If in doubt, throw it out!

Restock your emergency kit with any supplies used during the event.

If you think refrigerated medications may be spoiled, do not take them, and contact your doctor immediately.

SPACE WEATHER EVENT

BEFORE

It is difficult to predict a space weather event, but because of our dependence on technology, we should be aware and ready. A solar storm or geomagnetic storm could wreak havoc on our way of life. Most of the effects of space weather, such as geomagnetic storms, cause a decrease in F-region electron density. This means a lowering of the maximum usable frequency of a radio's path between two points on earth, resulting in communications difficulties even on shortwave radio. Other potential effects could tamper with power grids.

In case the power grid goes down, have candles, flashlights, and generators in your supply kit or pantry.

Keep a solar-powered cell phone charger, or get a ham radio license in case cell phone service is cut off. Also keep a stockpile of extra batteries for the phone and flashlights.

Monitor local news on radio, television, cell phone, or ham radio.

Stay indoors unless told otherwise by local authorities.

Keep your car gas tank at least half full at all times.

Know how to manually open your garage door if you need to leave.

If you own a traditional landline phone, have at least one corded receiver in case the power goes out.

Back up digital data often, at least on a weekly basis.

DURING

Listen to the Emergency Alert System instructions.

Do not use the telephone unless it is an emergency. Keep lines clear for emergency services.

Use as little power as possible to help the power company avoid a rolling blackout. If instructed to, disconnect and unplug all electrical appliances, computers, and other items to save power.

AFTER

If the power has been down for days, throw away food kept in the refrigerator and freezer.

Replenish water, food, and supplies used during the event.

(More on catastrophic space weather in the next chapter.)

TERRORIST ATTACK

Terrorist attacks can be a variety of scenarios, from active shooter events to bombings to receiving anthrax in the mail. It is hard to predict when they will occur, how they will occur, and where they will occur. Terrorists use the element of surprise for a reason, because it doesn't give victims time to react.

The most prevalent scenarios are shootings and bombings, and the *before, during,* and *after* plan for active shooters is almost identical. But because bombings are a consideration, there are some tips that can help you avoid becoming a victim.

If you are going to another country, it is critical you learn their customs, beliefs, and even their cultural etiquette to avoid doing something that might bring you unwanted attention. Because most terrorism occurs outside the United States, we forget that our behaviors and actions make a difference in other countries, and what may seem insignificant and normal to us can come across as offensive, even threatening, elsewhere in the world. Also know that most terrorist attacks occur in high-traffic areas, including tourist spots. It might behoove you to read up on news about the area you are traveling to so you can know which places to avoid.

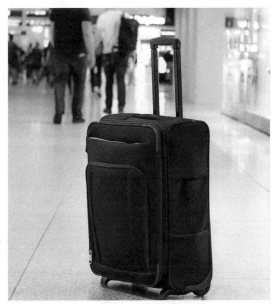

Here at home, it is all about being aware of your surroundings, especially in a crowd, such as at a sporting event, concert, or shopping mall. Knowing what normal is can help you spot something abnormal quickly. Knowing where the exits are, what hiding places are available to you, and what you might use as a weapon if you have to fight for your life can save your life. Take the time to look around and make some fast observations, because in an active terrorist attack, you have the choice to flee, fight, or hide, depending on the number of terrorists, the type of attack, and where you are when it happens.

An abandoned bag at an airport or other public place is an object for immediate suspicion. Always be aware of your surroundings and be vigilant of such potential dangers.

In order to do this, *you must be paying attention*. Too many of us are caught up in conversation with friends, burying our noses in our cell phones, or just not being aware of the potential threat in the first place. Being aware of the present surroundings is key, but how often are we?

Some tips for home and abroad:

- If it seems strange, report it.
- Look for packages and luggage left unattended and out in the open. Report them to authorities.
- Plan routes ahead of time, including exits, escape routes, and hiding places.
- Be aware of people carrying large backpacks or wearing oversized clothing.
- Use your gut instinct, and if something is out of place, get away from it.
- If a bomb goes off, hit the floor or get behind something sturdy. Report it immediately to 911.
- If you can run out an exit, do so, but be sure that exit doesn't lead you towards more terrorists.
- If you must fight, do it with everything you have, and use whatever you can as a weapon.
- If a grenade is tossed in your vicinity, run or hide behind a wall or sturdy cover.
- If caught in gunfire, run in a zigzag pattern until you can either get to an exit or a good hiding place.

Terrorist attacks often occur in waves, so just because you survived the first attack does not mean you are out of danger. Get out, hide, call for help, stay away from the area of the initial attack.

If you are taken hostage, do what you are told to buy time. This is a tricky situation, as you may want to try to escape or fight, but depending on how many terrorists there are, you may be better off submitting and staying quiet. If you have access to a weapon, such as a large shard of broken glass or chunk of wood, you can fight back, especially if you are in great shape, bigger than the terrorist, or can get others to fight with you against a small number of terrorists. This is a personal choice you must make in the heat of action! Can you survive if you fight? Do you have loved ones with you to protect as well? No book can make this decision for you. *Use your best and fastest judgment of the situation*. The same would go for being in a bank robbery or similar situation, which are terrorist attacks on a smaller scale.

If a shooting or bombing occurs indoors, get outside and away, and hide, then call 911. Try to avoid running away in the open as gunmen may see you and shoot.

Bomb Threat Stand-Off Distance

Threat	Explosive Capacity	Building Evacuation Distance	Outdoor Evacuation Distance
Pipe bomb	5 lbs/2.27 kg	70 ft/21 m	850 ft/259 m
Backpack/briefcase	50 lbs/22.7 kg	150 ft/46 m	1,850 ft/564 m
Compact car	500 lbs/227 kg	320 ft/98 m	1,500 ft/457 m
Sedan	1,000 lbs/454 kg	400 ft/122 m	1,750 ft/533 m
Van	4,000 lbs/1,814 kg	600 ft/183 m	2,750 ft/838 m
Small delivery truck	10,000 lbs/4,536 kg	860 ft/262 m	3,750 ft/1,143 m
Moving van/truck	30,000 lbs/13,608 kg	1,240 ft/378 m	6,500 ft/1,981 m
Semitrailer	60,000 lbs/27,216 kg	1,500 ft/457 m	7,000 ft/2,133 m

Courtesy of the National Counterterrorism Center (NCTC), Office of the Director of National Intelligence

If the danger is outside, stay in the building, and get to an interior room, closing and locking doors and windows on the way. Call for help immediately. Shut off vents to the room in case of a biological or radiation dispersal attack. Stay quiet.

THUNDERSTORMS AND LIGHTNING

BEFORE

When a storm is predicted for your area, make sure you have supplies of extra food, water, batteries, and candles for possible power failures.

Clear out rain gutters, cut down tree branches near the house, and check windows for leaks if heavy rains are expected. Use sandbags if flooding around your home is a possibility.

Secure outdoor furniture, planters, and other objects against potential high winds.

Rubber-soled shoes give you protection from lightning!

Never plan a trip to the beach if thunderstorms are in the forecast.

Use the 30/30 plan when a storm first begins. If you see lightning strike, but can't count to 30 before you hear thunder, then get indoors.

Listen for alerts on television, radio, cell phone, or ham radio, and keep abreast of the storm's intensity and location.

Have umbrellas in the car in case you need to travel during the storm.

DURING

When thunder roars, go indoors! Don't stay outside to watch for lightning, or you may end up being struck by it!

If You're Present during an Attack

Three rules of a terrorist attack or getting caught in a crime such as a bank robbery:

- Try to Identify the Threat Beforehand
- Locate Exits and Hiding Places
- Ascertain Whether You Can Run or Must Stay and Fight/Submit

Even in a bank robbery, you will have to engage in situation awareness. Does someone look out of place? Nervous? Anxious? Jittery? Are there several people that look as though they are scoping out the place, perhaps about to commit a crime or terrorist act? Does anyone have a package or backpack on them, or are they dressed in heavy clothing that could conceal weapons?

If something does happen, you may do everything in your power to submit to their orders, lie on the ground, and be quiet—and survive or not. You may run and hide and fight back—and survive or not. In such spontaneous situations, survival often comes down to immediate responses, so it is imperative to control panic and try to keep a clear mind. Many people report that during a crime or terrifying situation, they actually become very clear and focused and eerily calm. Use that to your advantage when deciding the best course of action to take based on the situation and your surroundings.

Often people freeze during a disaster. This is a natural neurological response to extremely fearful situations. You cannot afford the luxury of even a few seconds of paralysis and wasted time. Be ready to act and use the knowledge you have gleaned to do so with a purpose: surviving.

Remember. *Escape. Hide. Take out the threat.* Those are your choices.

Stay inside until thirty minutes after the *last* clap of thunder you hear.

Stay away from windows and doors.

Unplug items from electrical outlets that might be affected by a power surge from lightning. Do not use your computer during a severe storm with plenty of lightning.

Unplug appliances, and do not touch electrical equipment, even plugged-in cords.

Faucets should not be used during a storm, as they conduct electricity. Do not use sinks, bathtubs, and showers.

Do not do laundry or touch pipes, as they too conduct electricity.

Do not use corded phones or items being charged electrically. Use a cordless or cell phone if you must call for help.

If stuck outdoors, take cover in a safe area. Do not sit or lean against concrete walls, as they conduct electricity.

Do not wait out the storm under power lines or heavy tree branches that could break due to rains and winds.

Stay away from open fields, the beach, golf courses, and tall trees or objects such as flagpoles if you are in an open area. Lightning will strike the tallest target, and that might be something near you. It also might be you! Get down on the ground if you are stuck in an open area.

Avoid touching metal objects when outdoors.

Hide inside a hardtop car, not a convertible. You are much better off inside a car than outside one during lightning strikes.

If you are driving on the freeway, drive safely until you can exit and park. Stay inside your car, and turn your emergency flashers on. Try not to touch any metal objects in the car.

Do not hide inside a building or shed in an open field.

If you are out camping or hiking in the words, seek shelter in a low area, like a ditch or ravine, or underneath thick brush or small trees. Do not lean against the tallest tree, as it will act as a lightning rod.

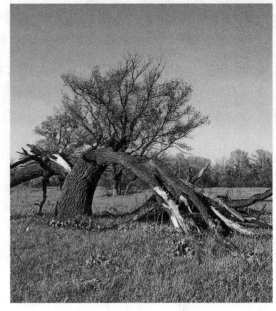

Hiding under a tree during a thunderstorm is a bad idea. Trees can serve as lightning rods, and branches can break off and strike someone standing underneath.

If you are in open water, try to get to land and shelter as soon as possible.

Try to comfort pets, and keep them indoors under your control.

AFTER

If you go outside, watch out for fallen branches, debris, and downed power lines.

Avoid waterways such as streams, creeks, and rivers that may have crested from heavy rains.

If someone has been struck by lightning, call 911 and check their breathing, heartbeat, and pulse. If they are not breathing, administer mouth-to-mouth. If there is no heartbeat, administer CPR. Check for burns at the entry and exit points the lightning may have taken. Observe the victim. There can be damage to their nervous system and eyes as well as internal injuries that are not obvious at first glance.

Avoid flooded roads if out on the road, and listen to the radio for weather updates. Storms can occur solo or as part of a cluster or line, and tornadoes are also a possibility.

Stormy Days

The average thunderstorm occurs during warm and humid conditions. It doesn't last long, usually a half hour to an hour, but can produce very heavy rainfall. Some storms produce hail and are accompanied by high winds and wind gusts. Other storms stall over one area and can produce flash flooding.

Approximately 10 percent of thunderstorms develop into severe storms that can spawn hail and tornadoes.

Lightning can occur up to ten miles (16 kilometers) away from actual rainfall.

The majority of lightning-strike deaths occur outdoors during summer afternoons and evenings, when people are likely to be outside.

Someone who is struck by lightning will not carry an electrical charge.

Your chance of being struck by lightning is about 1 in 600,000.

Lightning goes for the "rod" or tallest object in an open area.

TORNADO

Tornadoes may not strike as wide an area as hurricanes, but they can do amazing amounts of damage and cause loss of life. The United States experiences approximately 1,200 tornadoes each year, most of which occur east of the Rockies and mainly in the Midwest, the South, and the Gulf Coast area. But they can happen anywhere, even in California! Because they are often a part of a larger thunderstorm system, they can make an already dangerous situation even deadlier.

Tornadoes can strike fast, and you may not see one until it begins to pick up debris, dirt, and dust. They move fast and often in a southwest to northeast pattern. Winds can approach 300 miles per hour (48 kph) and can destroy buildings and bridges, uproot trees, and lift heavy vehicles.

Tornado season is mainly in the spring and summer, but they can happen at any time if weather conditions are ripe. The magic hours appear to be between 3:00 P.M. and 9:00 PM, but they can occur at any time. Tornadoes over the water are called waterspouts and can often touch down on shore and cause damage along beaches and coastal areas.

BEFORE

Find a safe room, or have a storm cellar that is fortified against tornadoes. Keep supplies there.

If you live in a tornado-prone area, check your school or office building for an emergency plan, shelter areas, and evacuation routes. Also know where emergency shelters are located.

Keep up on weather alerts if a storm is coming that could spawn tornadic activity. Watch for the signs of an imminent tornado:

- Dark grey sky, can have a greenish cast
- Large hail
- Large, dark, low clouds
- Cloud rotation
- A loud roar that sounds like a train coming towards you
- The beginnings of a funnel formation

DURING

Take cover immediately, preferably inside a storm cellar, safe room, or an interior room of the building. Avoid windows and doors.

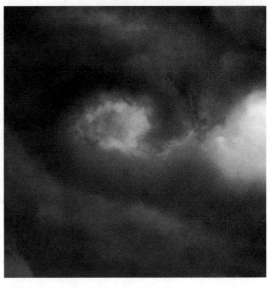

Clouds that are clearly moving in a rotating pattern are a sign that a tornado may soon form.

If in a high-rise, seek cover in an interior room or even a stairwell.

Get under a sturdy table or desk, cover your head, neck, and body as best you can, and if you have blankets or jackets, cover yourself with those. Protect yourself from falling debris.

If outside, get into a vehicle, and cover your head with your arms, coat, jacket, or blanket.

Never take cover under a bridge or an overpass as they do in the movies. You are actually safer lying down in a low, flat location. Look for a ditch or ravine.

If you are in a car and a tornado is almost upon you, don't try to drive away. Get out of the vehicle, and look for a sturdy building to hide inside of.

If you are stuck outside in a field or open area, lie down and avoid flying debris. Cover your head with your arms, a jacket, or whatever you have with you (backpack, laptop bag).

AFTER

If you are indoors, watch out for fallen power lines and debris when you go outside. Make sure the structure you are in is safe to move around in first!

If you are trapped by debris, call for help out loud or tap on a pipe. Do not move or you can make your injuries worse.

Stay away from damaged buildings, including your own home. Wait for help to arrive, and follow the instructions of authorities.

Once your home is said to be safe, photograph or videotape the damage for insurance purposes.

Do not attempt cleanup without first getting the approval of authorities. Wear an N95 face mask, heavy work gloves, long-sleeved shirt, long pants, and closed-toed boots or sneakers, and watch for sharp objects.

Replenish batteries and other supplies used during the storm or any power outage. Try to avoid candles, as there may be a gas leak nearby.

Let family and friends know you are okay. If phones are down, perhaps you can report in on social media.

VOLCANIC ERUPTION

This section focuses on volcanoes. We will address supervolcanoes in the next chapter. If you live near a volcano, especially an active one, you must be aware that volcanic eruptions can also result in earthquake activity, mudslides, fires, flash floods, mudflows, and of course lava flow.

BEFORE

Build your emergency supply kit. Be sure to include goggles and face masks for each member of the family, because ash fall will be a major hazard.

Have a plan if you and your family are going to be together, and a meeting place if you are apart when the eruption occurs. Go over evacuation routes that take you downwind of the volcano. You may have to travel by foot or bicycle if ash fall is heavy, as it can damage car engines.

Get a hazard-zone map from your local emergency services or from the U.S. Geological Service to learn the potential danger to your home's location.

Become familiar with your community's plan of action if you live near an active volcano. When the warning siren sounds, be ready to follow instructions. Most active volcano areas have designated shelters. Find out where they are.

Watch the local news if there are signs of an imminent eruption, and follow the instructions of local authorities, even if the volcano still looks peaceful and inactive.

DURING

Evacuate if told to. You will be dealing with the initial eruption, lava, and debris, and the falling ash afterwards. Often it is the ash that creates the most problems. It can cause major health issues if breathed in and can disable car engines. You may need to go on foot or by another method of travel. Watch for planes overhead during ash fall, as their engines may be disabled, causing them to crash.

If you live near a stream or creek, mudflow and heavy rains can become a problem. Mudflows travel faster than you can run, so watch your surroundings, and do not attempt to cross a bridge or waterway unless you can tell it is clear upstream.

Stay away from the path of lava flow, and avoid low-lying areas such as river valleys. Try to get to higher ground to avoid volcano-associated flash floods, mudflow, and lava flow.

Do *not* go into an open body of water, stream, creek, river, or pool during an eruption if near the volcano. The heat of the pyroclastic gases, such as sulfuric acid, can turn the water extremely hot in minutes.

Shield yourself if outdoors from pyroclastic flow, which is the blast of rock, sand, debris, and deadly gases that fly outward during an eruption. Pyroclastic flow can travel at speeds over 300 miles per hour (483 kph). The rocks can be dangerously hot, and they may rain down on you from the sky for miles. Protect your head and face, and get under some cover if possible (but nothing that can catch fire easily!).

If outdoors in an open area near the volcano, remember that lateral blasts can shoot chunks of rock sideways for miles. Get low to the ground, but out of the path of any lava flow, until the initial blast is over, then get to help or inside a sturdy building.

Try to get to cover as quickly as you can to avoid injury from lateral blast and hot gases. The poisonous gases released in the eruption can be deadly if breathed in directly. Use a mask, respirator, damp cloth, or if none of those are available, an item of clothing you can remove and wet down.

Keep your skin covered to avoid burns.

If indoors, shelter in place, and shut off all windows, doors, and ventilation systems such as air conditioning and heating as well as chimneys, furnaces, and fans to avoid getting ash inside.

Use a face mask or wet cloth to breathe, and do not breathe in air with visible ash fall!

If outdoors, use goggles, face mask, long-sleeved shirt, long pants, and sturdy boots or sneakers. Wear eyeglasses, and remove contact lenses.

Avoid the roadways unless it is an emergency. If you must drive, go slower than 35 miles per hour (56 kph), and be prepared for engine stalls from heavy ash fall.

Move downwind of the eruption, as ash will travel upwind.

Be aware of geothermal hot spots, mudflows, and geysers that can be deadly hot. Cooled ground may be nothing more than a thin cover over hot lava, so tread carefully, and try to avoid crossing any lava flows.

Watch for fires caused by falling embers and hot rocks and debris, especially if you are trapped inside a building with a shake-shingle or nontile roof, a wood structure (storage shed), or outdoors in an area with trees and dry brush.

AFTER

Stay in a designated shelter, if you have evacuated, until you are told by authorities it is safe to go back home.

Once home, clear ash from roof, gutters, and overhangs, being careful not to breathe it in.

Wash clothing thoroughly after exposure to ash, and wash your hair if it has been exposed.

Do *not* turn on the air conditioner or ventilation system until you know it is clear of ash.

Stay tuned to local news or NOAA Weather Radio (http://www.nws .noaa.gov/nwr.) to see if there is a chance of another eruption after the initial blast.

WILDFIRE

BEFORE

Have a family fire emergency plan that includes what to do if you must evacuate, evacuation routes, and what to do if it is too late to evacuate. Remember to consider pets and the sick or elderly.

Pick a predetermined area to meet after a fire if the family is separated. This can also be a designated shelter that can be texted to family members.

Have your emergency supply kits updated, and be sure to include face-masks, extra water, and first aid supplies.

Prepare defensible space around your home by clearing, reducing, or treating vegetation at least 100 feet (30 meters) from the structure. Clear out grass and brush, and cut trees back to a minimum of 100 feet (30 meters) from the structure. Within the defensible space, you can grow ground covers and other drought-tolerant and fire-resistant plants, or fill the space with rocks, pebbles, and stones. Contact your fire department for great suggestions of plant, ivy, and ground-cover choices.

Remove dead leaves and debris from rain gutters and roofs.

Replace rotten wood fencing around the home.

If building a home, use noncombustible materials for the exterior, such as

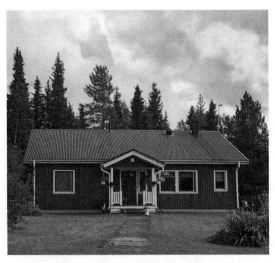

You should keep trees and bushes cleared away from your house to make it less vulnerable to wildfires, especially if you live in a wooded area.

stucco, metal, and composite siding and masonry. Limit the number of structures attached to the main home. Keep woodpiles for fireplaces at least 30 feet (10 meters) away from the home or other structures.

Make sure there is a clear access road to your home, and keep it free of overgrown vegetation and other blockages.

Tree branches should be at least six feet (two meters) above ground and at least ten feet (three meters) from the roof or chimney.

If the weather is hot and dry, and fire is possible, be sure to keep your car gas tank full and ready in case you need to leave.

Make sure your street address number is clearly visible from the street.

DURING

If the local news is reporting a wildfire near you, listen for instructions on television, radio, or via phone alerts. If you can see smoke and fire, begin gathering items for evacuation, and pack up your car. Don't wait until it's too late!

Evacuate immediately if told to. Don't try to stay and save your home or you may lose your life. Take your emergency kits and any personal items you have set by the house door or garage door ready to go. Don't go searching for items you forgot.

Go to the nearest designated shelter that is out of the path of the fire.

If anyone is having difficulty breathing due to ash and smoke nearby, get them to the hospital or call 911 if roads are still open to your home.

If you have more than one exit route from your home, take the one that will take you farthest away from the fire.

If a fire is very close, and you have not received evacuation orders, call 911 immediately for instructions.

Once at the shelter, listen to local news for instructions on when you can return home.

AFTER

Do not return home unless cleared by fire and emergency services authorities.

Since sparks can reignite a fire, check around your home property for hot spots, and put them out immediately. This includes the roof and attic.

Use extreme caution entering a burned area, and if you see smoke or a flare-up, leave immediately, as a small reignited area can soon turn into a new raging inferno.

Once back home, throw away any exposed food.

Wear a dust mask, and wet debris so that you aren't breathing in dust particles.

Do not drink any water that may have been exposed to smoke or high heat during fire.

Use work gloves when handling burnt objects.

Catalog damage with a cell phone camera or video camera for the insurance company.

Contact professionals to clean extensive smoke and fire damage inside and outside the home. Do not assume you can wash the smoke away. Smoke has a way of binding to materials for a long time, and you may need to throw away many items if the smell persists.

WHEN YOU ARE TRAPPED!

Chances are, you will have ample warning time and can evacuate safely from the path of an oncoming wildfire. But if the unthinkable should happen, and you are trapped, here is what you can do to increase your odds of surviving.

In Your Home

Stay calm. Get family members together in one area.

If you have time to wet down the exterior of the house, do so, but only if the fire is still a distance off. *Only do this if you absolutely cannot evacuate, even on foot!*

Call 911 and let them know you are trapped in your home.

Fill sinks and tubs with cold water. Fill buckets and containers, and put them around the perimeter of the home.

Close doors and windows, but keep them unlocked for firefighters. Close off any vents that bring air into the home.

Stay inside the house once the fire is close. Do not go outside to use garden hoses. The fire will win.

Stay away from outside walls, windows, and doors, and get inside an interior room of the house.

Try to cover your bodies with wet clothing or blankets. Use dust masks if the air is thick with smoke.

Wait for help, and do not try to escape once the fire surrounds your home.

If on Foot

Stay calm. Panic will cost you precious time.

If you are camping or hiking in an area, and a wildfire breaks out, get between the fire and a body of water such as a creek, river, or lake if you can.

Find a road leading away from the fire, and use it if it is clear.

If you are near a clearing free of vegetation, a ditch, or a cave, use it until the fire passes.

Call 911 and let them know your position and situation.

If there is thick smoke, protect your airways. Use a moist cloth or face mask, and do not take deep breaths. Try to stay low to the ground, and cover your mouth and nose with the cloth or mask.

Try to stay upwind of the fire at all times. Do not try to run uphill from a fire. Fire travels faster uphill because heat rises and causes the flames to spread faster!

If the fire is too close and you cannot outrun it, lie face down and cover your body. If you can wet your clothes, or find a muddy area to roll around in, do so, as the moisture will help.

If you are on a roadway, and the fire is upon you, look for a ditch away from the path of the fire, and get down, protecting your face.

If you can get behind the fire to where it has already burned, you will be safe, but only if there are no hot spots, so be aware of your surroundings. Kicking up ash can cause breathing issues, so use your face mask or cloth as you get out of the area.

In Your Vehicle

You may not have anywhere else to go but your car, or you may get caught in the path of a wildfire during evacuation. If you cannot flee on foot, then do this:

Stay calm. If you can keep driving, do so slowly. Keep headlights and hazard lights on so you can be seen through the thick smoke. Watch for other people, animals, and obstructions.

If you must stop, park the vehicle in an area clear of vegetation or behind a solid structure if possible.

Close windows and air-conditioning vents.

Keep the engine running, and put on the air conditioning on recirculation.

Cover yourself with a thick blanket or wool jacket, and get on the floor of the back seat. If the blanket or jacket is made of flammable materials, do not cover yourself with it!

If you have water in the car, wet some cloth, and keep that to your mouth and nose. Drink water too to stay hydrated against the hot, drying fire's effects.

Call 911 on your cell phone, and let them know your location and situation.

The car will get unbearably hot, and ash and smoke may enter the car. Hot air currents will rock the vehicle, often violently. Try to stay calm even if the engine stalls.

Once the fire has passed, call for help again.

Get out of the car and attend to anyone who may be in shock or have fainted during the fire's passing.

If the car starts up, drive away from the fire.

If the car is on fire or won't start, go away from the fire on foot to get to safety, but watch for overhead burning tree branches and hot-spot flare-ups.

SCAMS

After any disaster, there will be people who seek to benefit from the pain and suffering of victims. Whether it be an earthquake, tornado, or hurricane, scam artists will be ready to knock on your door and play on your anxieties and fears by promising you things they cannot and will not deliver.

Obviously, the first thing you should do in the cleanup period after an emergency is contact your insurance company. Only communicate with them and not any outsiders that may offer you help or try to convince you that your insurance company won't cover your damage. Keep in mind there will not be much in the way of federal assistance for rebuilding your roof or your home, so people who tell you they represent a government agency are probably scam artists.

Some tips to remember:

Be wary of contractors who are not licensed or do not have a good track record with references. Confirm their state registration, ask if they have a local office, and always get more than one quote for the work you need.

Do not sign anything with a company, other than your insurance company, that you feel forced or intimidated into signing.

Do not deal with door-to-door salesmen after a disaster. If you seek out contracting work or an insurance adjuster, use reliable sources that have been well vetted.

Demand that companies that call you after a disaster remove you from their call lists.

Never give a company bank, personal, or financial information over the phone, unless it is your legitimate insurance company representative.

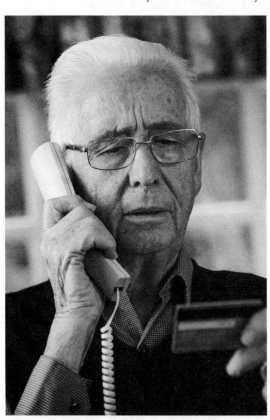

After a disaster, never give a contractor company your credit card or other financial or personal information over the phone unless it is through your insurance company.

STRUCTURE AND NON-STRUCTURE HAZARDS

No matter the type of disaster, being aware of hazards inside and outside can save your life. Structural hazards depend on the type of building you are in: a home, office building, skyscraper, or warehouse. Obviously, the first things to look out for are broken glass and ceiling panels that are loose or fallen. If the power is out, you have to tread carefully, looking for holes in the ground and sharp debris. Shopping malls and warehouses will be a mess of broken glass and collapsed walls, as will airport terminals and churches. The disaster will be one challenge. Surviving the hazards it leaves behind is another.

Trying to leave a building, you may encounter collapsed walkways and stairwells. Walls may be partially caved in, and there may be beams hanging from above. All of these are hazards that can cause injury if you aren't alert and careful.

If you are in your home, the type of construction makes a difference. Older brick homes that have not been retrofitted will be a big problem in a large earthquake but may offer protection in a wildfire or hurricane. If your home was built before 1940, it may not be bolted to the foundation and could be shaken, blown, or lifted off of its foundation as a result. You can spend the money to bolt your home to its foundation and be assured it will stand up to most hazards. If you live in a mobile home, think about strapping it to its concrete pad.

Also look around at what you have in the home and garage that might be potential "weapons." A water heater that is not strapped down, large bookcases, grandfather clocks, and refrigerators can all become deadly in a tornado or massive earthquake. You can buy industrial strength Velcro to keep them from flying around or bolt them to the wall. Cabinet doors should be fastened in a way they won't fly open and create a mess of broken glass and dishes. Appliances and office equipment such as printers and computers can cause electrical shock after a disaster.

Nonstructural hazards include downed power lines, ruptured gas lines, water main breaks, fallen bricks and cement blocks, and sinkholes outside the home. Look around the outside of the home for fallen trees or branches that are resting against the roof, holes in the roof, major cracks in the exterior walls, exposed wires from inside the home, and signs of water coming into the house around the foundation, which can undermine the floor and eventually the entire house.

After any disaster, an inside and outside assessment can identify problems that could be deadly. You may still be in a state of shock from the initial disaster, but don't wait until it is too late to see what other dangers lurk. Address them quickly so that you or someone else doesn't get hurt.

Because of all of the above hazards, it is unwise to go inside a building to try to rescue other people unless you can safely assess the exterior and interior. Professionals such as police, firefighters, and emergency workers know how to do a quick visual assessment as part of their job. You may not. People don't realize that floors may appear to be safe to walk on but are actually on the verge of collapse from the slightest shift in weight. The same applies for ceiling beams and walls that appear to be structurally sound, but can topple during another high wind or aftershock. If there are no emergency services personnel around, and you know someone is trapped inside a building or structure, you enter at your own risk.

EXPOSURE TO HAZARDOUS MATERIALS

Another post-disaster hazard is hazardous materials such as explosives, chemicals, flammable liquids, deadly gases, corrosives, oxidizers, and radioactive materials. These materials can be highly unstable and toxic to all living things and may not be identifiable except by their containers, which should be marked. Stored hazardous materials will feature a National Fire Protection Association (NFPA) 704 diamond. This diamond-shaped mark will feature four quadrants, each with a different color and number to indicate the type of hazard and the degree of risk. A red quadrant will indicate the material is *flammable* and can have any number. The higher the number, the greater the risk. A yellow quadrant indicates *reactivity*. Blue indicates *health hazards*. White indicates an unusual reactivity with water, so the material should never be mixed with water. Different letters in this quadrant will tell you why. For example, OX means the material possesses oxidation properties when mixed with water. ACID of course indicates an acid, ALK indicates that the material is a base, and COR means corrosive. A nuclear triangle means it is radioactive.

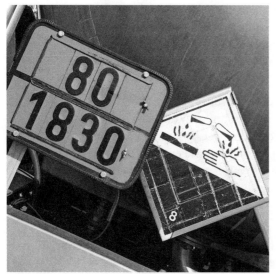

Trucks hauling hazardous materials are marked with signs explaining what they are carrying. This one indicates the truck is shipping sulfuric acid.

These indicators are mainly for firefighters and professionals, but it doesn't hurt to know what you might be dealing with. You can also learn to identify hazardous materials that are being transported by trucks and tankers. Any vehicle carrying hazardous contents will be marked with a Department of Transportation placard known as DOT. These diamond-shaped placards indicate by color what the hazardous material is. Orange is for explosives, red for flammable gas, yellow for inhalation hazard, blue for anything that is dangerous when wet, white for poison, and yellow for oxidizers. Yellow and white are for radioactive materials, black and white for corrosives, and red and white for spontaneous combustibles. We all know the skull-and-crossbones poison symbol, and often that will be on a toxic hazard container.

However, you cannot assume that an unmarked tanker is *not* carrying hazardous materials, as often drivers forget to change out or put on markers. If there is a big-rig crash or tanker overturn on the freeway, keep as far away as you can until it is determined what the cargo was. If there is any indication the cargo was toxic, try not to breathe it in without using a cloth or something over your mouth and nose. Your eyes may begin to burn if exposed. Leave the area as soon as possible, and keep car windows rolled up, with the air conditioner on recirculation only.

THE POWER OF PREPARATION

The key similarities in all of the above situations are: Be prepared. Be prepared. And—be prepared.

Having a supply of food, water, and other necessities, having a plan of action ahead of time, having evacuation routes identified, listening for news and information, doing what you are instructed to do, being careful, having common sense, looking out for your safety and the safety of others first, property later—it is all the same. The more of these steps you see fit to take, the more prepared you will be.

Watch the news during the next natural or man-made disaster that occurs somewhere else in the country. Notice how there are always people who blame everyone but themselves for not following instructions, not having supplies ahead of time, and not using their common sense. *Do not be one of those people*. Those people put their own lives at risk but also the lives of emergency services personnel who have to rescue them because they refused to listen to instructions.

A disaster or emergency is not a time to focus on protecting a painting or a house or a car. If doing so puts you in danger, *get out*.

In the next chapter, we will look at a handful of high-level impact events that may require more than just carrying out the basic plans for a short duration. These events may require that we do more than just the minimum to survive. Knowing what we *can* do before, during, and after will hopefully empower us not only to survive but also to rise out of the ashes and thrive.

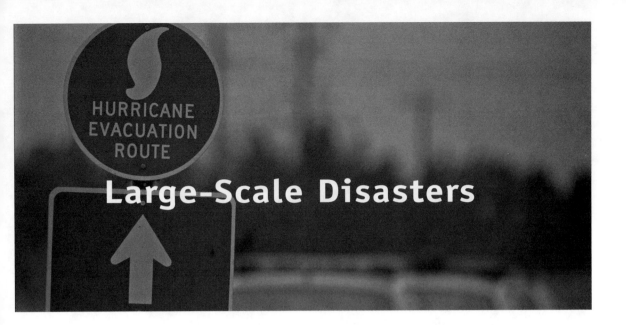

Large-Scale Disasters

There are local, regional, and national emergencies and disasters—and then there are those that affect us on a global scale. Massive, catastrophic, almost apocalyptic events that create their own challenges when it comes to surviving and thriving before, during, and after. In "How to Survive a Global Disaster" in the February 2016 *Guardian*, reporter Keith Stuart wrote, "Whether it's a natural disaster, bioterrorist attack or pandemic, experts reckon society as we know it will collapse within 13 days of a catastrophic event." That's right. Thirteen days. Not even two weeks.

That is not a lot of time, and the bigger the disaster, the longer the help will take to arrive. The article went on to say that the Johns Hopkins Center for Civilian Biodefense Studies organized a war game called Operation Dark Winter in June of 2001 to simulate the effects of a biological attack on the United States, and the results were jarring. "What they discovered was that the country was ill prepared to cope. Within two weeks there would be enormous civilian casualties, a catastrophic breakdown in essential institutions, and mass civil unrest. Food supplies, electricity and transport infrastructures would all collapse."

Basically, America would go medieval! Some of the key survival tips the study generated, though, could improve your chances of not being among those casualties.

Don't Go It Alone If You Don't Have To: Find others to join, and up your chances of survival. Others can be potential threats, so use discernment, but you are better off banding together than trying to be a lone wolf.

Get Out into the Rural Areas: But don't get too remote. Cities are more dangerous during disasters, when there is no rule of law and everyone is looting and marauding. But don't totally isolate yourself, because you might need others to work and cooperate with to create a small and sustaining community that can also offer better protection than you can solo.

Find Access to Running Water and Land Where Food Can Be Grown: Running water can be used to create a power source too. Growing your own food is also something you can do better when you team up with others.

Communicate: Try to get basic information about what is happening beyond your small area. You will also need to communicate with others in your group, other survivors, and emergency services once they come back on line and begin helping civilians re-establish order.

Beware of Government and Authorities: Can you trust them? Do you need them? Beware of authority figures, including the military exceeding their authority. But if they are trying to help, *take it*. When the proverbial SHTF, trusting in the government may be a hard thing to do, but it also behooves you to take what offers of assistance come your way.

Be Ready to Trade and Barter: Your cash won't last long. ATMs will be useless. What can you do or what do you have that might buy you more food, water, and supplies? Can you build things out of wood or make shelter out of leaves and branches? Use the skills you have to barter for the skills you don't. Not many people will be carrying around diamonds, gold bars, and fur coats to trade, so your food and water and your talents and gifts will be the hottest commodities out there for getting your own needs met.

Plan on Being Self-Sufficient for a Long Time: In the event of a massive global catastrophe, you have to plan on surviving long-term, and that means working with others to build some type of community and bring about some semblance of order.

What are the chances of something this big happening and shaking up every aspect of your life? Slimmer than smaller disasters, to be sure, but they can and do happen. While it is terrifying to consider having to resort to the above to survive, it is better to be prepared ahead of time with some ideas of how you will survive than to be left with only fear, confusion, and disorientation.

The following events must be addressed, for they are potential threats we all face living on this planet. These are some of the possible global catastrophes we face, along with some tips and ideas on how to increase your odds of living to talk about it with your grandchildren one day.

ASTEROID IMPACT

We already know the devastation an asteroid can cause, and of course the larger it is, the more deadly it will be to life on this planet. A huge asteroid would wipe out the planet itself. While there are not many things we can do to assist in our survival should that happen, we can have some tips in mind should we hear on the news tomorrow that a smaller chunk of space rock is heading for a face-to-face with Earth.

In September of 2004, an asteroid named Toutatis, named after the Gaulish god of thunder and destruction, passed within four lunar distances of Earth. It has passed by our way before, but this time it was to come much closer. Luckily, that's all it did. Back in 1989, another asteroid, with kinetic energy 5,000 times more powerful than the Hiroshima bomb, passed very close to Earth, and scientists didn't discover how close until after it happened.

We do face this threat. Space rocks that are hurtling towards our planet, big and small, are out there. Like comets, they are chunks of debris from explosions that occurred during the formation of our solar system over four billion years ago. Although an asteroid impact the size of the one that wiped out the dinosaurs is pretty unlikely, simply because something of that size would be recognizable and identifiable now and just isn't "out there," there can be many smaller impacts we need to worry about.

Even one that is about 600 feet (183 meters) in diameter could wipe out the entire East Coast of the United States within an hour if it were to blast

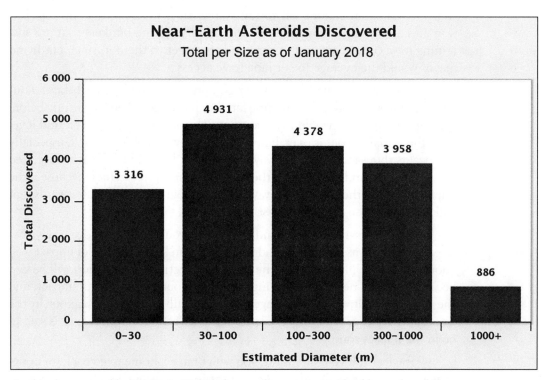

As this chart created by NASA in 2018 indicates, there are a considerable number of Near-Earth Asteroids that are a potential threat to our planet.

down into the Atlantic. Our atmosphere serves to protect us from smaller asteroids. Once they come into our atmosphere, because of their high speed, they tend to shatter from the pressure and then burn up from friction created upon entering the atmosphere, so we don't see them strike land.

But those that do make it through can cause major devastation, depending on where they land, ground or water. Ironically, smaller asteroids landing in the ocean can cause greater damage, and with many people now living in coastal regions, wipe out large amounts of life.

Tsunamis filled with broken-up debris from an asteroid create a deadly wall of water that can destroy anything in its path. Because we can't run away from a large impact—and going underground would do no good either, folks—we rely on government agencies such as NASA to come up with deflection methods to counter the orbit or trajectory of such killer rocks. Another method being tested is to blow the asteroid to bits while it is still out there in space, before it has a chance to strike Earth.

So can you survive such a thing *at all?* Well, to some extent. Large asteroids would render us extinct and most of life on Earth as well. Maybe being able to escape underground to some type of bunker would work for a while, but survival would only be possible for a couple of years, and you would not have any "outside" communications left to tell you when it was safe to go up top. Billionaires and wealthy governments can build biodome bunkers that are sustaining for a certain amount of time and try to get to them in time, but by no means would the average Joe or Jane have access.

Some preppers believe an underground bunker built to withstand a nuclear blast would work for protecting families if they get enough warning before the impact. Again, it would involve great risk coming back up to ground level once the initial impact is over, but you can survive the impact itself, especially if it occurs thousands of miles away. If you don't have a bunker, it is suggested you move far inland and up onto the highest ground you can find, because if the impact occurs in the ocean nearby, you might avoid the tsunami afterwards that will wipe out those along the coast.

Evacuation from an impending impact would hopefully occur days before the impact was to happen, and we might even know its path of impact well enough to get people moving in the opposite direction. Information will be key, because you may need extra driving time to get out of the zone of impact, and the later you wait, the more congested roads will be. You can bug out in the woods and try your hand at wilderness survival if the city you live in is said to be in the impact zone.

Tragically, if your city is hit, you won't have a home to go back to. Long-term survival needs will either be met by assistance from government agencies, or you may be on your own for a while. You may even end up in a FEMA detention camp for a while before life returns to normalcy and you can find a way to get to family and friends elsewhere.

Thankfully, solar system debris does vaporize before it can reach us, but it is out there and one day will come close—too close for comfort. In the year 2029, the asteroid Apophis is going to come pretty darn close to Earth, possibly even below the altitude of our communications satellites. It will return again in 2036, and that time it might decide to slam into Earth altogether. Others like Apophis are already identified and being watched as potential threats in the near future. Hopefully, by then we will have figured out the exact method for destroying or deflecting them.

ASTEROID/COMET SURVIVAL TIPS

Have your kit ready, and be sure to have over a month's worth or more of food, water, and supplies. A major impact will decimate infrastructure, and a smaller, localized one will cut off supplies from local stores for a while.

If an impact has been predicted, watch the news for updates on where it might strike and what to do. If in coastal areas, move inland days before impact to avoid congested evacuation routes.

If you don't have an underground bunker, consider building one, and make sure it has its own energy source. Understand that a direct impact could even destroy your bunker.

If you don't have a bunker, and impact is days away, look for possible areas nearby where you can take your family, such as a cave or high ground deep in the woods.

If you are stuck inside your home or office building, head to the lowest point in the house or building, and stay clear of windows.

Once impact occurs, you will need to ration food and water to make it last long enough for infrastructure to get back up and running.

Conserve generator fuel if you need to have it for the long haul.

LED lights use less energy and are great for conserving battery power.

The initial impact can trigger large earthquakes and volcanic activity, so be ready to deal with those hazards as well.

Keep listening to any communication source you can find to get the most current news.

Stay mentally and physically active and healthy, especially if stuck underground.

Do not go outside unless you are assured the air is clear of ash, soot, debris, and toxic gases. Impact will cause rain and soot and acidic rains for months to come, making living above ground a deadly option.

The sunlight may be greatly diminished by the soot, ash, and debris kicked up by the impact, so have many light sources available if you are above ground.

Scavenge for more food and water if you can, but be ready to defend yourself from others out doing the same.

Be aware that the impact may have greatly damaged water pipes and many above-ground facilities needed to supply fresh food, water, and fuel.

If there has been a great loss of life, find a place where you and your family can organize a new system of living with others who have survived.

An impact can send us back to the Stone Age, and the vast majority of us are not prepared physically or mentally to live off the land and fight for our survival. One of the greatest dangers we face in an event of these proportions is how our fellow humans will react and respond, and many smaller disasters have shown that, while we may initially all come together to help one another in good spirit, after a while, when food and water grows scarce, it becomes every man for himself. After the disorienting experience of an impact, one that could possibly even alter our planet's orbit, our humanity may not be the first thing we consider when wondering whether we will see the light of another day.

Let's hope we get nothing but fly-bys for a good long while.

ECONOMIC COLLAPSE

That's right. An economic disaster can be every bit as hard to survive as a natural disaster. Just ask anyone who lived through the Great Depression and the many recessions to follow. No matter how good the economy may be at any given time, what goes up can and often does come down, and it helps to be prepared, especially if you have a lot invested in the stock market.

How might economic collapse affect you directly? Well, do you use a credit card, a debit card, have a mortgage, an open line of credit? Do you have enough cash on hand to survive for a while if economic and banking infrastructures are useless? Is all of your wealth in stocks or real estate, and none of it in liquid investments you can get to quickly if needed? Are you living paycheck to paycheck, in a job that is in flux, and dependent on fuel for that long commute to work?

So many things factor into an economic meltdown. If the banks close their doors suddenly, and you cannot get to your money or even to an ATM, how will you pay for food and water? It is never too late to start planning for a money-related disaster on a national or global level. Many other nations have experienced such collapses, such as Greece, Venezuela, and Argentina, and it could happen in the United States just as easily if the right ingredients are thrown into the brew, especially if we were to go to war or experience a catastrophic event that would tap out government resources and shut down millions of jobs.

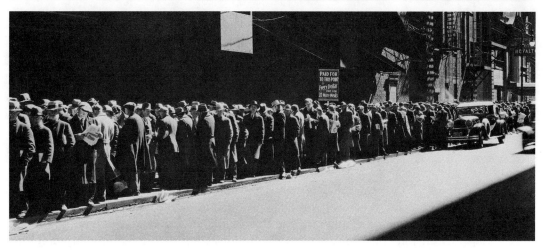

Unemployed men stand in a bread line in New York City during the Great Depression of the 1930s. The Great Recession of 2008 was nearly as bad in many ways, and some economists feel the U.S. economy is extremely vulnerable to another economic collapse.

In addition to having some cash on you at all times, in smaller bills, you can do a few things to prepare.

Stock up on food and water for well beyond the short term. Try to become somewhat self-sufficient by collecting rainwater, growing your own food, stockpiling food and extra water, teaming up with neighbors and friends to create collective gardens and food sources, and making your own food all move you towards more sustainability in a crisis. While shelf-stable foods are the best option, stock up on anything, and grow whatever you can with what you have. Times of economic stability are the right times for learning about growing food, stockpiling food, saving water, creating water sources, what supplies to have, finding shelter away from urban and populated areas, and setting aside cash for the rainy days to come.

Don't stop there, though. Stock up now, while prices are normalized, on nonfood items such as toiletries and medications, even clothing, cleaning products, pet foods, and anything else that you will need for a year or more should the SHTF, as preppers like to say. Also have plenty of firewood and fuels for grilling should the power go down from a collapse of infrastructure.

If you cannot stockpile and grow food where you are, perhaps consider buying a small tract of land away from urban areas, or use a vacation home as your survivor homestead. This is even easier if you go in with family members to buy land and build small homes and storage facilities. Sounds paranoid? Sure it does, until the disaster of all disasters occurs and you are wishing you had done it sooner.

Paper money may be worthless in a total collapse, so think about trading and bartering either products you have in excess or services and talents you possess, such as babysitting, cooking, woodworking, transportation, repair, construction, cleaning, and even things like trading your extra lemons for their extra squash. The more you can offer to others, the more valuable you become to them, and the more likely they will be to give you what they have that you need in return.

Look into spreading money between smaller banks or using credit unions in case larger banks experience difficulties. Community banks may be better in situations where larger chains are tumbling like dominoes, but also think about buying gold, silver, or other precious metals that may be worth more when the dollar becomes worthless.

Eliminate as much debt as possible. Increase assets as a goal, and consider putting valuable items up for sale and using the money to buy more emergency stockpile supplies for you and your family. You may not have considered this before, but think about taking courses on wilderness survival, CPR, and personal safety. These may come in handy for a variety of emergencies, not just economic collapse.

Self-sufficiency is the key. Can you grow your own food? Save up rainwater? Create other sources of drinking water? Make preserves and other food items that can be canned and jarred for the future? Raise chickens, rabbits, and goats for food?

This is when learning how to protect yourself, your home, and your family becomes critical. When a financial collapse occurs, people panic and become focused on getting what they don't have, which may be what you *do* have. Buy

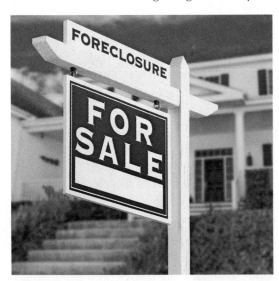

Foreclosures were rampant in the Great Recession because lenders had sold subprime mortgages like they were cheap candy and then lied about their stability to shareholders.

a gun, learn how to use it, find ways to secure your home, learn self-defense, and be ready for a fight. See the chapter on self-defense for more information.

Insulating yourself and your family against everything from a job loss to a company shutdown to a complete economic apocalypse will help buy you time in a situation where time is all you have on your side. The longer you can ride out a money-related disaster and be resilient enough to still feed yourself and your family, have access to water, and have a shelter over your heads, the easier the duration of the event will be until it changes or rectifies itself.

Recall, back in September of 2008, when the U.S. economy was on the verge of collapse thanks to investors withdrawing over $140 billion in investments from money

Economic Collapse Timeline

When the SHTF, banks will be the first to close. Without access to money, people won't be able to shop for food, water, and supplies.

Demand for food, water, fuel, and supplies will surpass supply.

Local water, power, and utility companies will close down.

People cannot get fuel for their cars and are stuck at home with what few supplies they have on hand.

People begin to go out and look for food and supplies and, because of panic, will turn on their neighbors and steal what they have.

Crime will skyrocket, including mass looting, raids, and violent assaults.

People will begin bartering for food and services, until they have nothing left to barter.

The demand for the dollar around the world will nosedive, and interest rates will soar.

Hyperinflation would set in, as the dollar loses all its value. Hyperinflation occurs when there is a huge increase in the supply of money that is not backed up by growth of the gross domestic product (GDP), resulting in an imbalance in monetary supply and demand. When this goes on for a long period of time, financial collapse will result as prices skyrocket and the dollar plunges in value.

Oil embargoes could stop fuel from getting across state lines in trucks. Other competing countries such as China and India would get the available oil if we couldn't.

Eventually, the supply of oil will not be able to keep up with the demand, and all transportation will shut down, including buses, trains, and planes.

Food would not be delivered anymore to local stores because of the shutdown of the trucking industry, which is responsible for moving over ten billion tons of goods every year in the United States alone.

Terrorism would run rampant because of the nation's vulnerable condition, and there would be little in the way of law enforcement and government agencies available to stop it.

The military would be busy policing the public, and anarchy would break out. Civil disobedience, mass uprisings, and the threat of martial law would prevail.

Our economy can withstand a lot of pressure and bounce back, but a massive hit would not only cripple every business that relies on money—and let's face it, that is every business—but also every individual who has taken for granted that they could always access their savings and go to the store to get what they need when they run out. Even the smallest of preparations can help you survive, instead of doing nothing and hoping the government will fix everything. The problem with economic collapse is this: it will be in great part the government that is broken and in need of fixing. So don't rely on it.

market accounts. This was the result of a short-term panic that, had it lasted longer than a week, could have crippled the country's economy for a long, long time. Luckily, it didn't. Saving money, budgeting, having a few hundred dollars cash tucked in your emergency kit, having an excess of survival food and supplies on hand, and even having a place to escape to in case of rioting and looting—these are small things you can do now to ensure your safety later.

Another possibility is to head to a family member's home and combine survival supplies and efforts. Relocating to a safer area that is remote and provides you with land to grow food on is best, but be ready to defend that land. If you do bug out, remember to take important documents with you, including valuable items such as jewelry, paintings, and collectables that you may want to sell or barter later for goods and services.

ELECTROMAGNETIC PULSE (EMP)

Twenty-first-century living means we are slaves to electricity and technology. When something catastrophic happens that knocks out our power grids, shuts down technology, and literally leaves us without the comforts we so take for granted, we react with terror. An EMP is just such a catastrophe, and one of the few that can cause chaos far beyond regional and even national boundaries.

An electromagnetic pulse is a burst of radiation that results from the detonation of a nuclear bomb in the atmosphere miles above the ground or from a coronal mass ejection. There are also eBombs that are meant to specifically cause an EMP and are smaller and more localized in their damage. Anything that pulses in a wildly fluctuating attack on the earth's magnetic field can create the kind of chaos we would see from an EMP. Imagine an EMP so powerful that it takes down the electrical grids of an entire nation, plunging the populace into darkness, with no power to computers, no cell phone service, no landline service, and dwindling supplies of food, water, fuel, and medical supplies.

An EMP can be carried through power lines and literally melt down transformers as it travels at the speed of light. Inside your home an EMP will fry semiconductors and anything plugged into an electrical circuit along with them. The further away the electronic source is from the EMP, the better off it will be, but a powerful burst will take care of just about everything that is connected to the grid or grids affected. This includes heaters, natural gas, and heat/cold thermostats, automobile engines, computers, lights, electronic panels, appliances, portable heaters, and anything else you can plug in.

A wood stove would be safe, as it does not rely on electricity to function.

In the early 2000s, the Senate Judiciary Subcommittee held meetings to discuss the threat of an EMP, especially in light of increased terrorism and how easy it would be for a terrorist group to detonate a small, cheaply made tactical EMP weapon. Senator Jon Kyl, who attended that meeting, later told the *Washington Post* in 2005 that the social disorder following an EMP would throw survivors back into the 1880s. The truth is, it might throw us back even further, thanks to our dependence on technology and computers, cell phones, and things that we plug in to make our lives easier, faster, and more comfortable.

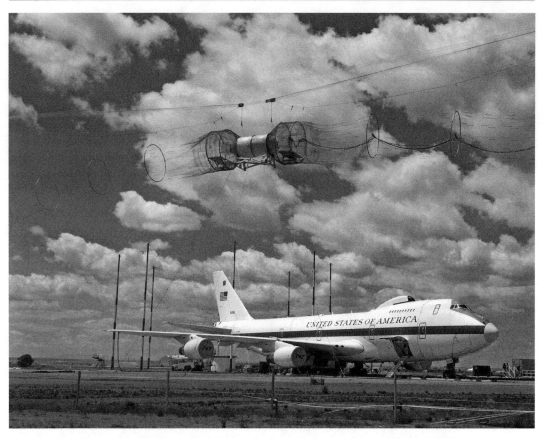

A test on the effects of an EMP on a 747 airplane is shown being run here at Kirtland AFB in New Mexico. Findings from such tests might help protect valuable equipment from future attacks.

Just to give you an idea of an EMP's potential for damage, a detonation at an altitude of 30 miles (48 kilometers) would affect everything within a 400-mile (644-kilometer) radius. Kick that up to a detonation at approximately 120 miles (193 kilometers), and the zone affected would have a 1,000-mile (1,610-kilometer) radius. A burst at an altitude of 300 miles (483 kilometers) in the atmosphere would affect a 1,470-mile (2,366-kilometer) radius. A full-scale detonation of more than one EMP would bring the entire continent to its knees, and the effects would eventually cause global economic and social chaos.

No one would actually die from the EMP itself. It would happen fast and be invisible but for the zapping of all electrical wires and semiconductor components as well as transformer boxes that would fry instantaneously. We might hear the pops and smell the burning before we realize what has happened. Once we are told an EMP has been detected—and there would be absolutely no warning if it were intentional—the real struggle to survive begins.

Within days, people would begin to panic, wondering when the power would be restored. Within weeks, people would begin attacking other people to get the things they are out of. Within months, people would begin killing other people to take what they need. Survival would be the only thing that matters, especially if the nation's infrastructure was crippled and it might be months before any semblance of normalcy returns.

If this sounds like a crazy science fiction movie, it isn't.

So, if we get no warning of a nuclear bomb bursting in the atmosphere, unless the terrorist group responsible warns us, and if we get very little warning during a highly active solar cycle, because such EMPs are rare, our own course of action is to *already be prepared* when it does happen. That means having our emergency supplies of food, water, and everything else we've discussed numerous times, but with a focus on stockpiling battery-operated devices and batteries, for they would not be affected by the EMP. This can include radios, cooking devices, clocks, walkie-talkies, cell phone chargers, etc.

There are ways to protect equipment and electronics from an EMP, although they may not be foolproof. One is to store it all inside a Faraday box or cage, which protects metal devices from electric fields. The box is made from metal, like filing cabinets, ammunition containers, cake boxes, and metal storage boxes. Do not let the appliances touch the metal container when placed inside, though, and you can insulate it with cardboard, thick paper, or any other type of insulation you have handy. If you don't have a Faraday cage, you can wrap appliances in good old aluminum foil for minimal protection.

You can also use shielding around components, loop antennas, self-contained battery packs, and even something called an Ovonic Threshold Device, a solid-state switch that will open a path to the ground when there is a massive EMP surge at a circuit.

After the EMP, you will have to decide whether to stay home or bug out. If you stay home, you will have to think about protecting your home and your supplies from eventual marauders and looters. It might be wise to team up with neighbors and watch out for each other as well as share supplies. Being a part of a small group may be safer than trying to go it alone, especially if you have no weapons or ways to protect yourself and your family. Think about all staying in one home as a main base and venturing out to other homes to get supplies. There is strength in numbers, and if everyone is in one place, you can better defend that one place than try to spread out and defend five or six separate homes.

The power may be back on within days, weeks, or months, so plan for the worst while hoping for the best. Once power is restored, there may still be an external threat from others who are roaming your neighborhood or out on the roads.

It may be safer to leave. Knowing that your car engine may be on the fritz, thanks to the EMP blowing out anything that operates with electronics and a computer, you may need to walk, ride a bike, or take horses if you have them. Take your bug-out bags with you and as much food and water as you can carry. Do not take main roads, as they will be clogged with abandoned cars and people looking for food and water in them. Stay hidden, and only travel when safe. This will be a frightening time, when other people will become the potential enemy, so be sure to keep quiet and explain to children the reason for the stealth.

If you find a place to settle in, whether another house, cabin, campsite, or clearing in nature, be sure you can defend yourself from others out looking to survive. Again, remember: strength in numbers, so perhaps travel with other neighbors who agree to leave as a unified group, or find people you know nearby, and become a part of their survival group. Yes, it might look like warring camps from an episode of "The Walking Dead," so operating within a larger community may be all that stands between you and certain death.

Surviving an EMP is possible, but it really depends on how much you have already done to stock up on the supplies you will need, your ability to defend your home and your family, and how long the electrical grids are down and authorities are unable to maintain control.

SOME TIPS TO GET THROUGH AN EMP

Have cash on hand, as there will be no working ATMs.

Be prepared to escape, and have a route planned out, with an alternative just in case.

Look for older cars that may not be affected by the EMP (non-computer panels), and see if they have keys or can be hotwired.

Buy a weapon and learn to use it properly.

Avoid large cities and highly populated areas.

Do not expect the government to have order restored within days.

If you bug out with bikes, be sure to take spare parts and tools you might need.

Do whatever it takes to survive and keep your family safe.

If you decide to hide, try to find a place that is hard to see from main roads.

Wear camouflage out in the wilderness to avoid being seen by marauders.

Learn ahead of time how to make a fire and hunt and fish for food.

An EMP may never happen in our lifetime, but it might behoove us to take some time to prepare just in case it does. Whether it comes in the form of a bombing or a natural coronal mass ejection, either way you will be responsible for your own survival, as it may be a while before emergency services can get to you and get things back to normal. Again, this is one disaster where it isn't the actual disaster that can harm you, but the reaction of people afterwards.

That alone makes something like an EMP terrifying, because it can bring out the worst in humanity and make an already bad situation much worse.

Be smart. Be aware. Be ready.

NUCLEAR ACCIDENT

Nuclear power plants dot the country, utilizing heat from nuclear fission to convert water into steam that provides a cheaper source of electricity and power to millions of people, approximately 20 percent of the population. But that very process is what makes living anywhere near a nuclear facility so dangerous. Over three million Americans live within ten miles (16 kilometers) of an operational nuclear power plant. Though there are very stringent emergency response plans at all nuclear facilities, and the U.S. Nuclear Regulatory Commission enforces strict regulations on all plants, they still pose a potential and devastating problem.

People who live within ten miles of a nuclear plant are at the greatest risk if there is a meltdown or accident. Those in the second, larger "danger zone" of about 50 miles (80 kilometers) from the plant will also be affected by the leaking of radiation into water, air, and food sources. Whether a partial meltdown,

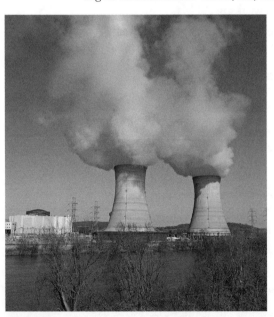

The worst nuclear accident in U.S. history occurred in 1979 at Three Mile Island in Pennsylvania. Faulty computer interfaces and human error combined to cause an operator to accidentally release radioactive coolant into an auxiliary building. Fortunately, the radiation did not escape outside the power plant.

as occurred at Three Mile Island in 1979, or an explosion resulting from a major quake and tsunami, as with the Fukushima Daiichi nuclear plant in Japan, or an accident on the level of 1986's Chernobyl, a nuclear plant is subject to minor, major, and catastrophic disasters, all exposing people to varying levels of radiation.

If you live near a nuclear power plant, three things matter: time, distance, and shielding. You must get to shelter quickly, you must get as far from the radiation source as possible, and you must know how to shield your body or more likely shelter in place, because you may not have time to evacuate in an accident. Accidents come without warning, as do terrorist attacks, and, yes, nuclear plants are prime targets.

There may be a little bit of warning time if an accident occurs. The nuclear plant will sound an alarm, and local and regional authorities will immediately act, so it is imperative that you listen and follow instructions. If told to evacuate, because a full meltdown may be imminent, don't waste time wondering if you should stay or go. Get out.

If you are told to shelter in place, be sure to cut off all air from getting into the rooms you are sheltering in. The dangers of radioactive fallout do decrease with time, but upon first exposure, you must get to safe shelter. But the longer you are *exposed* to radiation, the greater the negative effects will be, including serious illness and even death. Just because you cannot see, feel, or smell the radiation does not mean it is there. Inhaling and being exposed to radiation must be avoided at all costs until you are told it is safe to go outside.

Also take into consideration the weather and wind conditions that may carry radiation over larger areas. Rain does not "clean" radiation away, but rather the opposite: it will wash the fallout from the atmosphere and send it back down to the ground. Wind currents can carry radiation for hundreds of miles, so if you are in the path of the wind, get out and away.

News sources and authorities will monitor the radiation levels and report on them regularly, but it will be up to you and your family to stay safe until the air becomes safe and stable enough to breathe again.

BEFORE

Before a nuclear plant accident occurs, think about shelter, because that will be the most important protection you have against deadly radiation. In previous chapters, bunkers and underground shelters were discussed, but whatever you do, make sure it keeps a barrier between you and fallout.

If you live near a plant, contact the power company for its public emergency information materials and its emergency action plan. These are materials you should be receiving on an annual basis, so if you are not, make sure you get on the list.

DURING

Once a nuclear plant emergency alert is broadcast, listen for instructions and follow them.

Evacuate if told to in order to put as much distance as possible between you and the potential fallout. Keep windows and air-conditioning vents closed.

If at home, get into your shelter, interior room, or basement, and close all doors, windows, and vents to keep outside contaminated air from coming inside.

Wait for further instructions from the authorities about how safe it is to open windows or venture outside.

AFTER

If you were exposed to radiation, you must act fast and follow decontamination instructions from the authorities. Call 911 or go to a hospital, or do what you are instructed where you are if you are unable to travel, especially if you are experiencing nausea or dizziness.

Get out of exposed clothing, and put it all inside a plastic bag. Seal the bag and set it somewhere out of the way.

Do not go home, if you have evacuated, until told to do so. Throw out all food that was not in covered containers or in the refrigerator.

NUCLEAR BOMB

The dangers of a nuclear bomb come much faster and harder than a slow leak or exposure. If a nuclear bomb goes off nearby, the initial blinding light and intense heat of the blast will kill everything in its path. Thermal radiation will cause first-, second-, and third-degree burns on the body. Another threat is that of fires caused by the initial blast, which can also lead to explosions of buildings and toxic chemical sites nearby. Add to that the coming fallout, and it is one of the most deadly of all disasters, having an even global effect if it occurs in wartime and creates the dreaded "nuclear winter," a period of six years or more when the sun will be blotted out by ash and debris, and the ground will be toxic and contaminated. Think of it as an asteroid impact with radiation to boot.

The extent of the blast's powerful pressure wave is directly related to how far above the ground the bomb was detonated and also to the size of the bomb itself. Smaller, portable bombs will cause more local and regional damage, while missiles and massive warheads will take out much larger sections of land and population. If more than one bomb is detonated, a huge area of land can be directly affected. But the radiation will spread on the wind currents, and everyone will be at risk for thousands of miles.

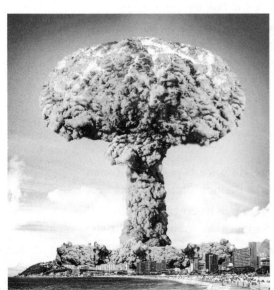

If you live in a large, urban area or near a military installation, you may be within a prime target for a nuclear attack.

The *before, during,* and *after* will be the same as for a nuclear accident, with a few exceptions to think about:

If the world is on the brink of war, there will be the threat of nuclear bombs being exchanged, so don't wait to act. Get your supplies, shelter, and action plan in order.

If you live near military bases and installations, you may be more of a target than most for a terrorist bombing, so be aware of the need to have an underground shelter or bunker, or something above ground that can withstand the blast and protect against fallout.

Symptoms of Radiation Exposure and Sickness

Common symptoms of radiation poisoning are:

- Nausea and vomiting
- Dizziness and disorientation
- Severe fatigue
- Bleeding from mouth, eyes, and nose and possibly from the rectum
- Diarrhea with blood
- Skin rashes and sloughing of skin
- Mouth ulcers
- Hair loss

Acute radiation syndrome, or ARS, happens when the entire body is exposed to a high dose of radiation in a very short period of time, as with a nuclear bomb blast. This can be a matter of minutes, with radiation dosages over 70 rads. It usually has an external source such as a bomb or nuclear plant meltdown. This type of radiation must penetrate the body, as with X-rays, gamma rays, and neutrons, and it penetrates the entire body, rather than just a smaller area, which would not lead to ARS.

There are three acute radiation syndromes:

Bone marrow—Dosage of 70–1,000 rads, causing destruction of the bone marrow, infection, hemorrhaging, and if not addressed quickly, death. An immediate bone marrow transplant can help the bone marrow cells repopulate, but it must be done immediately.

Gastrointestinal—600 rads or above, but usually over 1,000 rads of exposure. Causes disruptive and usually irreparable damage to the GI tract and bone marrow and can lead to death within two weeks, after a period of infection, dehydration, and electrolyte imbalances, if the symptoms are not treated.

Cardiovascular/central nervous system—As low as 2,000 rads, but usually 5,000 rads or more, causing death within seventy-two hours from circulatory system collapse, convulsions, coma, meningitis, and increased fluids in the brain, causing extreme cranial pressure. Symptoms in the early stage before death can include anorexia, severe dehydration, confusion, diarrhea, and major infections.

How do you know if you have ARS? The four stages of ARS are:

Prodromal—Nausea, vomiting, and diarrhea occurring within moments or days of exposure and lasting up to several days.

Latent—The patient may look and feel well for a few hours, days, or weeks, while damage is occurring within the body on a level dependent on the exposure.

Manifest illness—Symptoms show up based on the level of exposure and can last hours, days, or even months.

Recovery/death—Patients who are not treated immediately or suffered high exposure may die within weeks or months, except for cardiovascular/central nervous system syndrome, where death is inevitable. Recovery can last weeks or up to two years.

Know several evacuation routes to avoid the panicked roadway congestion that will occur.

If you work in a government building, you are also a target. Make sure there is a plan and that you know what it is!

Larger urban areas will be targets, so if you must bug out, head for a rural or wilderness area as soon as possible. Get as far away from the blast area as you can.

Learn about the symptoms of radiation sickness, and take action immediately to seek help if needed. Radiation sickness is not contagious, so help others who are showing symptoms.

Don't think that once the initial blast is over, the radiation has dispersed. Residual radiation, or fallout, can fall as "black rain," which burns the skin.

Symptoms of radiation sickness may not appear immediately, so continue to protect yourself from black soot and fallout.

Prepare to be in your shelter for at least two days, if not more. Make sure you have enough supplies to last. Ration supplies, if needed, if you are directed to stay indoors longer to avoid various "fission products" created by a nuclear blast, such as cesium, radioactive iodine, and strontium.

If you must go outside, cover yourself head to toe in protective clothing.

THERMAL BURNS

If you or someone you know has been burned from exposure, you can take steps to treat it. Minor burns are called "beta burns."

Immerse the burned area in cold water for a minimum of five minutes.

Wash blistered or charred skin with cold water to remove contaminants, and cover with a sterile compress, being careful not to break closed blisters.

Keep skin uncovered if there are no blisters, welts, or charring.

Major burns are known as "thermal burns" and are much more severe. The main cause of these will be the initial blast itself. These burns are deadly!

Protect existing burns from further contact with radiation.

If the burn is covered by clothing, cut the clothing away gently, trying not to take skin with it. If clothing is stuck to the skin, leave it and call for emergency help immediately.

Never put ointment on a thermal burn. You can gently wash with water. Do not use butter or oil or cream.

Use *only* a sterile pad specifically for burns.

Treat the victim for shock by lifting their legs above heart level. Allow them to lie still. Keep an eye on their breathing and pulse rate while help is coming. Signs of shock include rapid breathing, pale skin, nausea, extreme thirst, disorientation, fainting, and extreme sweating with cold and clammy skin.

A SCENARIO OF A BLAST

Once the bomb detonates, if you are within 50 miles (80 kilometers), you risk not only flash blindness from the brilliant white light, but instantaneous first- to third-degree burns. *Do not look at the blast.* If you happen to be caught outdoors, once you can actually see again, and if you are not so badly burned that you can't move, you must either lie flat on the ground and cover your head for at least thirty seconds or until the blast wave has passed, take cover behind a concrete wall or structure, or run away from the blast as fast and far as you can. If near buildings, get inside a sturdy building, preferably built from dense materials, and get to the basement, cellar, or bottom floor to hide out if there is no nearby bomb shelter you know of. You can also get to the center of the building, preferably where there are no doors or windows leading outside.

While you will still be exposed to some radiation, it won't be anywhere near the deadly levels out of doors. If you are at home and see the mushroom cloud and bright light, get into a basement or stay on the bottom level of the home. Wood homes don't offer much in the way of protection, but anything you can do helps lower the risk. The rule of thumb is, if you cannot find more adequate shelter within five to seven minutes of the blast, stay put and shelter in place for at least twenty-four hours, or longer if told to by authorities. Yes, you should have some way of getting news, such as a battery-operated radio or television set, but since power will go down with the blast, and not everyone carries around a radio, you may be relying on sketchy cell phone service, or local authorities coming down the street blaring instructions over a bullhorn.

Until help arrives, you can take a shower or wash over your body to remove possible contaminants. Wash with soap and use shampoo, but never rub skin that may have been exposed or skin that looks rashy or burned. Wash out your ears, blow your nose if you can, and wipe over your eyes with a clean, damp cloth to clean eyebrows and lashes.

Unlike a nuclear plant accident, where there might be a few moments of warning time, a nuclear bomb probably won't be announced by those responsible, and it will happen fast. Most people won't even understand what has happened until they see a mushroom cloud in the distance. This is a terrifying truth about nuclear explosions, whether the result of terrorism or outright war. The authorities may be able to provide a timetable for the arrival of fallout in specific areas of the region or country, but that is about all the warning we can expect.

Remember afterwards not to consume any food or water that was not in a sealed, plastic container. If in doubt, throw it out. Once the initial bombing or attack seems to be over (and be ready for additional bombs if it is not), you must stay out of the way of authorities and military personnel who might be coming through your area or on the roadways. The last thing you want to do is go out into the world and be exposed to more contaminants, so you'd better have a good hazmat-style suit handy, otherwise stay inside until told it is safe to go outdoors.

Potassium Iodide—Can It Save You from Radiation?

Potassium iodide (KI) is a salt made of stable iodine that blocks radioactive iodine from being absorbed by the thyroid gland. It is not the same as iodized table salt. Taking KI could help protect the sensitive and delicate thyroid gland from radiation during a nuclear event or an accident involving high levels of radiation. It *only* protects the thyroid, though, and not other parts of the body or internal organs. In order to receive the benefit, you must take actual KI and not a supplement that may contain KI. Taking KI if there is *no* present radiation threat to the thyroid can be dangerous.

KI comes in tablet and liquid form, both approved by the Federal Drug Administration, and many people buy it in advance to keep as part of their emergency supply kit. During a nuclear event, the government or emergency services will also give out potassium iodide to the public. But it does come with some risks for those who cannot take KI to begin with.

Those at risk are infants, children, pregnant women, breastfeeding women, and the elderly who may have existing thyroid conditions. Taking it when not needed or taking too high a dosage can lead to thyroid cancer. Check with your doctor to see if KI should be a part of your emergency survival plan.

According to the FDA, recommended dosages (if your doctor has okayed taking it) are as follows:

- Newborns to 1 month: 16 milligrams, or 1/4 of a 65-milligram tablet, 1/4 milliliter of liquid form

- Infants 1 month to children 3 years of age: 32 milligrams or 1/2 of a 65-milligram tablet, or 1/2 milliliter in liquid form

- Children 3 to 18: one 65-milligram tablet or one 1 milliliter in liquid form

- Adults: one 130-mg tablet or two 65 mg tablets, or 2 milliliters in liquid form

- Breastfeeding women: take adult dose

If the radiation threat continues beyond twenty-four hours, emergency ser-

Depending on the type of attack and the size of the bombs involved, you may be asked to stay put for days or possibly weeks. Emergency services and authorities will be trying their best to respond and get help where it is needed. Communications and power will be out for a while. Even when you are able to venture outside, know that local law enforcement, the military, and government agencies will be operating in major crisis mode, and they may enforce curfews and even martial law as they try to deal with the existing attack and prepare for a possible retaliation attack. Do not expect them to be able to deal with your individual problems for quite some time if the entire country is devastated.

There are two types of radiation from a nuclear blast. Exposure to either can cause death.

Prompt/initial radiation—This is released during the detonation, is short-lived, and travels for a shorter distance. However, because of the size of

vices officials and government officials will tell you to take a second dose if needed. You may be told to take one dose per 24-hour period for several days.

Side effects can include stomach pains, gastrointestinal upset, allergic rashes and reactions, and inflamed salivary glands. Newborns that are given more than one dose run the risk of developing hypothyroidism, which can cause brain damage if not treated correctly.

KI is a great item to have on hand and is very inexpensive. You can buy it online and in many survival stores and outlets. It does not require a prescription. During recent nuclear accidents and threats, supplies became scarce very quickly. Right after the 9-11 terrorist attacks, KI was near impossible to find online or otherwise and was back-ordered on most websites that normally had a full stock. Government and emergency services can pass out KI in the event of an emergency, but do you want to wait that long and run the risk of ex-

posure before you can reach a distribution site? It behooves you to have a good supply, and hopefully never have to use it, rather than not have any and need it. But please check first with your doctor to make sure the risks of taking it are worth it, not just for you but for your children too, and do *not* take it unless you are instructed by the authorities to do so.

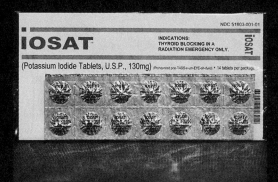

After the Fukushima incident in Japan, the government there distributed potassium iodide tablets to those in the area to help protect their thyroid glands from absorbing radioactive iodine.

many newer nuclear weapons, it can cause great amounts of death from the initial blast.

Residual radiation—This is the fallout that occurs if the bomb explodes near to the ground, creating a "rain" of gas, debris, radiated particles, and dust which is sent up into the atmosphere, then rains down upon the ground. Black soot, or black rain, is contaminated fallout materials that are extremely hot and incredibly deadly.

Avoiding as much fallout as possible can come down to the type of shelter you seek. About 20 percent of U.S. homes are built from materials that would offer little protection. Brick buildings offer more protection than wood structures. Going below ground into basements or lower levels of high-rises or apartment buildings would be best. For example, hiding out in a sub-basement of a five-story brick building would expose you to 1/200 of the amount of the fall-

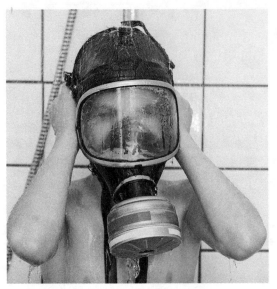

If you have water available for decontamination, remove your outer clothing, keep your mask on, and wash thoroughly without scrubbing or scalding the skin.

out radiation outside. Being in an underground bunker or nuclear fallout shelter built specifically for this purpose is best, but chances are you will need to seek shelter where you can at a moment's notice. Remember: thick as a brick, concrete is king, and stay away from windows and doors.

Some experts suggest staying in any shelter you can find for at least an hour, then seeking better shelter, but use your judgment if you are not able to get news from the authorities on radiation levels.

SELF-DECONTAMINATION STEPS

In the event of any kind of chemical, biological, or nuclear exposure, you must get the contaminants off your body as soon as possible. You can also decontaminate other people, even pets.

If there is still running tap water, you can use it for decontamination if there is no other source, as radioactive materials will be diluted by the time they reach the ground water sources.

Step One—Put on your face mask or face protection. Remove outer layers of clothing, which will remove about 90 percent of contaminants. Do this carefully to avoid shaking loose radioactive or chemical dust. Put clothing in a sealed plastic bag or container, and put it somewhere where there's no risk of someone opening it.

Step Two—Wash yourself off thoroughly. You can shower or use a sink or any faucet in the home or shelter area. Use soap. If you are nowhere near a sink or shower, you can wash off with damp, clean clothes or paper towels/napkins. Include the face and hair. Do *not* use hair conditioner, which will bind radioactive and other materials to your hair and scalp. Use shampoo only. Do not rub, scald, or scrub skin to avoid breaking the skin open and allowing contaminants in. If you have cuts, wounds, or abrasions on the body already, cover them as best as you can during washing so you don't contaminate the areas.

Step Three—Blow your nose, wipe your eyelids and eyebrows, and wipe out your ears with a moist wipe or towel. Throw *all* clothes, wipes, and towels used into a sealed bag or container, and set it out of the way.

Step Four—Find clean, unexposed clothing, and put it on. Clothes kept in a closet, drawer, or dresser will be unexposed. (If you do not have any other clothes to wear, you can remove an outer layer of the clothing you have on and brush off the next layer as best you can.)

You can wash pets with soap and shampoo, and be sure also to wipe down their eyes, ears, and noses.

PANDEMIC (GLOBAL)

A regional or national pandemic is far more likely to affect us than a global outbreak, simply because there are specific actions authorities overseas can take to stop the infectious disease from reaching our shores. But it can happen, and with new mutations of such viruses as avian flu breaking out every year, it may be only a matter of time before one becomes so virulent and so aggressive that international borders won't stop it.

It has happened before. According to "How to Survive the Next Catastrophic Pandemic," an article by George Dvorsky for Gizmodo, the twentieth century saw three global influenza outbreaks that killed over 100 million people. The HIV/AIDS pandemic, which began in earnest in the 1980s, killed over 35 million alone. Other viruses have posed grave threats in the last ten years, including SARS, MRSA, Ebola, and Zika. But influenzas appear to be the most likely to spread far and wide and fast enough to cause global chaos, as well as diseases that are seeing a rise in outbreaks due to climate change, an increase in the mosquito population, and urbanization.

In the event of a viral pandemic such as influenza, which mutates so easily that our attempts to create a vaccine are often months behind the current mutation, with air and boat travel it would be possible for the virus to appear in many countries of the world before we even identified it, at which time certain quarantines and bans on travel could be imposed. If a flu pandemic happened in the United States, there are ways to deal with it and survive as long as common sense is used. Ideally, it would be confined to our country, but chances are, other countries would find themselves doing battle with their own breakouts thanks to air and boat travel.

A pandemic here in the United States would result, no doubt, in a shutdown of workplaces, schools, and services in order to rein in the spread from person to person. The bigger the breakout, the longer the shutdown will be in effect, so running to the store for a gallon or two of water might be out of the question. Stocking up on food, water, and medical supplies, which should include antiviral medication if it is available, is a necessity, because in a global outbreak, emergency services and medical aid may be tied up with severe cases, and hospitals will be overloaded with patients.

Staying indoors, protecting yourself from those who might be infected, and listening for possible vaccine distribution plans by local authorities are at the top of your list, as well as washing your hands and expecting many services to be disrupted because of the large scale of the emergency.

The biggest problem arises when you or a loved one displays symptoms of the disease. Then it is imperative you stay away from others and call 911 or get to the nearest hospital. If that is not possible, you must do your best to treat the flu symptoms as best you can and not expose anyone else in the process.

A pandemic will overload the medical response and healthcare systems we usually take for granted, so think about getting a flu shot every year to at least protect yourself from the "standard" flu going around, even if it may fall short of the most current mutations. Try to avoid people who have the flu, and if you get it, don't go to school or work and spread the disease to others. You don't want to become a spreader of the disease in an already troublesome situation. Instead, self-isolate and wait until the outbreak is under control. Public health officials will most likely impose a "cease assembly."

Some pandemics may be weaponized anthrax or other agents that are not contagious or communicable, but still need to be avoided, as exposure can be deadly, so it is critical you listen to the news and get the most current information on whether there is a vaccine available or some other way to offset exposure. With some diseases, you need to stay away from certain kinds of birds, mosquitoes, and standing water where carriers can breed. West Nile virus in the Southwest, where this author lives, has caused several deaths and alerted residents to the dangers of standing water and certain types of dead birds that need to be reported to the authorities. Learn what the facts are for the disease involved, and don't spread conspiracies, rumors, or misinformation to an already frightened community.

The biggest problem during a pandemic is public panic. Civil unrest can occur when there is not enough information about what the virus or agent is, how it affects us, and how contagious it is. That is when people begin filling in the blanks themselves and often turn to violence to protect themselves or get supplies they may be short of. People also cause trouble when they show up at hospitals and demand attention, even worse when they do it armed with weapons. Be ready to deal with the contagion of fear that a pandemic can cause.

SUPERVOLCANO ERUPTION

We know the power and potential devastation of a volcanic eruption, but a supervolcano would have global effects that last long after the "big blowup." In the United States, there are two supervolcanos that could erupt at any time. Yellowstone caldera, as stated earlier, is highly active, with earthquakes and geyser activity and even some carbon dioxide–related tree kill, all of which are parts of the puzzle that is a supervolcanic eruption. Long Valley caldera in the Central California region is a major threat to surrounding urban

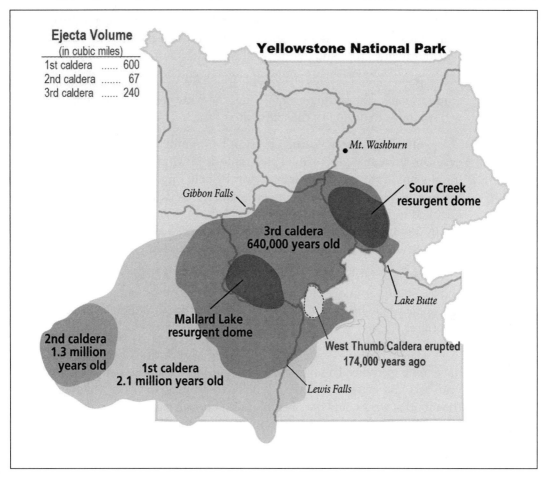

Ejecta Volume
(in cubic miles)
1st caldera 600
2nd caldera 67
3rd caldera 240

Yellowstone National Park

Mt. Washburn

Gibbon Falls

Sour Creek resurgent dome

3rd caldera 640,000 years old

Lake Butte

Mallard Lake resurgent dome

2nd caldera 1.3 million years old

1st caldera 2.1 million years old

West Thumb Caldera erupted 174,000 years ago

Lewis Falls

Yellowstone park sits on four calderas that have had massive explosions over the last two million years. It is possible that an eruption of global significance could happen soon.

areas, including Southern California, and is especially frightening because of its potential to trigger a major earthquake along the central or southern San Andreas Fault—and vice versa. If either one of these erupts, the western half of the United States will be reduced to rubble.

Because of the sheer amount of pyroclastic flow, ash, and debris sent into the atmosphere in a supervolcanic eruption—enough to block out the sun and create a nuclear winter for up to six years—the damage would be widespread, even outside of the United States. All infrastructure would be shut down, including trucks, cargo ships, railroads, and planes. People and goods would not be able to move about the country for a long time, which means running out of food, water, and other supplies long before the emergency lifts enough to get the nation up and running again. The Midwest agriculture belt would be severely compromised because of inches of ash and no clean water for irrigation. Sulfur dioxide in the gases produced by the eruption could cause years of acid rain, destroying crops and livestock all over the country.

But we could survive a supervolcano, if we are not within the immediate eruption zone. The further away we are, the better our chances, but again, we will still have to deal with the aftermath of the initial blast.

Should a supervolcanic eruption be imminent, people would have to evacuate as far away as possible, preferably downwind to avoid the overwhelming amount of ash and debris sent skyward. Sheltering in place would be a given, because being outside would mean exposure to deadly ash which could, if breathed in, kill you. That ash could create some gorgeous skies and sunsets, but in the lungs it is nothing more than pulverized glass. It can fall six inches thick and literally change the atmosphere and weather patterns for years.

Because of the massive scale of the disaster, not only would local stores and gas stations run out of supplies in a matter of hours, but all over the country people would be scrambling to stock up on what they didn't have before the eruption.

There might be some warning time to work with, but the problem is, we have not experienced a supervolcano in our lifetimes. The last one was 28,000 years ago, and so we don't have all the boxes to check off as to what happens in the months, weeks, and days before. But if enough signs prompt the U.S. Geological Service and authorities to issue a warning, there will be little time to take action.

If a supervolcano erupts in the United States, what might it look like? As far as earth scientists can tell, it might look something like this:

Vents in the caldera floor crack and explode open, shooting gas and debris upward. Eventually, the caldera floor could succumb to moving magma and implode, then explode upward 30 miles (48 kilometers) high or more into the atmosphere as white hot debris, gases, and ejecta. Pyroclastic flow would devastate everything within a 500-mile (800-kilometer) radius, and ash would fall for thousands of miles away, carried on the jet stream and other wind currents, first across the Northern Hemisphere, then to the Southern Hemisphere.

The sun would be blocked out for years, creating a "nuclear winter" that would cripple the nation and destroy most of the agriculture needed to feed people. All travel would be shut down for months as ash and debris are cleaned off of streets. Planes would stop traveling to avoid ash getting into engine blocks. Eventually as the ash spread, global agriculture would be decimated, and mass starvation would be the order of the day. Drinkable water would be a scarce commodity, thanks to falling ash and debris.

Global temperatures would drop by as much as 20 degrees or more, and we would enter a mini ice age. Sure, it would offset some of our global warming, but not in a positive way.

All in all, the world would be brought to its knees.

Some people may be so intimidated by the scope of a supervolcanic eruption that they give up on any attempts to survive. But like an asteroid impact, it is possible to survive, just as our ancestors survived several supereruptions in the past. The most important things again will come down to adequate shelter (a full-on fall-out shelter is best), extended supplies of water, food, and other items, and a source of energy, because the power grids will be inoperable for a long, long time.

Food grown outside as well as water collected outdoors would be ash-covered and useless, so stocking up on things that can be kept in the home, garage, a supply shed, or an underground shelter or bunker would be better in this situation. Once the eruption occurs, roadways will not be open, so staying put is the only option (unless you are within 500 miles (800 kilometers) of the supervolcano—if so, get the hell out at the first sign of a warning!). You will be required to shelter in place as long as ash is falling to avoid it getting into the home or building.

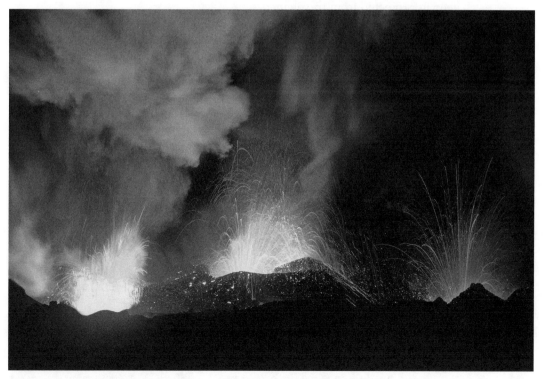

A supervolcano eruption—such as what will one day occur at Yellowstone—would change the climate of the planet for years.

You may want to add respirators and chemical or hazmat-style suits to your supply kits or storage areas. If you do have to go outside, these items will protect your lungs and skin from the ash and from any burning debris that could be falling after the initial eruption. Unfortunately, the air quality may be compromised for years afterwards, which may drive more people underground to try to ride it out.

Like an asteroid impact, your chances of survival may have a lot to do with location, location, location. Being 3,000 miles (4,828 kilometers) away will be a much better scenario than living within the eruption zone. Living upwind or in the opposite direction of the jet stream and other large wind patterns might help keep ash moving away from you, but eventually it will come around and encircle the entire planet.

The people who survived supervolcanoes of the past did so by getting inside caves, riding out the aftermath, and basically using their primitive skills of hunting and finding water and shelter to up their odds. Today, we have billions of people on the planet, and a major dependence on ease, comfort, and technology, all of which will be gone the second the caldera explodes skyward. It might behoove us to study some more primitive techniques for making fire, acquiring food, cooking it, finding water we can drink, and building shelter to keep us protected from the elements.

But unlike our primitive ancestors, we do have organizations on a global scale that can assist in rebuilding the broken parts of our nation. We have emergency services personnel and law enforcement agencies and government agencies that, to some extent, may be operational enough to help begin the process of rebuilding infrastructure like roads, railways, and bridges and get utilities up and running again, even if it takes months to do so. We have so many people on the planet today that there is little chance of wiping out the species, even if Yellowstone gave its best shot at a supereruption. Our best hope is that people will come together in the aftermath.

In the book *Supervolcano: The Catastrophic Event That Changed the Course of Human History*, written by this author and her father, Dr. John M. Savino, we wrote that those living on the perimeter of the initial impact zone have the best chance of survival, depending on many things, "including pro-activity before the disaster strikes, and the ability to get as far away from the event area as possible in as quick a time period as possible. Even then, it may not be enough." But it may, and this will be no time to hem and haw over what to bring if you have to evacuate. You grab what you can and you get out.

"Surviving a supervolcano will come down not to the survival of the fittest, but of the smartest and most prepared, not to mention the most psychologically resilient," we wrote in *Supervolcano*. A major factor after every disaster, as stated in the chapter on first aid and disaster psychology, is trauma and the ability to act despite panic, fear, and confusion. A volcanic eruption will scare the pants off you. A supervolcano may send you and your loved ones into a state of shock, so you have to find the inner strength to work alongside your outer strength to improve your chances of survival.

WAR

Yes. War. Even here in the United States, we must be aware of the possibility of a war, whether on our soil or in another country. War may also break out on a global scale. We have come a long way from the "duck and cover" air and bomb raid drills of yesteryear, when the most we were taught to do was get under a desk and cover our heads until the sirens ceased.

Chances are that an invasion of the United States would be hard to mount, but it can occur. More likely, our experiences of war will come in the form of terrorist acts, bombings, nuclear and biological attacks, EMP, and other methods that are a bit more insidious than a full-on invasion with foot soldiers, tanks, and planes by a foreign military.

So can we be prepared? Obviously, the same rules apply here as with other disasters. Be prepared with food, water, and supplies. Have a strong shelter, preferably underground. Know first aid. Evacuate when and where told to. Follow the instructions of the authorities.

But war brings its own challenges that go beyond simply trying to stay alive. There is extreme mental stress and trauma that must be addressed for those affected and those who witness violence, death, and destruction. Post-traumatic stress disorder will skyrocket, as it did after the 9-11 terrorist attacks, and it will become a medical crisis. Soldiers who come back from war bring with them the mental trauma of what they experienced overseas, and PTSD will become the greatest challenge of wartime and post-wartime.

Running out of food, water, and fuel as well as necessities of life such as toiletries, medical supplies, and pharmaceuticals is another byproduct of war. It behooves us all to stock up, stock up, stock up.

Perhaps the only way to avoid the consequences of war is to not have wars, but they are a reality. Though we may be limited as to what we can do, we can do something.

Stock up on food, water, and supplies, and look for ways to become self-sufficient, such as growing food, raising food animals, saving water, and creating energy sources.

Buy firearms and learn how to use them properly.

Create a safe and strong shelter; below ground is better, but a panic room will do.

Have cash on hand in small bills.

Learn wilderness survival skills, first aid, triage, and self-defense.

Have methods of communication with loved ones and preferably more than one.

Fuel will run out fast, so keep a full tank of gas and several gas cans full. Do not store gas cans in the home!

Have propane tanks full, and store them away from the home.

Buy generators, batteries, flashlights, and portable cooking devices.

Does all of this sound familiar? The way to survive any emergency, big or small, even war, comes down to being prepared and having knowledge as well as staying connected to information sources.

War presents a terrifying prospect. For many people living in high-risk target areas such as urban centers and coastal areas (ports, harbors) as well as near major military bases and installations, nuclear silos, and government buildings and offices, the best bet might be bugging out, way out, into the wilderness. Own a cabin in the woods? Go there and shore up the place. Try to go with others, as there is strength in numbers, especially if you are not familiar with rural areas to begin with. You may be able to ride out the duration of the conflict, until hopefully clearer heads in positions of power prevail. But until then, getting out of the way of the conflict is best.

Analyze the threat and your location and proximity to it. If trapped in an urban area, you must do your best to find protective shelter that can withstand bombs and gunfire. Band together with others to create a stronger force. If you have weapons, keep them with you, but be aware of the risk of others wanting your weapons if their survival depends on it. The same applies to food, water, and other emergency supplies. Often during war and times of extreme duress, we turn allies into enemies and forget about the greater enemy we came together over in the first place. Know that during the war and even afterwards, there will be looters and raiders looking for supplies. Sometimes, they will be your former neighbors and friends. You may, in fact, have to become one of them to survive.

They say all is fair in love and war, and that may be terrifyingly true.

If it comes to fighting, the more people you are with, the greater your chances of surviving against a small-scale assault. Going solo during a wartime situation is taking a huge risk with your life.

MASS PANIC AND RIOTS

The stories fill the news: a major attack at a large event, and suddenly thousands of human beings turn into wild, stampeding bulls. Or perhaps a news event sends people out into the streets in a riot or protest, and you are stuck in the middle of it all. Either way, you suddenly become very much aware of how fear, panic, and anger can kill as much as any disaster can, and that sometimes the gravest danger we face is our fellow man.

Imagine a situation where a small number of people, say employees in an office, must evacuate a building immediately due to a fire in the supply room. The employees, if low in numbers, could easily get out quickly through several exits. But even if there were only one exit, they could easily file out one at a time, calm and clear-headed. If the entire building is on fire, then we have more people trying to get out the same number of exits, and if there is only one exit, it creates what is called a "bottleneck"—a small area through which a large number of bodies must pass to get out of the bottle.

Think of a bottle containing a handful of marbles. You turn the bottle upside down, and the marbles line up to come out of the neck one by one, or perhaps two at a time if they are smaller. But fill that bottle with marbles, and you have a clogged neck as they all try to get through at the same time. It's that way with people too, especially when they are in shock, terrified, immobilized and just being pushed along, or desperate.

Panic is normal in an extreme situation, but only those who can snap out of it and think, observe, and act will survive, because extreme panic causes

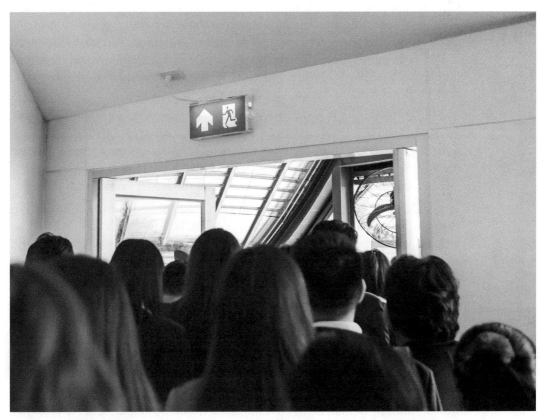

When panic takes over in a crowded room such as a theater with limited exits, bottlenecks can form and people can be injured or even killed by trampling.

people to make bad decisions or no decision at all. Often a herd mentality takes over, and individuals just stop thinking for themselves. On September 20, 2016, ScienceDaily featured a story called "What Causes Mass Panic in Emergency Situations." Researchers at the Max Planck Institute for Human Development, along with Rutgers University and other research groups, decided to see if people would act the same way in a virtual environment. They wanted to understand why mass herding took place in an emergency. So they performed a virtual experiment with subjects that simulated an evacuation from a complex building that had four exits, only one of which was usable.

The group did not know which exit was which, although some were given an arrow pointing to the proper exit. The stress level was increased by timing the group to escape within fifty seconds or lose points, which would be converted into money bonuses at the end. They also threw in bad lighting, fires blocking exits, and flashing lights.

The result was clear. There was more pushing and shoving as the stress escalated. Bottlenecks occurred in areas in which a decision had to be made, with the greatest stressors caused by having to turn around at a bad exit under even more time pressure. The individuals in the study were exposed to stronger social signals and were more aware of where the group was going and thus more influenced by group or herd behavior. Perhaps they felt there was truly safety in numbers. Or perhaps they just had no clue what to do and felt so helpless that they let the current of the crowd take them.

Add to the stress of an extreme emergency someone screaming or crying loudly, and the stress level can become explosive as panic spreads and people are sent "over the edge." If there is someone who steps up as a strong group leader, it can alleviate some of the panic and discombobulation. Now the herd has someone to focus on, listen to, and follow as long as the leader knows what to do.

Our knee-jerk panic default can kill us, as pointed out in "Why Do We Panic in Emergencies?" in the October 5, 2016, issue of *Psychology Today*. The article opens with a recollection of a December 24, 1913, Christmas party on the second floor of a hall in Calumet, Michigan, for the Western Federation of Miners and their families. The workers were facing a strike, but they wanted to enjoy the festive atmosphere. But when someone yelled, "Fire!" it triggered a panic, and suddenly all four hundred partygoers rushed downstairs searching for exits out of the building.

Seventy-three men, women, and children died in the ensuing herd panic, mainly crushed to death during the rush for an escape. There was no fire.

This and other stories like it show how easily we can go from being rational, thinking human beings to rampaging hordes so desperate to survive that we don't think twice about who we kill on the path to survival. It is as if something snaps inside of us, and we stop using our brains, or at least the higher parts of the brain, and we run entirely on instinct and primal fear. That is not to say instinct and primal fear do not ever serve us. They do. But when it comes to logical decision making, that is more the realm of the left analytical brain, which seems to shut down during extreme duress.

When there is no emergency, and we must leave a building, say at closing time, we do so easily and without pushing and walking over others. Yet the moment our survival is at stake, a switch goes off that turns us into colliding bodies operating solely from fear.

How do we prevent this from happening? The best thing to do is look around and get a good grip on the environment you are in before anything happens. Situational awareness is key. Where are the doors? Are there windows that can be used as exits? Can you sit close to the end of an aisle in case you need to evacuate quickly? Are there emergency exits, fire hydrants, axes, and fire hoses nearby? Getting a solid visual when you attend an event can give you the edge if all hell breaks loose and you need to act fast, and in the right direction.

You want to get to cover if bullets are flying overhead, or find a place to hide and be out of sight. Even a strong wall can be a good spot to hide behind, but look for a structural pillar, telephone pole, thick tree, car or truck, or thick hedges or brush. If you are caught in the fray, just keep moving, and keep your arms crossed over your chest as you work through the crowd, all the while looking around for an exit point.

Don't forget that many buildings and offices have back doors, side exits, and other potential places where you can break away from the main herd and get out safely. The last thing you want to do is get backed up into a wall or pressed against a locked door and be crushed by bodies. Try to make your way around the edges of the horde of people to where the crowd thins out. Always keep your eye on the situation around you. If you know where the threat is coming from, get away from it, hide from it, get behind it, and stay out of its way, but also don't risk your life while doing so, going against a massive crowd of panicked people or falling to the ground and being trampled.

RIOTS

As social unrest becomes a part of the fabric of our society, the threat of a riot persists in almost every area, unless you live out in the country. The best way to avoid a riot is to watch the news and stay out of the area it is happening in. This also applies to avoiding streets around a sports arena or stadium during a huge playoff game. If your team wins, expect crowds to flood out into the streets, and many will be drunk.

If a riot springs up while you are out, and you are stuck in it, you must remain calm and survey the scene. Again, situational awareness is key. If you are with others, keep everyone close together. Do not get involved in any way, and try to find back streets or paths away from the crowds. You want to stand out as little as possible and not draw attention to yourself. In a riot, people are not thinking clearly, and violence becomes the major response to anything or anyone, whether it is provoked or not.

If you are on foot, get away from the area, but if you are in your car, and the mob is forming all around you, honk your horn and drive. Keep driving even if people threaten you, because in this kind of situation, you want to get *out* of the area alive. If your car is swarmed, you may want to decide whether it is better to get out and join the crowd and let them have the car to tip over or burn as they may. As soon as you can, get out of the area. Your life means more than your car.

If you cannot escape the crowd, try to move with them until you spot an alley, path, hiding place, or other way out. Don't go against the flow of the crowd. You can slowly work your way to the edge of the crowd as you go along and then make a run for safer ground. If police begin using chemical sprays or any other weapons, cover your mouth and nose, and protect your face as best you can as you work your way to the edge, but don't get right up front where the police line is, or you will get the brunt of their weapons. Most weapons will be non-lethal, but if the riot is getting out of control, police may resort to lethal methods, and you don't want to be the first one hit.

Speaking of police, don't drive your car towards them, because they won't look at you as someone just trying to get away. They will see you as a potential threat and respond accordingly.

Try to get inside a building or room that you can secure against the outside. This is especially important if rocks and bottles are being thrown and bullets are being fired. Look for an interior room that doesn't lead directly back out to the street where the riot is taking place. Also watch for fire, as rioters will set buildings ablaze as they pass by. If you are already in an office, apartment building, or store when the riot begins, try to secure the door and board up the windows to the street with anything you can find. Hunker down until the riot has petered out, but be careful when emerging that you don't alarm police. Come out with arms raised overhead so they know you are not out to cause trouble.

If it is a sporting event, the situation can be just as dangerous as a social protest. Maybe even more so, because sports fans will be intoxicated. Hopefully, you aren't wearing the other team's jersey. If so, you may want to take it off. It is better in this situation to blend in and cheer for the winning team than stand out as "the enemy" and risk being injured.

Look at what the crowd is doing and where they are headed and if there are fights breaking out. Do your best to get away from this activity, and if you can safely reach your car, get inside it and head towards the nearest exit. If there are police around, don't think you can let down your guard, as police can be outnumbered by a huge crowd. If you have others with you, everyone stick together until you are all at a safe point away from the riots, and then wait it out to get to your cars. Or pile into the car nearest a clear exit and get out. You can go back later to fetch other cars.

Obviously, staying away from large crowds helps you avoid these situations. But we all enjoy going to a football game, a rock concert at the stadium, or a show downtown. Anywhere there are large numbers of people present, the potential for rioting and mob behavior exists. Be aware, and be ready.

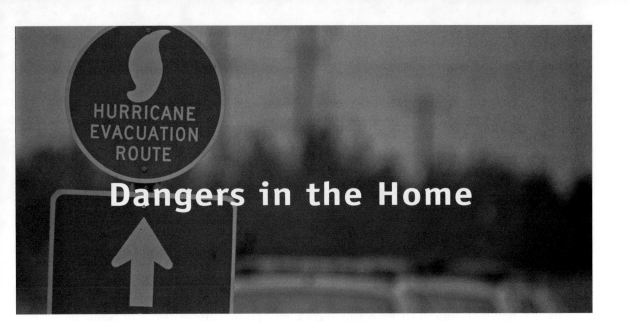

DOMESTIC AND CHILD VIOLENCE,
DRUG OVERDOSE, AND SUICIDE

Sometimes emergencies occur that test us both physically and mentally. Domestic violence is a national disaster and a national disgrace. It can happen in any household, to the elderly, adults, and children alike. Victims often feel helpless and hopeless. You may be, in fact, a victim. Abuse can occur at the hands of a spouse, loved one, or family member, and there may be threats of death that compound a victim's inability to act on their own behalf.

Violence can take the form of physical abuse, beatings, even rape, but it can also be psychological and verbal abuse that breaks down the victim and immobilizes them with shame and fear. Sometimes the abuser threatens to kill a beloved pet, a child, or a family member as a power play to get the victim to accept the abuse and keep quiet about it.

According to the Centers for Disease Control and Prevention, one in four women and one in seven men will experience physical violence at the hands of their partner in their lifetimes.

One in ten women will be raped or sexually assaulted and abused by their partner in her lifetime.

Eight percent of all men will experience sexual abuse at the hands of an older person, even a relative.

Approximately 10 percent of all women and almost 3 percent of men have been stalked.

Nearly half of all women and men in the United States alone will experience some form of psychological abuse in their lifetime.

Domestic violence of every kind occurs to whites, people of color, lesbians, gays, heterosexuals, all ages, all creeds, all nationalities. There don't seem to be any boundaries or exemptions when it comes to this type of crime. Intimate-partner sexual abuse can turn into murder or murder-suicide. Family members, friends, and neighbors may have no idea of the turmoil that goes on behind closed doors until it makes the nightly news.

With adult domestic violence, the abuse often begins slowly and builds up over time as a systematic pattern of control and power. Frequency of abuse can vary and often is hard to predict, even if the abuser is drunk or abusing drugs. Anger and rage seem to be a predecessor, and abusers often take out their own deep problems using others as their punching bags. What makes abuse so difficult is that often the abuser will apologize profusely for their actions and beg forgiveness, promising never to do it again. In addition, if the abuser is the "breadwinner," the spouse will take the abuse because they simply don't have anywhere else to go, especially if they have no supportive friends or family to turn to. Or the victim will be so afraid they will be killed, they give in to the abuser's every whim. Even when an opportunity to escape presents itself, they are numb and blind to it because of how they have been conditioned and weakened to a state of absolute helplessness.

Often people comment on how strange it is that victims of abuse stay and don't leave sooner. Unless you have experienced the pervasive and often insidious types of abuse to body, mind, and spirit, you cannot possibly know what keeps victims from acting on their own behalf, and often it comes down to just not knowing there is the option of escaping the abuse. Psychological torture may not be as visible as bruises on the skin or a broken arm, but the aftereffects are agonizing and soul-destroying to the already terrified victim. Some signs of abuse are:

- Showing extreme jealousy if the victim goes out with friends
- Telling the victim they are worthless and cannot do anything right
- Controlling who the victim sees and what they wear
- Taking the victim's money from a job and keeping it
- Shaming the victim in public with put-downs
- Forcing sex on the victim
- Stalking and monitoring the victim's every move, including cell phone use
- Threatening to kill the victim's pet, child, mother, father, friends
- Not permitting the victim to leave the house
- Not allowing the victim to have a say in anything
- Pressuring the victim to use alcohol or drugs
- Destroying the victim's personal property

Abuse can range from subtle pressure to outright brutal beatings. The only way for a victim to survive is to get out and get help. It is easier said than done, but if you are the victim, call a friend or loved one who can come and help you pack up your things and your children when the abuser is not home and get you to a safe place. If you have been beaten, call the police and press assault charges. Do not be taken in by false apologies.

If you have children, you must get them to safety. Do not confront your abuser. Work behind the scenes to get out and get to a safe place.

If you cannot call anyone, try to text someone or alert a neighbor that you are in trouble and need help.

Do not call the abuser later and tell them where you are, no matter how much you miss them.

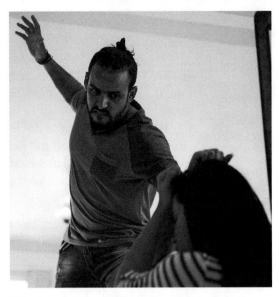

Whether it is outright beatings or psychological abuse, you have an obligation to yourself and your sanity and health to leave someone who is hurting you and find a safe place.

The National Domestic Hotline Number is available twenty-four hours a day, seven days a week, for anyone who is not sure what steps to take to get out and get safe. Call 1-800-799-7233 (SAFE).

Don't wait for things to get better. They won't. If the abuser isn't getting help, you can be assured the abuse will not only continue, but possibly get worse, and you may end up dead.

Don't depend on a restraining order to keep the abuser away. Protect yourself, and buy a weapon if you feel you need to. Learn how to use it properly. Many victims end up dead after leaving an abusive relationship because they get back in contact with the abuser or let the abuser know where they are.

If you suspect someone else is being abused, ask them directly. If you get the feeling they are being evasive, offer to help them get to safety. They may still refuse your help out of fear for their own life, and possibly even fear for yours if you get involved. Let them know you are willing to help and that they can come to you when they feel safe doing so.

If someone has bruises and broken limbs, and you know they are from domestic abuse, call the police. Too often we ignore the signs or brush them under the rug so as not to make waves, only to find out later the victim was beaten to death. Make the waves and let the police step in.

If you take someone in, realize you may be putting yourself in danger. It is best that you get the victim away from the abuser, but get them to a domestic violence shelter where they are equipped to deal with threats you may not be.

Child abuse is even more challenging. Often we see other people being abusive to their children in public, and we don't know whether it crosses the line. If a child looks terrified, has bruises and broken bones, and cowers when struck by the adult, it might be safe to assume they are being abused at home too. It is hard to know what to do in this situation. You can step in and tell the parent you are going to call the police, or if you know the child, keep a record of times you've suspected abuse, and make a case. You can go to a child's teacher in confidence and discuss your concerns.

Child abuse often goes unreported, so actual accurate statistics are difficult to find. Children between the ages of 4 and 7 and between 12 and 16 are at the greatest risk, according to the National Child Traumatic Stress Network. However, very small children, including infants, are the most susceptible to serious, if not grave, injuries.

Like adult domestic abuse, child abuse can be physical, sexual, psychological, or a combination of all three. Children will often be covered in bruises beneath their clothing, but sometimes the bruises are visible enough to concern someone. If a child ever tells you they are hit at home or being abused in any way, call the police and child protective services in your area immediately. Do not confront the parents. Get the child help so an authority figure can take the child away from the abuser before it is too late.

Some signs of abuse include:

Physical marks and bruises, bite marks, burns, lacerations, abrasions, loose and missing teeth, broken teeth and bones, black eyes, split lips, difficulty sitting or walking, and excessive crying.

Psychological marks include withdrawal, not speaking, cowering when touched, cringing when touched, not looking you in the eye, not looking away from the abusive parent, staying home from school often, and general anxiety and fear.

Children who are being hit by their parents will not in general want to implicate their parents and may lie. They also fear more abuse if they tell an adult what is happening. Often parents excuse abuse as "spanking" or disciplining a child, but abuse is abuse and often involves a parent's lack of patience and inability to control anger and temper. But sometimes the parent is just cruel and vicious.

Ask a child open-ended questions about any bruises or marks you see. Look for inconsistencies in their answers, and see if their explanation matches the injury. Ask them if they sleep well or have nightmares. Often abused children suffer from nightmares and night terrors and appear very sleepy during the day. They may also act out aggressively, especially against pets and other children they feel they have some power and control over. Abused children have trouble concentrating and often worry excessively, to the point of paranoia, about themselves and their parents, especially if the parents are not the abusers. The child may feel that they need to know where the parents are at all times and feel unsafe and vulnerable when they are not protected, such as at school or a friend's house.

A child will not open up to you if you are a stranger or they feel unsafe around you. They may not even open up to close relatives such as aunts and uncles. But the signs of abuse are there if you are alert and aware, and if you see the child all the time, patterns will reveal themselves in their behaviors, actions, and reactions. If you think a child you know may be a victim of abuse and are not sure what to do, contact the Childhelp National Child Abuse Hotline at 1-800-422-4453. In imminent dangerous situations, call 911.

Be careful if you try to get the child out of the home yourself. Parents don't give up their children easily, and you may be mistaken about the situation in the first place. Even if you aren't, the parents may resort to violence against you.

DRUG AND ALCOHOL OVERDOSE

Millions of Americans are addicted to alcohol, hard drugs, and prescription drugs. Addiction has become a pandemic that grows in size and scope every year. Because many people don't seek treatment, we have no real way of knowing just how many people are out there drinking and drugging to extremes until something happens. They bottom out and end up on the side of the street, beaten up and robbed, in detox in the downtown police station, or worse.

Drug abuse plagues all age groups, genders, and nationalities. Drug dependency is considered a disease and requires serious treatment at a rehab facility or hospital or even a twelve-step program. But too many drug and alcohol abusers continue to believe they can handle their addictions and get better either by going cold turkey or slowing it down a bit. It doesn't usually work out well.

Drugs can be taken orally as pills and liquids or inhaled or injected. There are al-

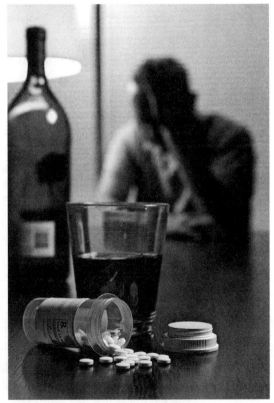

In a society in which going out for drinks or using prescription drugs is considered normal, it can sometimes be difficult to assess if someone is descending into addiction.

ways signs that someone is abusing drugs and alcohol, but in our society, where we go for drinks at the drop of a hat and consider popping prescription pills for every symptom imaginable, it can be hard to distinguish between someone who has a problem and someone who doesn't.

Overdoses occur after the fact, sadly, and sometimes it is too late to save a person by then. But the best prevention for overdosing is helping yourself or a loved one or friend get help for their addiction before things go too far. You can assist them in seeking an outpatient or inpatient rehab facility, preferably one their insurance will cover or partially cover, and even go with them to twelve-step meetings and encourage them to speak and tell their stories. You can remove drugs and alcohol from the home, but expect a real abuser to find them elsewhere.

If someone is abusing drugs or alcohol and becomes violent, you can call the police and have them taken in, usually to an overnight detox. Don't ever allow violence of any kind to exist in your home, especially when children are involved. Turning someone in is often the best thing that could happen to them, as most abusers need to "bottom out" in order to admit they have a problem and seek help.

Whatever you do, don't let anyone drink or drug and get behind the wheel of any vehicle.

If someone overdoses, you will either find them conscious or unconscious. If they are unconscious, begin checking their ABCs, and call 911 immediately. Give rescue breathing and CPR as needed. If you have help, have the other person look around for signs of the drug used, such as needles, cocaine powder, heroin residue, spoons, tinfoil and matches, prescription bottles, and empty alcohol bottles and containers. Have those ready for the emergency responders when they arrive so they know the cause of the overdose.

If the person is conscious, keep them awake, and elevate their legs above heart level to avoid shock. Do not move them, and keep them as calm and quiet as you can. If they can speak, ask what happened. Often the victim took an accidental overdose of too many prescription pills. But sometimes they were having suicidal thoughts. Do not leave them alone until help arrives, and let EMS know what the person's intentions were. Often a medical sensitivity can cause symptoms of an overdose, so the more information you can give EMS, the better.

In the case of chemicals, plants, or toxic substances inhaled or ingested to get a "high," the higher the dose and the longer the body is exposed to the toxin, the worse the poisoning will be. Act quickly to get help. If you can identify what was inhaled or ingested, be ready to report that to EMS.

Young children can overdose on drugs too, and it is imperative that medications be kept out of their reach. Toddlers often find bottles of pills and share them with other kids, thinking they are candy. Children put everything into their mouths, so this is playing with danger in the most extreme way. Sticking pill bottles on a high shelf may not be enough, because children are curious and will find a way to get to something that catches their eye. If a child overdoses, get help *immediately*. Their bodies are smaller, and the toxin will act more powerfully.

Effects of alcohol poisoning are:

- Seizures
- Vomiting
- Loss of consciousness
- Low body temperature
- Bluish tint to the skin
- Irregular or slow breathing

Effects of cocaine or crack:

- Sweating profusely
- Fast and irregular heartbeat
- High blood pressure
- Jitters

Effects of heroin/opiates:

- Slow breathing
- Difficulty breathing
- Weak pulse
- Low blood pressure
- Tiny, pinpoint pupils
- Disorientation
- Loss of consciousness

Effects of methamphetamine (meth):

- Confusion
- Jitters
- Aggression
- Convulsions
- Extreme paranoia
- Rapid heart rate
- Rapid breathing
- High body temperature

Even before an overdose, an abuser may display changes in their sleep patterns, the way they dress, their hygiene, behavioral changes that border on the extreme, withdrawal from family and friends, talk of suicide and death, lying

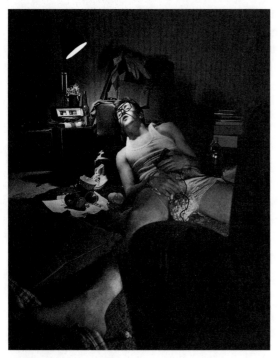

One possible sign of drug addiction is when you notice a family member or friend no longer cares about their appearance or keeping their living space clean.

and stealing, violent or criminal behavior, and extreme mood swings. These are all indications that something is wrong and needs to be addressed in order to avoid an even worse situation. As with domestic violence and child abuse, there are many red flags with drug and alcohol abuse. It is just a matter of being aware enough to see them.

Often teenagers who are using drugs and alcohol to try to cope with life will become strangers to their parents. They may even stop seeing their friends and participating in school activities they once loved. They no longer care if they shower, how they look, and even their eating patterns may change. Their rooms are a mess, and often a parent with hawk eyes will find evidence of substance abuse. If you suspect your teenager is using, confront them but do it with care and compassion. Ask to see their phones if you think they are buying from friends. Check into their Web use, and breach privacy boundaries, because you might be saving their lives by doing so.

Teens do drugs and drink alcohol to feel better, but also to fit in, so watch the behavior of their friends, and if you suspect one of their friends is using drugs and encouraging your child, confront the other child's parents. Don't be an ass. Believe it or not, they may be asking the same questions about your child. Try to find the source of the drugs and alcohol, and refuse to allow your child to interact with those persons.

If someone appears to be overdosing, call for help and try to keep them calm. If they are having seizures, move dangerous objects out of the way so they don't injure themselves. Keep them calm, and try to keep them still until help arrives. Try to find out what the substance is and how much of it they consumed. Keep the person warm and watch for possible shock. Someone who is on meth will be all over the place. If you can safely keep them somewhat restrained, it will keep them safe until help arrives, but if you are alone, simply do the best you can, and always protect your own health and safety first and foremost.

If the victim overdosed on prescription drugs, there may be instructions on the pill bottle for what to do in the event of an overdose. There should also be a number for poison control: 800-222-1222. Don't call your local doctor or pharmacist to ask what you should do. Call 911 so that the victim will get help quickly, as you don't know what they took or how much or how it will interact

Prescription Drug Abuse

Prescription drug abuse is a growing problem in this country. Most people don't bother to keep their prescription medications out of the reach of children, teenagers, and anyone who might be having suicidal thoughts. But how can we safely dispose of meds we don't need to use? Throwing them away is the easiest thing to do, but is it the best?

According to "How to Safely Dispose of Unused Medication" in the Fall 2017 issue of *Lifelines*, the magazine of the American Association of Retired Persons (AARP), some medications will actually include disposal instructions on their labels or on the dosage information sheet that comes with the medication. Follow those instructions, because not doing so could cause unintentional harm to others.

Flushing medications is no longer suggested, because of the overwhelming amounts of prescription drugs found in our nation's water sources. This is becoming a big medical problem as drugs containing hormones, sedatives, and painkillers get flushed into our wastewater and then out into rivers and even the ocean. You are better off throwing the pills away, but first take the pills out of their original packaging, and place them in a small bag with dirt or cat litter covering them. Seal the bag, and then throw it in the outdoor trash bin so that children and pets cannot dig the pills out of the trash inside the house.

Last, but not least, you can participate in a local Take Back program. Your pharmacist will know of these programs. This allows you to drop unwanted medications off at various local collection sites, usually at clinics or hospitals, where they can be safely disposed of. You can find a local Take Back program by calling the Drug Enforcement Administration at 1-800-882-9539.

with their metabolic system. They may have even mixed drugs intentionally or by accident.

Be aware that under the Good Samaritan law, if someone is in a life-threatening situation, you must call 911 immediately, so do that first before anything, unless you have help who can do that while you try to administer life-saving techniques. Some states may not have this law, so know the rules in your area. In any event, if you have any reason to fear getting involved, just get away, and call for help. If it's a drug deal gone bad or the abuser is out of control, it could put your life at risk or put you in a very dangerous situation.

After the person gets immediate help, and they are treated by a hospital, encourage them to get professional rehab help. You may even want to do an intervention if it is a family member and the pattern of abuse continues. Ongoing drug and alcohol abuse take a toll on more than just the abuser. Users and addicts are adept at trying to downplay their diseases and won't ask for help unless they hit bottom, and maybe not even then. If they don't get help, they risk not only their own lives, but the lives of innocent others they may harm in a DUI or a bad drug deal.

SUICIDE

It is one of the top ten leading causes of death in the United States, with over 44,000 people dying each year. It can happen to anyone, regardless of race, color, creed, social status, gender, or age. It costs the nation over $50 billion annually, and for every one suicide, there are approximately twenty-five more failed attempts.

Suicide is a topic nobody wants to talk about, but it is pandemic, and statistics show it is on the rise. According to the American Foundation for Suicide Prevention, approximately 13 in 100,000 people take their own lives, with men three times more likely than women to die, but women three times as likely to attempt suicide. There are on average 121 suicides each day, almost half of which involve the use of firearms. The rate of suicide is highest in middle age, and white men are hit the hardest. In 2015, 19.6 percent of suicides were among adults between the ages of 45 and 64, with the second highest percentage, 19.4 percent, being people over the age of 84. We think of suicide as a teenage crisis, and it indeed is, but it truly does affect everyone. Suicide is the second highest cause of death in children and young adults between the ages of 15 and 34.

The method of suicide is often firearms, almost 50 percent in 2015, with suffocation (including hangings) second at 26.9 percent, and poisoning third at 15.4 percent. Attempted suicides sent over 500,000 people to local hospitals from injuries due to self-harm, and these were only those who chose to seek help. So many others suffer, or die, in silence.

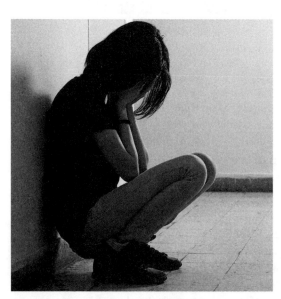

Suicide is pandemic in the United States. It affects people of all ages, not just troubled teenagers, with about 44,000 dying annually in America alone.

Suicide is rampant, and now with cyberbullying, it is something we need to pay even closer attention to with our children, who may be influenced by total strangers to go out and end their lives.

Ninety percent of those who die by suicide have some type of mental health disorder at the time of death, and had they been able to seek or receive treatment, it might have spared their lives. When it comes to preventing suicide, it is critical we all learn the signs of behavior that may be leading up to such a drastic cry for help and often an attempt to end suffering and pain we may not even know the person was in.

According to the National Institute of Mental Health, some of the risk factors we can look for (in ourselves and others) are:

• Depression and anxiety disorders

- Prior suicide attempts
- Family or marital problems
- Drugs and alcohol abuse
- Family history of suicide
- Guns and firearms in the home
- Family violence and past abuse
- Incarceration
- Chronic health issues and chronic pain
- Prolonged stress from job, bullying, school, expectations of others, abuse

Someone who may have just suffered a huge personal loss, such as the death of a loved one, a bankruptcy, loss of a job, or a natural disaster, can be at high risk as well. This is especially true for seniors who are mourning the passing of a spouse.

Signs someone may be contemplating suicide include:

- Direct threats
- Veiled threats
- Withdrawal from normal activities
- Loss of interest in hygiene and eating and sleeping
- Sleeping disturbances
- Behavioral changes
- Depression and despair
- New behavior patterns
- Drinking and drugging
- Isolating themselves from friends and family
- Acting out aggressively
- Contacting people to say goodbye
- Aggression
- Purchasing guns
- Feelings of humiliation and worthlessness
- Rage
- Mental health symptoms such as bipolar, or manic-depressive, behaviors, conduct disorder, and even antisocial personality disorder
- Excessive use of the Internet, which can indicate possible cyberbullying and attempts to stop it

Getting treatment means first getting help. Whether you fear that you may take your own life or that someone you love may take their life, get help immediately. You can start by calling the toll-free National Suicide Prevention Lifeline at 1-800-273-TALK (8255), which is available twenty-four hours a day, seven days a week, and is free and completely confidential. There is also a crisis text line, 741741. You can also talk to your doctor about getting mental health treatment set up, which can involve medications for depression and anxiety, talk therapy, cognitive behavioral therapy, or other kinds of healing modalities such as psychotherapy, electroconvulsive therapy, alcohol and drug abuse counseling, and more. If an at-risk person is given a medication, they need to be monitored for possible side effects that might increase their desire to end their lives.

To start, here are five steps recommended by the National Institute of Mental Health:

1. Ask the person if they are thinking of suicide. This does not increase their desire to do so, and may open the door to allow them to express the feelings that are making them feel hopeless.

2. Keep the person safe by removing anything they can use to commit suicide, such as guns, knives, pills, etc.

3. Be there for them if they want to talk, and listen carefully. Just acknowledging suicidal thoughts can help reduce the thoughts.

4. Help them connect and get help by giving them the suicide hotline number and naming other trusted individuals they can turn to if you are not available.

5. Stay connected even after they have gotten help and are back home feeling better. Studies show that suicide deaths decrease when someone follows up with an at-risk person.

Going beyond suicide, we need to be aware of the dangers of mental illness that is not being addressed or treated, as it can make the victim feel alone, vulnerable, ashamed, and worthless. Knowing the signs can help us help others and possibly give them the hope they are missing and the feeling of being cared for. Suicide is a double-edged sword that not only takes the lives of those we love, but in a way, destroys our own lives as well. If someone you love or know commits suicide, be sure to reach out for the help you may need to process and heal from the sudden and shocking death. You may suffer from the guilt and shame that comes from feeling as though you should have known or you could have stopped it. Know that if someone is determined to take their life, they will do so no matter what in many instances, and it is impossible to know the innermost thoughts going through someone's mind, especially if they are acting normal on the outside.

Grieving the death of a loved one is hard, but even harder when they died by their own hand and those left behind are wondering how and why. Be gentle with yourself, reach out and talk about it with trusted friends, and get professional help if you are having trouble moving on from the tragedy.

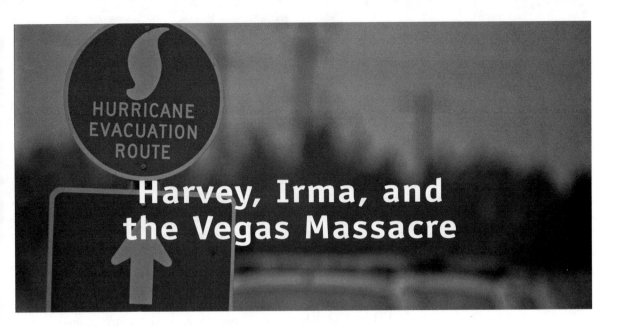

THE LESSONS OF EXPERIENCE

The months of August, September, and October of 2017 proved to the nation, indeed the world, that natural and man-made disasters happen all the time, often in clusters, and can be devastating. Within just this three-month period, the United States would experience several hurricanes that would break flooding and rain-total records, wildfires across the entire West, including sixty different fires burning at one given time, and the worst mass shooting in the country's history. People would barely recover from one situation, only to be dealt another blow, and another. The nation would be sent reeling into an emotional black hole, trying to deal with the physical and financial losses of these three months alone.

Emergency Management Services, the Federal Emergency Management Agency, the Department of Homeland Security, the U.S. government and military—all would be taxed to the maximum and faced with lessons on what to do and not do, when catastrophic events tax services and test the fabric of human resilience. The lessons learned from the past would be applied, only to fall short with this new onslaught of mega-disasters.

It would begin with Hurricane Harvey in late August. This massive Cat 5 would make landfall and break the record for the most extreme rainfall ever on the U.S. mainland. Houston, Texas, would see over 50 inches of rain, breaking the record of 48 inches held by Tropical Storm Amelia back in 1978. The flooding and damage to the United States would be astounding, and that didn't include the horrendous damage inflicted on the islands in the Caribbean it crossed before making landfall. As the rain continued, flooding would be beyond catastrophic, so deep that in many areas rain sensors would stop working and measuring water depth.

Rivers would overflow their banks. Lakes would too. Major roads would be closed for days, some for weeks, and even as Harvey closed in on Louisiana on the twelfth anniversary of Hurricane Katrina, which devastated that city, the rains did not let up. Desperate victims and families in other states would swarm social networking sites, trying to connect, to report in safe, and to locate loved ones.

There were so many emergencies for responders to attend to, many people would die. Then, in early September, Irma came. Hurricane Irma seemed like the two in a one-two punch, striking the already shattered Caribbean, but this time aiming its power at Florida. It made landfall as a Cat 1 before becoming a tropical storm, after causing absolute chaos as hundreds of thousands evacuated inland and shelters reached capacity. The state was already suffering from a limited supply of gasoline, thanks to Harvey and the inability to import fuel from Houston. New shelters had to be set up, as people were stuck in town, unable to get out before the storm hit.

Then Hurricane Jose would threaten, although with less of a punch, as it chose to take a different route. But then there was Kate, and Maria, which obliterated the Commonwealth of Puerto Rico just over a week after Irma, to the point where over one million people were left without power. Maria was a monster, making landfall on the island as a Cat 4 with sustained winds of 155 miles per hour (249 kph). Just before it made landfall, the island's three million plus residents were warned by local radio and told to shelter in place.

And then, on the night of October 1, 2017, just before midnight, a lone gunman would open fire on a country music concert at Mandalay Bay Resort and Casino in Las Vegas, Nevada, killing over 50 people and injuring over 500 others. He would shoot down on the crowd from the thirty-second floor while country music superstar Jason Aldean performed at the three-day Route 91 Harvest Festival. Before police could find him, he would shoot himself dead, leaving behind a world in absolute shock. It was the worst gun-related massacre in U.S. history, worse than the previous record holder, the shooting of 49 people at the Pulse Nightclub in Orlando, Florida, in June of 2016. When will the next one occur?

One week later, around October 9, over 3,500 structures had been damaged or destroyed in a massive wildfire in California's wine country. Eventually, over seventeen fires would burn down homes, buildings, and wineries and take the lives of over 29 people. As hot, dry winds blew through California, much of the state was on high red-flag alert for fires. The firestorm of October 2017 would become one of the worst natural disasters in California state history.

As the nation and the world mourned and dealt with their horror and grief, with losses of life and losses of homes and personal histories, we would once again be reminded that these disasters and emergencies can occur at any time, anywhere. We must always be prepared. We must always be ready. We can no longer say that it happens only in big cities or suburbs or out in the country, because it happens everywhere. No place is immune to its share of catastrophes big and small.

Also during the same time period, Mexico City reeled from a 7.1 earthquake that killed dozens of people and injured so many more, leaving buildings and villages in ruins as rescue workers searched for the living and the dead. It was a stark reminder to the states to the north of their own pending, even imminent, quake disasters. Are we ready? There are many faults in the United States capable of an 8 or much bigger, and we won't have much, if any, warning. Can we survive?

The spate of mega-hurricanes alone was enough to manage, and a warning of what may come as climate change is factored into existing weather patterns. Recent computer modeling suggests that global warming may result in fewer tropical cyclones because of heated oceans, but the ones that do form will be more intense than ever. Scientists actually began discussing the possible need to revise the number of categories describing a hurricane's power by adding on a Cat 6. Perhaps a year from now, they will be wondering if they need to add on

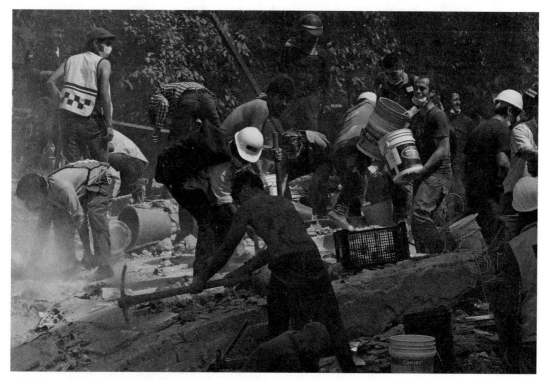

The 2017 earthquake in Mexico City measured 7.1 on the Richter scale.

a Cat 7 and Cat 8. With hurricanes that unimaginably powerful, will our infrastructure hold up? Will anyone survive? Not to mention the billions upon billions of dollars required to clean up and rebuild as well as pay insurance claims to victims.

No matter how much of this book you take to heart and put into practice, at the very least do what you can to protect yourself and your family. You don't have to be a hero to your city or country, although if you can help after a disaster, there will most definitely be a need for it. But take the time to sit down now and go over your plan, and put that plan to the test. Stock up now, because in Hurricane Harvey and the storms that followed, stores ran out within *minutes* in many cases of essentials like nonperishables and water. If you live far from the nearest grocery store, it behooves you even more to stock up at home.

With the Internet and cell phones, there is really no excuse for not signing on and learning about what is happening in your city and country and how you might need to respond in the days to come. Some disasters come with a long warning period, such as storms that can potentially become hurricanes. Others, like mass shootings, bank robberies, and hazardous chemical spills, come without warning, and you must know what to do immediately. Even with today's technology, there is no warning before a large earthquake hits, and we now understand that they can strike in most every state of the nation.

"With preparation comes confidence." This applies not just to job interviews, but to being in a stronger position to survive emergencies big and small, local and national, even global. No doubt, by the time this book reaches your hands, there will be more disasters to contend with. In "How to Survive a Global Disaster: A Handy Guide," an article for the UK *Guardian*'s February 10, 2016, issue, writer Keith Stuart says how important it is that we forge a community as survivors, even if all we have are walkie-talkies or ham radios to do it with. He also emphasizes the importance of working with others to grow food and find water after a major global event. The problem is, many of us are not even able to do these things for ourselves and for our families, let alone contribute to the larger community that may need us to help rebuild.

Planning is essential, and if the back-to-back horrors of late summer and early fall 2017 are a sign of things to come, you may not be able to wait until next month or next year. You don't put off buying groceries or paying the power bill, so why on earth put off doing what is necessary to save your life? Since you have to go grocery shopping each week anyway, why not add a few items for your emergency food stock each time you go? Maybe add a few gallons of water too. Before you know it, you have everything you need to get you through two weeks on your own.

But just as we fail to plan, we also fail to think. In a January 28, 2015, article titled "In a Catastrophic Event, Most People Fail to Do the One Thing That Would Save Their Life" for BBC.com, Michael Bond writes about a cruise ferry disaster in 1994 when the MS *Estonia*, hit gale force winds and broke apart, sending its 989 passengers into the water as it sank. Experts who studied the event were stunned by the high death toll, even taking into account the stormy waters and time it took rescuers to arrive on site.

The official report stated that people drowned because they basically did nothing to save themselves! "A number of people ... seem to have been incapable of rational thought or behavior because of their fear," the report stated. They froze up, unable to move, or went into a panic state and didn't even respond to other passengers trying to help them. Paralysis, even for just a few seconds, can be deadly. But it is purely natural. Perhaps the best way to overcome it is with the confidence that comes from knowing you can act in beneficial ways when the SHTF.

The article included an interview with John Leach, a military survival instructor working at the University of Portsmouth. He studies actions and behaviors of survivors and victims, and he found that in a life-threatening situation, approximately 75% of people will be unable to think clearly or plot their escape because they are so mentally bewildered and paralyzed by the event. Only 15% of people know how to remain calm and rational in the face of fear and panic, and the other 10% become so dangerous they hinder everyone's survival.

Think about which of those categories you would prefer to be in. The ones who are so afraid, they die without a fight. The ones who are so freaked out, they cause everyone to die. Or the ones who can stay clear and focused and find a way to *survive*. This is why we worship heroes so much, because we believe they alone have that extra-sharp mental edge to save us from our woes. We don't realize that we possess the very same ability if we can retrain ourselves to react differently, and not from some default setting based in fear.

In an emergency there will be people who simply do not have the capacity to help themselves, even if the thing they need to survive is right in front of them. Instead, they will stampede for one exit, when many are available, killing others beneath their own feet. Or they will cower in a corner despite an open window they can crawl out of or an emergency exit lit up with an alarm sounding. The article goes on to state that there is an actual psychological explanation for this kind of behavior. It is caused by a "failure to adapt to a sudden change in environment." The environment of a disaster or emergency is unfamiliar, and we fear the unknown. Things are also usually happening faster than normal day-to-day events, or at least they appear to be happening at ultra-high speed. A disaster also increases our emotional arousal, which can give us a kind of tunnel vision about our options and alternative courses of action. We get so caught up in what we are feeling, we forget to use our brains to think our way through. Feelings are a great indicator that something is wrong, but they don't work well when it comes to finding viable options to save yourself and others.

Just think of how crowds behave at major sporting events or concerts when something goes wrong. They stampede and become killers themselves just trying to get away from the threat. They act without thinking. Many people just go into a deep state of shock and move as if robotic, reacting with the crowd. The problem arises when the crowd is not reacting in the best of ways. Think of the proverbial lemmings falling off a cliff because they are following other lemmings. Nobody ever bothers to ask why they are going off a cliff in the first place.

In *The Unthinkable: Who Survives When Disaster Strikes—and Why*, Amanda Ripley states, "In life or death situations, people gain certain powers, and lose others." She refers to some people having crystal-clear vision during an emergency and others having tunnel vision. Their field of sight can literally be diminished by up to 70 percent. This can also happen with hearing, where suddenly some sounds are muted and others are louder. This may be a mechanism of the brain to help us focus on what we need to see or hear to survive, but it can also hamper us from seeing and hearing important information we need.

Have you ever been in a car accident and felt time suddenly slow to a crawl? Maybe you couldn't hear things like the car radio anymore—just the sound of skidding tires and crashing metal. Maybe all you could see was the front of your car about to smash into a wall. Time was like molasses, maybe to allow you more "thought processing time" to react properly. Then upon impact, you were shocked back into reality, and everything looked and sounded normal again. Ripley writes, "Time distortion is so common that scientists have a name for it: tachypsychia, derived from the Greek 'speed of the mind.'" This kind of time distortion also occurs during violent crimes, major disasters, and terrorist attacks.

Studies show that time did not actually slow down of course, just our perception of it, and it may indeed be all about involving more parts of the brain, such as the amygdala, which reacts to fear, to lay down memories in a much richer, deeper way because of the intensity of the situation. Therefore it feels like time has slowed. But the cutting out of extraneous sights and sounds can indeed help the brain to focus on what it needs to by removing distractions.

We cannot count on our brains to respond perfectly in a dangerous situation. But we can feed them enough input in the form of knowledge and information to improve our odds. We may also be fighting our body's reflexes, which happen without thinking. It takes a lot of control to get it together at the times when we most feel we are falling apart. Nor can we count on others to respond well. They may panic, but in more cases than not, they will become paralyzed and do nothing to help themselves, others, or the situation. You may have to work around them.

In disasters and emergencies, we do see many more examples in the media of people coming together to help one another. Humans are not loners by nature. We thrive in groups, and we flourish in communities. We join forces when a neighboring city is decimated by a tornado outbreak, and we give blood,

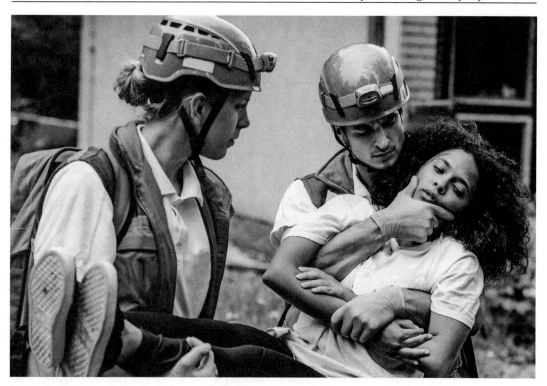

It is human nature to come together in a crisis and help one another—most of the time. As long as we don't let fear, panic, hate, and despair overwhelm us, human beings can be incredibly noble and kind when disaster strikes.

time, and money when a neighborhood is devastated by a Cat 3 hurricane. We are good and we are humane, most of the time. We become extra kind and courteous and sometimes put our own lives at risk for total strangers, and we become heroes to others. But it helps to recognize the human capacity for fear, panic, anger, shock, numbness, and despair, as we will feel it. We will experience it. The more we know that we can still move past it and take action to save ourselves, the stronger we will be alone or together.

Perhaps it helps to watch videos of disasters and see how survivors acted. Perhaps it helps to watch disaster movies and think about how you might do things differently in the same situation. Perhaps it helps to read books like this and watch documentaries. The more you can teach yourself how you should respond when the SHTF, the better chances you have of actually overcoming that initial terror and *responding* that way. Engage your family members. Look for videos online that are sponsored by organizations such as the Federal Emergency Management Agency, CERT, law enforcement, and the Department of Homeland Security. There are live shooter training videos and videos that show you how to put out a kitchen fire. There are videos that walk you through building a storm cellar or underground bunker and videos that show how to remove a bee's stinger. You can find just about anything in video form as well as book form for those who prefer to read.

This author was surprised to find a number of disaster video games, disaster simulators, and disaster preparedness interactive games online during a basic search. There are games that put you right into the heart of a major earthquake, a zombie attack, a tsunami, and many other scenarios. While these are games, they are also great ways to vicariously deal with a variety of situations and even compete against others, all the time learning key survival basics. "Look for Disaster Hero" and "Stop Disasters!" are the two most popular, but there are several others. Other good online resources are disaster simulations for high school and college students as well as emergency preparedness videos that offer a particular scenario involving actors role-playing in a disaster.

There is no excuse anymore. Information is everywhere. Gone are the days of saying, "I don't know how to...." Keep a copy of this book or any other in your emergency kit. Read it first, though.

Learn. Practice. Visualize.

Just do something to be proactive, because disasters happen, and emergencies lurk around every corner. Someone, maybe you, will break a leg on a camping trip. Your house may be robbed while you are at home. You might get bitten by a rattlesnake or burned in an office building fire. Disasters and emergencies don't have to be the fodder of schlocky movies where everything happens but the kitchen sink, and sometimes the kitchen sink is thrown in for good measure. They can be common events that happen in common places to common people. It's a part of life, but it doesn't have to result in death.

Few of us will ever have the harrowing experience of being in a situation where our life literally hangs in the balance and we must fight to survive. More than likely, we will be exposed to smaller situations throughout our lifetimes that will test our resilience and strength. Few of us, if any, will escape this life unscathed by personal and collective tragedies. Even if we go into the mountains to live as hermits far from the terrors of modern society, we still face wildfires, mudslides, flash floods, wild bears, and heart attacks.

Today we can go online and buy any number of survival kits and items without ever leaving home. We can buy apps for our phones and Road ID cards, dog tags, and bracelets that give our personal and medical information if we are found collapsed on a hiking trail or in the woods. We can buy food, water, and first aid kits that have been put together for us and have them delivered directly to our door. It is only a matter of time before technology allows us to chip ourselves with ID information under our skin, as we do with our pets (and some children!). It is so easy to be prepared today, it's a wonder there are still so many people who aren't.

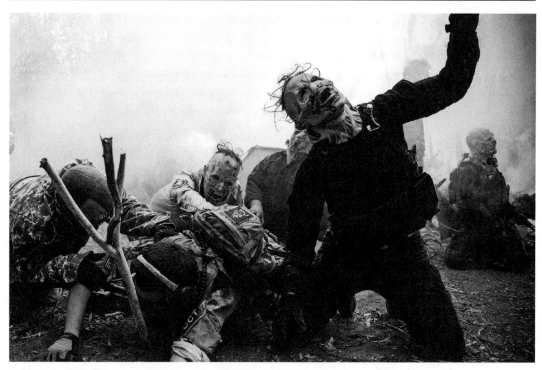

Although the U.S. military doesn't believe that there will actually be a zombie apocalypse, they created a scenario about flesh-eating humans gone mad as an effective training scenario for disastrous circumstances.

In the year 2011, the U.S. Defense Department did what many thought was the unthinkable. They drafted a plan called CONPLAN 888-11, Counter-Zombie Dominance. While it sounded more like a video game script, it was an actual working government document. According to the plan's disclaimer, "This plan was not actually designed as a joke. During the summers of 2009 and 2010, while training augmentees from a local training squadron about the Joint Operation Planning Process (JOPP), members of the U.S. Strategic Command found out (by accident) that the hyperbole involved in writing a 'zombie survival plan' actually provided a very useful and effective training tool."

You read that correctly. The idea was to use the backdrop of a zombie invasion, ripped right out of pop culture and television shows like *The Walking Dead*, to assist Pentagon trainees to look at new ways of thinking about disaster preparedness and response. The zombie element gave the plan's creators a way to break out of old and stuck mindsets and become open to more options for dealing with all aspects of a potential major emergency.

The plan suggested that, in order to better respond to huge threats, we must get out of comfort zones and get uncomfortable with our thought processes. They had some suggestions for how even members of the public can do this:

1. Identify our own zombies or potential threats to our businesses, our families, our neighborhoods. Basically, who are the "enemies" we might be facing off against?

2. Dump our inner circle for a day and look at differing perspectives. Hang out a bit with those who don't agree with us to see what their thought processes are and how they view things. Know your opposition.

3. Find the opposites and opportunities. Consider reversing stereotypes, exploring the outlandish, coming up with innovative ways to bring totally opposite sides together.

The Department of Defense document fully laid out the basic concepts of military plans and order development, all via the fictional scenario of a zombie invasion. It covered everything from initial response to operation phases to contingency plans for dealing with hospitals and medical facilities overrun by zombies, as well as the possible deployment of remote-controlled robots to man critical infrastructure stations if the zombie threat became overwhelming. There was even a chain of command set up from the president on down to members of the intelligence community, indicating the roles each would play.

Though it sounds comical, we are reminded of one of the reasons why we flock to disaster television shows, novels, and movies. As fantastical and out of this world as the scenarios they present may be, we can vicariously react and respond and even identify all the ways the characters failed to respond properly. Nothing is more powerful than watching a disaster movie and asking, "What if?" What if that were me, how would I respond, what would I do, how would I protect my family? Perhaps it isn't enough to ask people to do this when threatened with something real, like a hurricane or an earthquake. But if you can engage them while they are being entertained, they might begin asking what needs to be asked and identifying what their own plans of action would be as they live vicariously through their favorite heroes and villains.

The Pentagon zombie plan appealed not only to the left analytical brain but also to the right creative brain, and it worked to give trainees ideas on what wouldn't work, what would work better, and how to improve existing contingency plans from the local to the national level. They got to think inside and outside the existing boxes of what they had always been taught and were able to identify problems and solutions they had never paid attention to before or had to think about. Besides, isn't it good to know that our military would be ready to respond to a zombie invasion at any time?

Zombies can be a valuable learning tool. If you don't like zombies, replace them with aliens. Or hordes of bigfoot creatures. The point is, whatever gets people thinking more about how to survive a potential emergency works, and if it leads to new ways of viewing old standard rules that may no longer work in this day and age, even better. Whatever it takes to prompt people to ask "what if" is a positive thing in getting them to consider their options in a disaster. So the next time you tune in to a zombie movie or alien invasion television show, pay close attention to the reactions and responses of the characters, and ask yourself what you would do in the same situation.

There is no escaping this darker, scarier side of life. So it behooves each one of us to be as well prepared as we can be. For ourselves. For our loved ones. For our communities. Much of the material in this book may have sounded repetitive, but repetition helps create habits, and many of the things that keep us safe in one disaster work in others too. Hopefully, the advice was strong enough, and repeated often enough, that it has moved you to take action.

Safe journeys.

FURTHER READING

Ackerman, Antonio, et al. *The Complete Illustrated Handbook of Survival*. New York: Anness Publishing, 2015.

"Acute Radiation Syndrome: A Fact Sheet for Clinicians." CDC. Accessed March 20, 2018. http://emergency.cdc.gov/radiation/ars/asp.

"Addressing Threats to the Nation's Cybersecurity." FBI. Accessed April 22, 2018. https://www.fbi.gov/file-repository/addressing-threats-to-the-nations-cybersecurity-1.pdf/view.

"All About Snow." National Snow and Ice Data Center. Accessed April 22, 2018. https://nsidc.org/cryosphere/snow.

Allan, Patrick. "Where to Hide If a Nuclear Bomb Goes Off in Your Area." Life Hacker. August 10, 2017. https://lifehacker.com/where-to-hide-if-a-nuclear-bomb-goes-off-in-your-area-1793493053.

Amadeo, Kimberly. "U.S. Economy Collapse: What Will Happen, How to Prepare." The Balance. April 4, 2017. https://www.thebalance.com/u-s-econ omy-collapse-what-will-happen-how-to-prepare-3305690.

"Amateur Radio Clubs Monitor Weather, Events." Emergency Management. Accessed April 22, 2018. http://www.govtech.com/em/disaster/Hams-Mon itor-Weather-Events.html.

Anderberg, Jeremy. "How to Recognize Poison Ivy, Oak and Sumac and Treat Their Rashes." The Art of Manliness. August 27, 2015. https://www.artofmanliness.com/2015/08/27/how-to-recognize-poison-ivy-oak-sumac-and-treat-their-rashes/.

"Animal Bites: First Aid." Mayo Clinic. April 1, 2018. https://www.mayoclinic .org/first-aid/first-aid-animal-bites/basics/art-20056591.

"Annual Disaster Statistical Review 2014: The Numbers and Trends." Centre for Research on the Epidemiology of Disasters, September 17, 2015.

"Bad News Bears." Mountain Nature. Accessed April 12, 2018. http://www.mountainnature.com/wildlife/bears/bearencounters.htm.

Bagley, Mary. "Volcano Facts and Types of Volcanoes." LiveScience. February 20, 2013. https://www.livescience.com/27295-volcanoes.html.

Barnwell, Jack. "When Natural—or Any—Disaster Strikes, Being Prepared Matters." *The Daily Independent*. September 16, 2017.

"Bear Encounters." Bear Smart Society. Accessed April 22, 2018. http://www.bearsmart.com/play/bear-encounters/.

"Bear Repellent—Preventing a Grizzly Bear Attack." Survival Grounds. January 13, 2009. http://www.survivalgrounds.com/bear_mace.php.

Bell, Terena. "An Incident Action Plan for Total Darkness." *Emergency Management Magazine*, July 21, 2017.

Bennett, Jessica. "Rise of the Preppers: America's Newest Survivalists." *Newsweek*. December 27, 2009.

Berkowitz, Bonnie, et al. "The Math of Mass Shootings." *Washington Post*, June 6, 2017.

"Big Five Mass Extinction Events." BBC Nature. October 2014. http://www.bbc.co.uk/nature/extinction_events.

"Bioterrorism." Ready.gov. Accessed April 20, 2018. https://www.ready.gov/bioterrorism.

Black, Chris. "3 Primary Steps to Survive a Terrorist Attack." Survivopedia. May 3, 2014. http://www.survivopedia.com.

"Boat Safety Tips." International Insurance. Accessed April 1, 2018. https://www.internationalinsurance.com/articles/boating.php.

"Bomb Threat Stand-Off Distance." Office of the Director of National Intelligence. April 22, 2018. https://www.dni.gov/index.php/nctc-newsroom/nctc-resources/item/1731-bomb-threat-stand-off-distance-chart.

Bond, Michael. "How to Survive a Disaster: In a Catastrophic Event, Most People Fail to Do the One Thing That Would Save Their Life." BBC.com. January 26, 2015. http://www.bbc.com/future/story/20150128-how-to-survive-a-disaster.

Bradley, Dr. Arthur T. *The Disaster Preparedness Handbook: A Guide for Families*, 2nd edition. New York: Castle Books, 2013.

Brennan, Charlie. "Boulder Author Warns of More 'Megafires' On Nation's Horizon." *The Daily Camera*, August 6, 2017.

Brockaway, Kevin. "Lessons Learned from Irma Will Help for Future Storms." Gainsville Sun, September 18, 2017.

Brouhard, Rod. "Spider Bites: Symptoms, Treatment & Identification." VeryWell Health. December 12, 2017. https://www.verywell.com/spider-bites-1298281.

"Camping Health and Safety Tips." Center for Disease Control and Prevention. Accessed April 20, 2018. https://www.cdc.gov/family/camping/.

Careless, James. "Emergency Communications Driving Increase in Amateur Radio Operators." *Emergency Management Magazine*, April 11, 2017.

"Choking: First Aid." Mayo Clinic. Accessed March 3, 2018. https://www.mayoclinic.org/first-aid/first-aid-choking/basics/art-20056637.

Christensen, Tom. "Residents Urged to Take Precautions in Extreme Heat." County of San Diego Communications Office. August 28, 2017.

Cowan, Jill. "When 911 Was Overloaded, Desperate Harvey Victims Turned to Social Media for Help." Dallas Morning News, August 26, 2017.

Crawford, Jamie. "Pentagon Document Lays Out Battle Plan Against Zombies." May 16, 2014. CNN.com. https://www.cnn.com/2014/05/16/politics/pentagon-zombie-apocalypse/index.html.

Cunha, John P. "Choking." eMedicineHelp. Accessed April 13, 2018. https://www.emedicine-health.com/choking/article_em.htm.

Dahlberg, Nancy. "Will My Phone Work During and After the Storm?" Miami Herald, September 7, 2017.

Davidson, Nick. "12 Outdoor Survival Skills Every Guy Should Master." Accessed April 21, 2018. Men's Journal. https://www.mensjournal.com/health-fitness/12-outdoor-survival-skills-every-guy-should-master/.

Dolce, Chris. "The Most Devastating Hurricanes in U.S. History." The Weather Channel. April 7, 2014. https://weather.com/tv/shows/hurricane-week/news/most-devastating-hurricanes-20130713.

———. "Six Things to Know About the 2017 Hurricane Season." The Weather Channel Online. May 31, 2017.

Dvorsky, George. "How to Survive the Next Catastrophic Pandemic." Gizmodo. April 5, 2017. https://gizmodo.com/how-to-survive-the-next-catastrophic-pandemic-1793487027.

"Economic Collapse." Happy Preppers. Accessed April 22, 2018. http://www.happypreppers.com/economic-collapse.html.

"8 Tips on How to Survive a Riot." Urban Survival Site. Accessed April 12, 2018. https://urbansurvivalist.com/8-tips-on-how-to-survive-a-riot/.

"Electromagnetic Pulse." Disaster Survival Resources. Accessed January 4, 2018. http://disaster-survival-resources.com/emp.html.

"Emergency Alert System Fact Sheet." FEMA. Accessed February 3, 2018. https://www.fema.gov/media-library/assets/documents/26975.

"Emergency and Evacuation Planning for Guide for Schools." California Department of Public Health. Accessed March 2, 2018. https://www.cdph.ca.gov/Programs/EPO/Pages/BP_Schools_Emergencies_Emergency-and-Evac uation_Planning-Guide.aspx.

"Emergency Bags Every Prepper Needs to Have." Prepper Journal. April 15, 2017, http://www.theprepperjournal.com/2017/04/15/emergency-bags-every-prepper-needs-to-have/.

"Emergency Survival Prepping Checklist." Survivalist Prepper. Accessed April 20, 2018. https://survivalistprepper.net/spal/emergency-prepping-checklist/.

Emerson, Clinton. "Run-Hide-Fight: Former Navy SEAL Reveals How You Can Survive a Terrorist Attack." Sofrep News. November 17, 2015. https://sofrep .com/44561/run-hide-fight-former-navy-seal-reveals-can-survive-terrorist-attack/.

"Evacuation Plan." American Red Cross. Accessed February 23, 2018. https://www.redcross.org/images/MEDIA_CustomProductCatalog/m12140138_Evacuation_Plan.pdf.

Fance, Charnita. "What to Do During an Armed Robbery." Life Hack. Accessed March 20, 2018. https://www.lifehack.org/articles/lifestyle/what-during-armed-robbery.html.

"50 Survival Tips and Tricks for Outdoors." Authorized Boots. Accessed March 12, 2018. https://authorizedboots.com/2015/07/50-survival-tips-and-tricks-for-the-outdoors/.

"Fire and Burn Prevention for Seniors." Burn Institute. Accessed April 3, 2018. http://www.burninstitute.org/fire-and-burn-prevention/senior-fire-safety-smoke-alarm-program.

"Flooding Risk: America's Most Vulnerable Communities." Science Daily, June 21, 2017. https://www.sciencedaily.com/releases/2017/06/170621114013.htm.

"4 Absolutely Necessary Things Every Prepper Must Realize." *The Prepper Journal*. June 17, 2014.

"Fukushima, Chernobyl and the Nuclear Event Scale." *Nuclear Energy Insight,* Summer 2011.

Gibson, Dusty. "How to Choose a Carry Gun with the 5 C's of Concealed Carry." *Handgun Magazine*, August 27, 2014.

"The Golden Hour: What to Do in the First 60 Minutes of SHTF." The Prepper Journal. August 2, 2016. http://www.theprepperjournal.com/2016/08/02/the-golden-hour/.

Graczyk, Michael. "Rescuers Pluck Hundreds from Rising Floodwaters in Houston." *USA Today*, August 28, 2017. https://www.usnews.com/news/best-states/texas/articles/2017-08-27/at-least-2-dead-as-harvey-slams-texas-coast-causing-floods.

"A Guide to Foraging Wild Edibles." Wild Edible. Accessed May 13, 2018. https://www.wildedble.com/foraging.

Guillen, Darla. "Las Vegas Attack Is the Deadliest Mass Shooting in Modern U.S. History." *Houston Chronicle*, October 2, 2017.

Hall, Shannon. "Volcanoes May Have Triggered the Last Unexplained Mass Extinction." *Scientific American*, August 2, 2017.

Harding, Mary. "Animal and Human Bites." Patient. June 16, 2014. https://patient.info/doctor/human-and-animal-bites.

Harper, Jim W. "Are Category 6 Hurricanes Coming Soon?" *Scientific American*, August 23, 2011.

"Hazardous Materials Incident." Ready.gov. Accessed April 20, 2018. https://www.ready.gov/hazmat.

Henry, Pat. "Preppers Are the Modern Survivalists." The Prepper Journal. November 24, 2014. http://www.theprepperjournal.com/2014/11/24/preppers-modern-survivalists/.

"Here Comes the EMP Blast—Will You Survive?" Off the Grid News. Accessed January 3, 2018. http://www.offthegridnews.com/grid-threats/here-comes-the-emp-blast-will-you-survive/.

Holland, Kimberly. "Internal Bleeding: Causes, Treatments and More." Health Line. June 26, 2017. https://www.healthline.com/health/internal-bleeding.

Horman, B. Gil. "Choosing a Home Defense Gun." *American Rifleman*, October 16, 2015.

"How Strong Can a Hurricane Get?" LiveScience. September 5, 2017. https://www.livescience.com/32179-how-strong-can-a-hurricane-get.html.

"Hurricanes, Cyclones, Typhoons." ATMOS News. Accessed March 3, 2018. https://www2.ucar.edu/news/backgrounders/hurricanes-typhoons-cyclones.

Jarvie, Jenny, and Molly Hennesey-Fiske. "Tropical Storm Harvey Breaks Historic Record for Rainfall on U.S. Mainland." *Los Angeles Times*, August 29, 2017.

Johnson, Terrell. "Super-Powerful Solar Storms Could Knock Out Communcations, GPS, Power Systems with Only a Few Hours' Warning." The Weather Channel. July 11, 2015. https://weather.com/science/space/news/solar-storm-1859-less-than-day-to-prepare-global-disruption-impact.

Jones, Marie D., and John Savino. *Supervolcano: The Catastrophic Event That Changed the Course of Human History*. Revised edition. CreateSpace, 2015.

Jorgustin, Ken. "Could We Survive a Super Volcano?" Modern Survival Blog. April 16, 2010. https://modernsurvivalblog.com/volcano/could-we-survive-a-super-volcano/.

———. "4 Simple Self Defense Techniques." Modern Survival Blog. September 25, 2013.

———. "People Who Panic in Emergencies." Modern Survival Blog. December 15, 2014. https://modernsurvivalblog.com/survival-skills/people-who-panic-in-an-emergency/.

Just in Case Jack. "How to Survive a Riot When All Hell Breaks Loose." Skilled Survival. Accessed April 22, 2018. http://skilledsurvival.com/ready-riots-social-unrest.

Kaste, Martin, Brittany Mayes, and Eunice Esomonu. "Most Mass Shootings are Smaller, Domestic Tragedies." NPR.com. June 5, 2017. https://www.npr.org/2017/06/05/530519844/most-mass-shootings-are-smaller-domestic-tragedies.

"Know Your Environment." Emergency Management Magazine, Summer 2017.

Lackey, Katherine. "Deadliest Air Disasters in Recent World History." *USA Today*, May 19, 2016.

"Learn How to Find Food in the Wilderness." Survival Grounds. May 29, 2009. http://www.survivalgrounds.com/finding_food.php.

Macwelch, Tim. "5 Tips to Help You Escape a Mob or Panicked Crowd." *Outdoor Life.* March 28, 2106.

Magid, Larry. "10 Lessons from Having Wallet Stolen While Traveling Abroad." *Forbes.* October 22, 2012. http://www.Forbes.com.

"Make a Plan." Ready.gov. Accessed March 16, 2018. http://www.ready.gov/make-a-plan.

"Making a G.O.O.D. Plan: Get Out of Dodge." The Prepper Journal. June 2, 2017. http://www.theprepperjournal.com/2017/06/02/making-a-g-o-o-d-plan-get-out-of-dodge/.

McNab, Chris. "Special Forces Survival Guide." New York, New York: MJF Books, 2008.

Mercola, Joseph. "Psychological Aftermath of Natural Disasters." Dr. Mercola. September 28, 2017. https://articles.mercola.com/sites/articles/archive/2017/09/28/natural-disasters-psychological-aftermath.aspx.

Michael, Paul. "10 Things You Should Do Immediately after Losing Your Wallet." Wise Bread. April 30, 2012. http://www.WiseBread.com.

Mosher, Dave, and Andy Kiersz "If a Nuclear Bomb Is Dropped on Your City, Here's Where You Should Run and Hide." *Business Insider*, March 18, 2017.

Munger, Sean. "We Interrupt This Program: The Terrifying EBS False Alarm of 1971." SeanMunger.com. February 20, 2014. https://seanmunger.com/2014/02/20/we-interrupt-this-program-the-terrifying-ebs-false-alarm-of-1971/.

"Natural Disasters Caused $175 Billion in Damage in 2016." Charles Riley. CNN.com. January 4, 2017. http://money.cnn.com/2017/01/04/news/natural-disaster-cost-insurance2016/index.html.

Nordqvist, Christian. "Pandemics: Past, Present and Future." *Medical News Today*, January 11, 2016.

Paris, R. Ann. "Prepping with Pets—Evacuating with Animals." The Prepper Journal. March 28, 2017. http://www.theprepperjournal.com/2017/03/28/prepping-with-pets-evacuating-with-animals/.

"Passenger Rail Safety." Operation Lifesave: Rail Safety Education. Accessed April 4, 2018. http://oli.org/about-us/passenger-rail-safety/.

Passi, Peter. "Shelter from the Storm for Pets, Too." *Duluth Union Tribune*, June 19, 2017.

Pietrangelo, Ann. "Allergic Reaction First Aid: What to Do." Health Line. August 25, 2016. https://www.healthline.com/health/allergies/allergic-reaction-treatment.

Pinola, Melanie. "Basic Self-Defence Moves Anyone Can Do and Everyone Should Know." Life Hacker. July 28, 2011. https://lifehacker.com/5825528/basic-self-defense-moves-anyone-can-do-and-everyone-should-know.

"Preppers Paradise: Basics to Build a Backyard Bunker." Seasoned Citizen Prepper. October 22, 2013. http://seasonedcitizenprepper.com/preppers-paradise-basics-to-build-a-backyard-bunker/.

Pritchard, Justin. "What to Do in a Bank Robbery." *The Balance*, September 3, 2017.

Puleo, Stephen. *Dark Tide: The Great Boston Molasses Flood of 1919.* Boston, MA: Beacon Press, 2004.

Pyzyk, Katie. "Surviving a Tsunami in the United States." *Emergency Management*, July 12, 2017. http://www.govtech.com/em/disaster/EM-Summer-2017-Surviving-the-Tsunami.html.

Rayburn, Rosalie. "Local Ham Radio Operators Step Up in Good Times and Bad." *Albuquerque Journal*, August 6, 2017.

Rice, Dovie. "Asteroid Flyby in October: A Drill For the End of the World?" *USA Today*, August 2, 2017.

Richardson, Robert. "Survival Vocabulary: Prepper Terms, Abbreviations and Acronyms." Off Grid Survival. March 7, 2017. https://offgridsurvival.com/survivaltermsabbreviationsacronyms/.

Ripley, Amanda. *The Unthinkable: Who Survives When Disaster Strikes—And Why*. New York: Crown Publishing, 2008.

Roberts, James. "Severe Danger of an EMP Attack and How to Survive." Secrets of Survival. https://www.secretsofsurvival.com/survival/emp_attack.html.

Robinson, Melia. "This 15-Story Underground Doomsday Shelter for the 1% Has Luxury Homes, Guns and Armored Trucks." *Business Insider,* April 7, 2017.

"Safety Officials Recommend 4 Tips for Using Uber." *USA Today*, October 26, 2015. http://college.usatoday.com/2015/10/26/uber-safety-tips.

"75 Bug Out Bag List Essentials." BOBA: Bug Out Bag Academy. Accessed January 13, 2018. https://bugoutbagacademy.com/free-bug-out-bag-list/.

"Shelter: Generating Power." National Geographic Channel. October 16, 2012. http://channel.nationalgeographic.com/doomsday-preppers/articles/gener ating-power/.

"Shut the Doors on Hurricane Irma." Insurance Institute for Business and Home Safety. September 6, 2017. https://disastersafety.org/ibhs-news-release/.

"Situational Awareness: The First Line of Defense." The Prepper Journal. March. 27, 2017. http://www.theprepperjournal.com/2017/03/27/situational-awareness-the-first-line-of-defense/.

"Snow, Ice, Freezing Rain." MoDOT. Kansas City District. Accessed April 22, 2018. http://www.modot.org/kansascity/winter_driving/ifyoubegintoskid .htm.

Snyder, Michael. "20 Things You Will Need to Survive When the Economy Collapses and the Next Great Depression Begins." *Business Insider*, May 7, 2010.

Spector, Dina. "Here's How Many Days a Person Can Survive without Water." *Business Insider,* May 9, 2014.

Stark, Lisa. "What If You Had Only 30 Seconds to Save Your Life?" ABC News. March 25, 2013. http://abcnewsgo.com/US/30-seconds-save-life/story?id=18776142.

Steen, Margaret. "Nightmare Scenario: A Flu Pandemic Is Coming, But When, and How Bad Will It Be?" Emergency Management Magazine. Summer 2017.

Stuart, Keith. "How to Survive a Global Disaster: A Handy Guide." *The Guardian*, February 2016.

Sturt, David, and Todd Nordstrom "A U.S. Government 'Zombie' Plan?" Forbes. May 29, 2014. https://www.forbes.com/sites/davidsturt/2014/05/29/a-u-s-government-zombie-plan/#6ee 16e494dce.

Tamblyn, Thomas. "The Earth Had a Near Miss with an Asteroid That Was Completely Undetected." *Huffington Post*, July 29, 2017.

Tervooren, Tyler. "Pulled Over? Here's the Right Way to Handle a Traffic Stop." Riskology.com. Accessed February 14, 2018. https://www.riskology.co/traf fic-stop/.

"This Is How to Survive a Plane Crash, According to a Flight Attendant." Fox News Travel. January 24, 2014. http://www.foxnews.com/travel/2017/01/24/ this-is-how-to-survive-plane-crash-according-to-flight-attendant.html.

"12 Top Safety Tips for the International Traveler." International Insurance. Accessed April 3, 2018. https://www.internationalinsurance.com/advice/12-tips-for-staying-safe-while-travel ing.php.

"20 Largest Earthquakes in the World." United States Geological Survey—Earthquake Hazard Program. Accessed March 3, 2018. http://www.usgs.gov.

Tyrell, Fred. "How to Survive a Wildfire." Survivopedia. March 16, 2016. http://www.survivopedia .com/how-to-survive-a-wildfire/.

Tyson, Neil DeGrasse. "We Can Survive Killer Asteroids—But It Won't Be Easy." *Wired*, April 2, 2012. https://www.wired.com/2012/04/opinion-tyson-killer-asteroids/.

"Using Social Media for Emergencies." *Fergus Falls Daily Journal*, August 30, 2017.

Vicinanzo, Amanda. "Biological Terrorist Attack on US an 'Urgent and Serious Threat.'" *Homeland Security Today*, April 23, 2015.

Vitelli, Romeo. "Why Do We Panic in Emergencies?" *Psychology Today*, October 5, 2016. http://www.psychologytoday.com/blog/media-spotlight/201610/ why-do-we-panic-in-emergencies.

"West Marine's Safe Boating Checklist." West Marine. February 13, 2018. https://www.westma rine.com/WestAdvisor/Safe-Boating-Checklist.

"What Is the Best Bunker Design?" The Prepper Journal. May 8, 2015. http://www.theprepper journal.com/2015/05/08/what-is-the-best-bunker-design/.

Whitman, Elizabeth. "How To Survive a Plane Crash: 7 Simple Tips on How to Prepare, What to Do, Before, During, After a Plane Accident." International Business Times. March 25, 2015. http://www.ibtimes.com/how-survive-plane-crash-7-simple-tips-how-prepare-what-do-during-after-plane-accident-1858970.

"Who, What, Why: How Long Can Someone Survive without Food?" BBC. com. February 20, 2012. http://www.bbc.com/news/magazine-17095605.

Wong, Kristina. "Could US Handle Biologic Attack?" *The Hill*, October 21, 2014.

Yago, Jeffrey. "Prepper Power!" *Backwoods Home Magazine*, July/August 2012.

Resources

AMERICAN RED CROSS: www.Redcross.org (local chapter locator www.redcross.org/find-your-local-chapter)

ARES—AMATEUR RADIO EMERGENCY SERVICE: www.arrl.org/ares

ARRL—AMATEUR RADIO RELAY LEAGUE: www.arrl.org

BURN INSTITUTE: www.burninstitute.org

CDC—CENTERS FOR DISEASE CONTROL: Hotline: 800-CDC-INFO, www.cdc.gov

CERT—COMMUNITY EMERGENCY RESPONSE TEAMS: www.citizencorps.fema.gov

CHILDHELP NATIONAL CHILD ABUSE HOTLINE: 1-800-422-4453

DEPARTMENT OF HOMELAND SECURITY: www.dhs.gov

DEPARTMENT OF STATE: www.state.gov (to call overseas citizens, or report a lost or stolen passport, from the United States and Canada, call: 1-888-407-4747; from overseas, call +1-202-501-4444)

DISASTER ASSISTANCE: www.disasterassistance.gov

DISASTER RESOURCES NETWORK/AMERICAN PSYCHOLOGICAL ASSOCIATION: www.apa.org/practice/programs/dm

FBI—FEDERAL BUREAU OF INVESTIGATIONS: www.fbi.gov

FCC—FEDERAL COMMUNICATIONS COMMISSION: www.fcc.gov

FEMA—FEDERAL EMERGENCY MANAGEMENT AGENCY: www.fema.gov

HUD DISASTER RESOURCES: www.hud.gov/info/disasterresources_dev

MANMADE DISASTER SURVIVAL RESOURCES: www.manmade-disasters.html

NATIONAL DOMESTIC VIOLENCE HOTLINE: 1-800-799-7233; http://www.ncadv.org

NATIONAL FIRE PROTECTION ASSOCIATION: http://www.nfpa.org

NATIONAL HURRICANE CENTER: http://www.nhc.noaa.gov

NATIONAL OCEANIC AND ATMOSPHERIC AGENCY (NOAA): http://www.noaa.gov; weather radio www.nws.noaa.gov/nwr

NATIONAL SUICIDE PREVENTION HOTLINE: 1-800-273-8255; text to 741741

NATIONAL WEATHER SERVICE: www.weather.gov

NATURAL DISASTER SURVIVAL RESOURCES: www.natural-disasters.html

POISON CONTROL—AMERICAN ASSOCIATION OF POISON CONTROL CENTERS: 1-800-222-1222; www.aapcc.org; Animal Poison Control—888-426-4435 (ASPCA)

SALVATION ARMY: www.salvationarmyusa.org

SKYWARN: www.skywarn.org

STATE GOVERNMENT WEBSITES/INFO: www.usa.gov/states

STEP—SMART TRAVEL ENROLLMENT PROGRAM: https://step.state.gov

SUNSPOT/SPACE WEATHER WATCH: Sunspotwatch.com

TRAVELER'S HEALTH/VACCINES: wwwnc.cdc.gov/travel

UNICEF USA EMERGENCY/DISASTER RELIEF: www.unicefusa.org

USDA DISASTER RESOURCE CENTER: www.usda.gov

USGS—UNITED STATES GEOLOGICAL SURVEY: www.usgs.gov

U.S. NATURAL HAZARD STATISTICS: www.nws.noaa.gov/om/hazstats.shtml

VOLCANIC HAZARDS PROGRAM: volcanoes.usgs.gov

WHO—WORLD HEALTH ORGANIZATION: www.who.int/en/

WOUND CARE CENTERS: www.woundcarecenters.org

To locate the nearest designated public shelter during an emergency, text SHELTER and your zip code to 43362 (FEMA). (Example: SHELTER 90278.)

FEMA/Emergency Management Agencies by State

Contact your state emergency services agency for questions about what you need to be ready for in an emergency. The telephone numbers listed are office numbers and toll-free numbers, when available, or you can visit their websites for valuable and often downloadable lists and information to guide you in getting your plan together.

ALABAMA EMERGENCY MANAGEMENT AGENCY
205-280-2476
http://ema.alabama.gov

ALASKA DIVISION OF HOMELAND SECURITY AND EMERGENCY MANAGEMENT
907-428-7000
http://www.ready.alaska.gov

AMERICAN SAMOA TERRITORIAL EMERGENCY MANAGEMENT COORDINATION
011-684-699-6415

ARIZONA DIVISION OF EMERGENCY MANAGEMENT
800-411-2336
http://www.dem.azdema.gov

ARKANSAS DEPARTMENT OF EMERGENCY MANAGEMENT
501-683-6700
http://www.adem.arkansas.gov

CALIFORNIA GOVERNOR'S OFFICE OF EMERGENCY SERVICES
916-845-8506
http://www.caloes.ca.gov

COLORADO DIVISION OF HOMELAND SECURITY AND EMERGENCY MANAGEMENT
720-852-6600
http://www.coemergency.com

CONNECTICUT OFFICE OF EMERGENY MANAGEMENT
860-256-0800
http://www.ct.gov/demhs

DELAWARE EMERGENCY MANAGEMENT AGENCY
302-659-3362
http://www.dema.delaware.gov

DISTRICT OF COLUMBIA EMERGENCY MANAGEMENT AGENCY
202-727-6161
http://www.dcema.dc.gov

FLORIDA DIVISION OF EMERGENCY MANAGEMENT
850-413-9969
http://www.floridadisaster.org

GEORGIA EMERGENCY MANAGEMENT AGENCY
404-635-7000
http://www.gema.ga.gov

GUAM HOMELAND SECURITY/OFFICE OF CIVIL DEFENSE
671-475-9600
http://www.guamhs.org

HAWAII STATE CIVIL DEFENSE
808-733-4300
http://www.scd.hawaii.gov

IDAHO BUREAU OF HOMELAND SECURITY
208-422-3040
http://www.bhs.idaho.gov

ILLINOIS EMERGENCY MANAGEMENT AGENCY
217-782-2700
http://www.state.il.us/iema

INDIANA DEPARTMENT OF HOMELAND SECU-
RITY
317-232-3986
http://www.in.gov/dhs/emermgtngpgm.htm

IOWA HOMELAND SECURITY AND EMERGENCY
MANAGEMENT DEPARTMENT
515-725-3231
http://homelandsecurity.iowa.gov

KANSAS DIVISION OF EMERGENCY MANAGEMENT
785-274-1409
http://www.kansasstag.gov/kdem_default.asp

KENTUCKY EMERGENCY MANAGEMENT
800-255-2587
http://www.kyem.ky.gov

LOUISIANA OFFICE OF EMERGENCY PREPARED-
NESS
225-925-7500
http://www.gohsep.la.gov

MAINE EMERGENCY MANAGEMENT AGENCY
207-624-4400
http://www.maine.gov/mema

MARYLAND EMERGENCY MANAGEMENT AGENCY
877-636-2872
http://www.mema.state.md.us

MASSACHUSETTS EMERGENCY MANAGEMENT
AGENCY
508-820-2000
http://www.state.ma.us/mema

MICHIGAN STATE POLICE, EMERGENCY MAN-
AGEMENT AND HOMELAND SECURITY DIVI-
SION
517-333-5042
http://www.michigan.gov/emhsd

MINNESOTA HOMELAND SECURITY AND EMER-
GENCY MANAGEMENT DIVISION
651-201-7400
http://www.hsem.state.ms.us

MISSISSIPPI EMERGENCY MANAGEMENT
AGENCY
866-519-6362
http://www.msema.org

MISSOURI EMERGENCY MANAGEMENT AGENCY
573-526-9100
http://sema.dps.mo.gov

MONTANA DIVISION OF DISASTER AND EMER-
GENCY SERVICES
406-324-4777
http://montanadma.org/disaster-and-emer
gency-services

NEBRASKA EMERGENCY MANAGEMENT AGENCY
402-471-7421
http://www.nema.ne.gov

NEVADA DIVISION OF EMERGENCY MANAGE-
MENT
775-687-0300
http://www.dem.state.nv.us

NEW HAMPSHIRE GOVERNOR'S OFFICE OF
EMERGENCY MANAGEMENT
603-271-2231
http://www.nh.gov/safety/divisions/bem

NEW JERSEY OFFICE OF EMERGENCY MANAGE-
MENT
609-882-2000, ext. 2700
http://www.ready.nj.gov

NEW MEXICO DEPARTMENT OF HOMELAND SECU-
RITY AND EMERGENCY MANAGEMENT
505-476-9600
http://www.nmdhsem.org

NEW YORK STATE EMERGENCY MANAGEMENT
OFFICE
518-292-2275
http://www.dhses.my.gov/oem

NORTH CAROLINA DIVISION OF EMERGENCY
MANAGEMENT
919-825-2500
http://www.ncem.org

NORTH DAKOTA DEPARTMENT OF EMERGENCY
SERVICES
701-328-8100
http://www.nd.gov/des

OHIO EMERGENCY MANAGEMENT AGENCY
614-889-7150
http://ema.ohio.gov

OKLAHOMA DEPARTMENT OF EMERGENCY MAN-
AGEMENT
405-521-2481
http://www.ok.gov/OEM

OREGON EMERGENCY MANAGEMENT
503-378-2911
http://www.oregon.gov/OMD/OEM/index.sht
ml

PENNSYLVANIA EMERGENCY MANAGEMENT
AGENCY
717-651-2001
http://www.PEMA.pa.gov

PUERTO RICO EMERGENCY MANAGEMENT
AGENCY
787-724-0124
http://www2.pr.gov/Directorios/Pages/
InfoAgencia.aspx?

RHODE ISLAND EMERGENCY MANAGEMENT
AGENCY
401-946-9996
http://www.riema.ri.gov

SOUTH CAROLINA EMERGENCY MANAGEMENT
DIVISION
803-737-8500
http://www.scemd.org

SOUTH DAKOTA OFFICE OF EMERGENCY MAN-
AGEMENT
605-773-3231
http://www.oem.sd.gov

TENNESSEE EMERGENCY MANAGEMENT AGENCY
615-741-0001
http://tnema.org

TEXAS DIVISION OF EMERGENCY MANAGEMENT
512-424-2138
http://www.txdps.state.tx.us.dem

UTAH DIVISION OF EMERGENCY MANAGEMENT
801-538-3400
http://www.publicsafety.utah.gov/emergency
management/

VERMONT EMERGENCY MANAGEMENT AGENCY
800-347-0488
http://www.dps.state.vt.us/vem

VIRGIN ISLANDS TERRITORIAL EMERGENCY
MANAGEMENT
340-774-2244

VIRGINIA DEPARTMENT OF EMERGENCY MAN-
AGEMENT
804-897-6500
http://www.vaemergency.com

STATE OF WASHINGTON EMERGENCY MANAGE-
MENT DIVISION
253-512-7056
http://www.emd.wa.gov

WEST VIRGINIA OFFICE OF EMERGENCY SER-
VICES
304-558-5380
http://www.dhsem.wv.gov

WISCONSIN EMERGENCY MANAGEMENT
608-242-3232
http://www.emergencymanagement.wi.gov/

WYOMING OFFICE OF HOMELAND SECURITY
307-777-4900
http://www.wyo.gov

P.E.A.P.
PERSONAL EMERGENCY ACTION PLAN

As you sit down to work out your P.E.A.P., here are some guideline questions you can answer to get started. Do this with your family!

WHAT ARE THE HAZARDS SPECIFIC TO MY REGION (I.E., EARTHQUAKE, WILDFIRE, HURRICANE ...)? _____

WHERE CAN I GET NEWS OF AN EMERGENCY? _____

MY EMERGENCY KIT: _____

BASICS: _____

OTHER: _____

CASH: _____

MY BUG OUT KIT: _____

WHERE IN MY HOME CAN I SHELTER-IN-PLACE? _____

WHAT DO I NEED? _____

WHERE CAN I GO IF I HAVE TO EVACUATE? _____

ROUTES _____

DESIGNATED SHELTERS _____

FAMILY AND FRIENDS _____

WILDERNESS _____

OTHER _____

MY PETS—HOW MANY? _____

WHERE WILL I TAKE THEM? _____

HOW WILL I COMMUNICATE WITH OTHERS? _____

WHAT ARE MY FAMILY MEMBERS' CELL PHONE NUMBERS? _____

WHAT APPS DO WE ALL HAVE? _____

CAN WE REACH ONE ANOTHER VIA SOCIAL NETWORKING? _____

WHO IS MY/OUR OUT OF STATE CONTACT PERSON? _____

WHERE WILL OUR FAMILY MEETING PLACE BE IF WE GET SEPARATED? _____

WHAT SPECIAL NEEDS TO I HAVE TO ACCOUNT FOR? (I.E., MY DISABILITY, DISABLED FAMILY MEMBERS, ELDERLY, ILL) _____

IF THERE IS A FIRE OR CHEMICAL EMERGENCY IN MY HOME, WHAT EXITS ARE AVAILABLE TO ME/MY FAMILY? _____

WHERE ARE THE FIRE EXTINGUISHERS AND DETECTORS LOCATED IN MY HOME? _____

ARE MY FIRE EXTINGUISHERS STILL FULL AND USEABLE? WHEN WERE THEY TESTED LAST?_____

WHEN IS THE LAST TIME FIRE AND CARBON MONOXIDE DETECTOR BATTERIES WERE TESTED? _____

REPLACED? _____

WHAT TYPES OF BATTERIES DO THEY REQUIRE? _____

WHERE IS THE SHUT-OFF VALVE FOR GAS IF TOLD TO SHUT IT OFF?_____

WHERE IS THE SHUT-OFF VALVE FOR WATER?_____

WHERE IS THE CIRCUIT BOX LOCATED FOR MY HOME? _____

ARE CIRCUIT BREAKERS LABELED?_____

WHAT ARE THE NUMBERS TO MY GAS COMPANY, ELECTRIC COMPANY, AND WATER COMPANY? _____

WHERE IS THE NEAREST HOSPITAL?_____

WHAT IS THE NUMBER FOR LOCAL LAW ENFORCEMENT? _____

INSURANCE COMPANY HOME INVENTORY LIST

If you have home or renter's insurance, you must document everything of value you have, including clothing and smaller items you might not think about, because it is all going to be included on an inventory you will do after a fire, flood, or other disaster. While it is best to go around your home and photograph every room in detail, keeping a written list is also invaluable in helping you recall what you owned at a time when your memory may not be at its best. In addition to structure and dwelling coverage, you will have a certain number of personal items covered. Check your policy and make sure you have enough coverage, preferably at the level of current replacement value so you can be reimbursed the actual amount it would cost you to buy the very same items.

The cost to rebuild your home can end up different than the actual market value. Size, type of construction, and unique features factor into the amount of coverage you will receive. Your insurance agent can help you find the right level of coverage for both structure and personal items that makes sense for you and offers you the deductible you can work with. Adequate insurance is your responsibility as a consumer, but your agent will be helpful in deciding what that level is. You also want to make sure you adjust the coverage amount when you buy new furniture, add on an additional room to your home, or purchase expensive new computers or electronic equipment. In many cases, things like furs, jewelry, and expensive cars will be listed as luxury items and require more insurance coverage.

Keep receipts for all major purchases with your inventory list so that you can prove you owned the item if you did not take the time to photograph it. This is especially important if you want to make sure the replacement value will be enough to get the same item in a newer version.

Basically, you can go from room to room and take a simple inventory in writing, but it is absolutely best to have photos or video to go along with the written records.

What is a "schedule"? A schedule is a detailed list of the items you want covered under your insurance. By scheduling luxury and expensive items with their brand names, dates of purchase, and cost, you can be assured of having enough coverage should you lose beloved items such as an expensive guitar or your grandmother's wedding ring. You don't want to be overinsured, but you also don't want to find out that the most precious belongings you lost in a fire or flood are not covered because you never took the time to schedule them.

Your state department of insurance probably has a great downloadable list on their website or an actual paper list you can print out and fill in like the ones above. Or use this list below as a template and keep the book with your emergency kit!

LIVING ROOM

Furniture Type	Brand Name/Model	Date Purchased	Purchase Price
Sofa			
Chairs			
Television(s)			
End Tables			
Lamps			
Other Furniture			
Piano/Organ			
Window Treatments			
Art			
Collectibles			
Flooring			
Books			
Sound System			
Other			

KITCHEN

Furniture Type	Brand Name/Model	Date Purchased	Purchase Price
Stove/Range	_____	_____	_____
Refrigerator	_____	_____	_____
Cabinets	_____	_____	_____
Oven	_____	_____	_____
Microwave	_____	_____	_____
Trash Compactor	_____	_____	_____
Dishwasher	_____	_____	_____
Dishes	_____	_____	_____
Glasses	_____	_____	_____
Window Treatments	_____	_____	_____
Faucets	_____	_____	_____
Sink	_____	_____	_____
Utensils	_____	_____	_____
Appliances	_____	_____	_____
Telephone	_____	_____	_____
Cookbooks	_____	_____	_____
Other	_____	_____	_____

MASTER BEDROOM

Furniture Type	Brand Name/Model	Date Purchased	Purchase Price
Bed	_____	_____	_____
Dresser(s)	_____	_____	_____
Armoire/Wardrobe	_____	_____	_____
Chairs	_____	_____	_____
Sofa/Loveseat	_____	_____	_____
Fan	_____	_____	_____
Lamps	_____	_____	_____
Bedside Tables	_____	_____	_____
Telephone	_____	_____	_____
Television	_____	_____	_____
Art	_____	_____	_____
Collectibles	_____	_____	_____
Clothing	_____	_____	_____
Shoes	_____	_____	_____
Accessories	_____	_____	_____
Closet Built-Ins	_____	_____	_____
Jewelry	_____	_____	_____

MASTER BEDROOM (cont.)

Furniture Type	Brand Name/Model	Date Purchased	Purchase Price
Wall Hangings			
Window Treatments			
Alarm/Radio			
Sound System			
Other			

BEDROOM 2

Furniture Type	Brand Name/Model	Date Purchased	Purchase Price
Bed			
Dresser(s)			
Armoire/Wardrobe			
Chairs			
Sofa/Loveseat			
Fan			
Flooring			
Lamps			
Bedside Tables			
Telephone			
Television			
Art			
Collectibles			
Clothing			
Shoes			
Accessories			
Closet Built-Ins			
Jewelry			
Wall Hangings			
Window Treatments			
Alarm/Radio			
Gaming System			
Sound System			
Toys			
Books			
Other			

BEDROOM 3

Furniture Type	Brand Name/Model	Date Purchased	Purchase Price
Bed	_____	_____	_____
Dresser(s)	_____	_____	_____
Armoire/Wardrobe	_____	_____	_____
Chairs	_____	_____	_____
Sofa/Loveseat	_____	_____	_____
Fan	_____	_____	_____
Flooring	_____	_____	_____
Lamps	_____	_____	_____
Bedside Tables	_____	_____	_____
Telephone	_____	_____	_____
Television	_____	_____	_____
Art	_____	_____	_____
Collectibles	_____	_____	_____
Clothing	_____	_____	_____
Shoes	_____	_____	_____
Accessories	_____	_____	_____
Closet Built-Ins	_____	_____	_____
Jewelry	_____	_____	_____
Wall Hangings	_____	_____	_____
Window Treatments	_____	_____	_____
Alarm/Radio	_____	_____	_____
Gaming System	_____	_____	_____
Sound System	_____	_____	_____
Toys	_____	_____	_____
Books	_____	_____	_____
Other	_____	_____	_____

MASTER BATHROOM

Furniture Type	Brand Name/Model	Date Purchased	Purchase Price
Appliances	_____	_____	_____
Vanity	_____	_____	_____
Countertops	_____	_____	_____
Flooring	_____	_____	_____
Lighting	_____	_____	_____
Sink/Faucets	_____	_____	_____
Shower Tile/Accessories	_____	_____	_____
Towels and Linens	_____	_____	_____

MASTER BATHROOM (cont.)

Furniture Type	Brand Name/Model	Date Purchased	Purchase Price
Toiletries	_____	_____	_____
Window Treatments	_____	_____	_____
Jacuzzi/Tub	_____	_____	_____
Decorative Items	_____	_____	_____
Hamper	_____	_____	_____

BATHROOM 2

Furniture Type	Brand Name/Model	Date Purchased	Purchase Price
Appliances	_____	_____	_____
Vanity	_____	_____	_____
Countertops	_____	_____	_____
Flooring	_____	_____	_____
Lighting	_____	_____	_____
Sink/Faucets	_____	_____	_____
Shower Tile/Accessories	_____	_____	_____
Towels and Linens	_____	_____	_____
Toiletries	_____	_____	_____
Window Treatments	_____	_____	_____
Jacuzzi/Tub	_____	_____	_____
Decorative Items	_____	_____	_____
Hamper	_____	_____	_____

BATHROOM 3

Furniture Type	Brand Name/Model	Date Purchased	Purchase Price
Appliances	_____	_____	_____
Vanity	_____	_____	_____
Countertops	_____	_____	_____
Flooring	_____	_____	_____
Lighting	_____	_____	_____
Sink/Faucets	_____	_____	_____
Shower Tile/Accessories	_____	_____	_____
Towels and Linens	_____	_____	_____
Toiletries	_____	_____	_____
Window Treatments	_____	_____	_____
Jacuzzi/Tub	_____	_____	_____
Decorative Items	_____	_____	_____
Hamper	_____	_____	_____

DEN/OFFICE

Furniture Type	Brand Name/Model	Date Purchased	Purchase Price
Sofa	_____	_____	_____
Chairs	_____	_____	_____
Flooring	_____	_____	_____
Lighting	_____	_____	_____
Window Treatments	_____	_____	_____
Office Desk	_____	_____	_____
Computer(s)	_____	_____	_____
Gaming Systems	_____	_____	_____
DVD Player	_____	_____	_____
Art	_____	_____	_____
Collectibles	_____	_____	_____
Coffee Tables	_____	_____	_____
Bar Items	_____	_____	_____
Other Furniture	_____	_____	_____
Television System	_____	_____	_____
Sound System	_____	_____	_____
Books	_____	_____	_____
Toys	_____	_____	_____
Other	_____	_____	_____

FAMILY ROOM

Furniture Type	Brand Name/Model	Date Purchased	Purchase Price
Sofa	_____	_____	_____
Chairs	_____	_____	_____
Flooring	_____	_____	_____
Lighting	_____	_____	_____
Window Treatments	_____	_____	_____
Office Desk	_____	_____	_____
Computer(s)	_____	_____	_____
Gaming Systems	_____	_____	_____
DVD Player	_____	_____	_____
Art	_____	_____	_____
Collectibles	_____	_____	_____
Coffee Tables	_____	_____	_____
Bar Items	_____	_____	_____
Other Furniture	_____	_____	_____
Television System	_____	_____	_____

FAMILY ROOM (cont.)

Furniture Type	Brand Name/Model	Date Purchased	Purchase Price
Sound System			
Books			
Toys			
Other			

GARAGE/LAUNDRY ROOM

Furniture Type	Brand Name/Model	Date Purchased	Purchase Price
Washing Machine			
Dryer			
Built-Ins			
Tools			
Crafting Items			
Flooring			
Lighting			
Appliances			
Generators			
Cleaning Items			
Other			

OUTDOOR EQUIPMENT

Furniture Type	Brand Name/Model	Date Purchased	Purchase Price
Grills			
Chairs			
Tables			
Bars			
Lighting			
Pool Supplies			
Other			

FINE ART_____

_____

COLLECTIBLES_____

_____

FURS_____

_____

COMPUTER EQUIPMENT_____

_____

SPORTING EQUIPMENT_____

_____

CAMPING GEAR_____

_____

MUSICAL EQUIPMENT_____

_____

Index

Note: (ill.) indicates photos and illustrations.

Boston Marathon [Massachusetts] bombing (2013), 72, 119
Boulder, Colorado, 53
"Boulder Author Warns of More 'Megafires' on Nation's Horizon" (Brennan), 53
brake failure, 211–12
breathing, rescue, 166
Brennan, Charlie, 53
British Columbia, Canada, 56
broken bones and fractures, 178–79
broken-down car, 209–10
Buckhorn [California] wildfire (2008), 56
bugging out, 154–56
bug-out bags, 106–8, 107 (ill.)
Burbank, California, 84
Burbank Fire Department, 84
Burbank Police Department, 84
burns, 180–81, 181 (ill.)
burns, thermal, 336
Business Insider, 141

C

Cabazon, California, 57
Cairo, Egypt, 66
Cal Fire, 8
California
 air disasters, 66
 bombings, 72
 disaster planning for families, 97
 earthquakes, 21, 23–24, 282
 economic impact of disasters, 11
 lessons of experience, 368
 mass shootings, 75–76
 psychological trauma, 204, 206
 readiness for disasters, 84
 recent disasters, 7 (ill.), 8
 role of amateur radio, 120
 storms and superstorms, 43
 supervolcanoes, 51–52, 342–43
 tornadoes, 306
 tsunamis, 32
 volcanoes, 49
 wildfires, 54, 56–57
California Siege (2008), 57
California wildfire (2016), 8
Calumet, Michigan, 350
Camille, Hurricane (1969), 46
Camp Funston, 34 (ill.)
camping and hiking, 247–51
Canada, 11, 15–17, 39, 53, 56–58, 115
Canada blackout (1989), 39
carbon monoxide, 278, 278 (ill.)
care, wound, 197–98

Careless, James, 121
Caribbean, the, 367–68
carjacking, 232–34, 233 (ill.)
Carnegie Institute of Washington, 52
Carrington, Richard, 39
Carrington event (1859), 38–39
cars
 accidents, 210 (ill.), 210–11
 being trapped in fires in, 313–14
 broken-down, 209–10
 readiness, 122
 safety, 209–17
 sinking, 213 (ill.), 213–14
 stuck, 212
 using as shelter, 164
Cascades, the, 51
Cedar [California] wildfire (2003), 11, 57
Center for Environmental Journalism, 53
Centers for Disease Control and Prevention (CDC), 35, 195, 219, 223, 248, 355
Central America, 20
Centre for Research on the Epidemiology of Disasters, 6
CERT (Community Emergency Response Team). See Community Emergency Response Team (CERT)
Chelyabinsk event (2013), 37, 38 (ill.)
chemical disasters
 evacuating at work or school, 160
 floods, 29
 hazardous materials, 316
 hazmat, 291
 lessons of experience, 370
 manmade disasters, 64–65
 masks and respirators, 105
 nuclear disasters, 334, 340
 preparing for and surviving disasters, 277–80
 readiness for disasters, 84
 staying put, 163
 supervolcanoes, 51
 worst natural disasters ever, 1
chemicals, household, 280, 280 (ill.)
Chernobyl nuclear disaster (1986), 22, 32, 63 (ill.), 65, 69, 332
chest wounds, 187
Cheyenne Mountain, 93
Chiapas, Mexico, 249
Chicago, Illinois, 64
child, CPR on a, 167–68, 168 (ill.)

child, Heimlich Maneuver on a, 184
child and domestic violence, 355–59, 357 (ill.)
Childhelp National Child Abuse Hotline, 359
children, involving in disaster preparedness, 112–14, 113 (ill.)
Chile, 8, 22
China
 air disasters, 67
 droughts and famines, 19–20
 earthquakes, 23–24
 economic collapse, 327
 economic impact of disasters, 11
 floods, 28, 30
 pandemics, 35
 recent disasters, 6
 top disasters globally, 9
Chinese drought (1876-1879), 20
Chinese drought (2006), 20
Chinese famine (1907), 20
Cho, Seung-Hui, 76
choking, 182–84, 183 (ill.)
choosing a route out, 156
Christchurch [New Zealand] earthquake (2011), 11
Christianity, 70
Christmas, 111, 129, 350
CIA, 80
Ciaccia, Jack, 121
Citizens Corps, 117
Cleveland National Forest, 57
Climate Communication, 25–26
Cloquet [Minnesota] wildfire (1902), 57
Coast Guard, 153
Cokeville, Wyoming, 72
Cokeville [Wyoming] hostage situation and bombing (1986), 72
cold, keeping cold things, 141
Cold War, 123
collapse, economic, 324–28, 325 (ill.), 326 (ill.)
Colombia, 8, 22
Colombia earthquake (1906), 22
Colombia mudslide (2016), 8
Colorado, 24, 53–54, 56–58, 76, 93, 121
Columbine [Colorado] shooting (1999), 76
comet survival tips, 323–24
communication in a disaster, importance of, 151–52
Community Emergency Response Team (CERT)
 lessons of experience, 373
 protocol at the shelter, 160, 162
 readiness for disasters, 84